BEHAVIOUR OF MICRO-ORGANISMS

BEHAVIOUR OF MICRO-ORGANISMS

Based on the Proceedings of
the 10th International Congress
of Microbiology held in
Mexico City

Publication co-ordinated by

A. Pérez-Miravete
Apartado Postal 4-862
Mexico

PLENUM PRESS · LONDON - NEW YORK · 1973

Library of Congress Catalog Card Number 72-77045

ISBN-13: 978-1-4684-1964-1 e-ISBN-13: 978-1-4684-1962-7
DOI: 10.1007/978-1-4684-1962-7

Softcover reprint of the hardcover 1st edition 1973

Plenum Publishing Company Ltd
Davis House
8 Scrubs Lane
Harlesden
London NW10 6SE
Telephone 01-969 4727

U.S. Edition published by
Plenum Publishing Corporation
227 West 17th Street
New York 10011

CONTRIBUTORS

J. Adler	University of Wisconsin, Departments of Biochemistry and Genetics, Madison, Wisconsin 53706,USA.
R.D.Allen	State University of New York at Albany, Departemt of Biological Sciences, Albany, New York 12203,USA.
P.B.Applewhite	Yale University, Biology Department, New Haven, Connecticut 06520. USA.
H.J.Blair	Michigan State University, Department of Biophysics, East Lansing, Michigan 48823,USA.
V.G.Bruce	Princeton University, Department of Biology, Princeton, New Jersey 08540,USA.
D.Davenport	University of California, Department of Zoology, Santa Barbara, California 93106,USA.
M.L.DePamphilis	Stanford University Medical Center, Department of Biochemistry, Palo Alto, California 94305,USA.
B.Deihn	The University of Toledo, Department of Chemistry, Toledo, Ohio 43606,USA.

K. Dimmitt — University of California at San Diego,
Department of Biology,
La Jolla,
California 92057, USA.

S.Dryl — M. Nencki Institute of Experimental Biology,
Department of Cell Biology,
Polish Academy of Sciences,
3 Pasteur Street,
Warsaw 22, Poland.

R.Eckert — University of California,
Department of Zoology,
Los Angeles,
California 90024, USA.

E.M.Eisenstein — Michigan State University,
Department of Biophysics,
East Lansing,
Michigan 48823, USA.

S.Emerson — University of California at San Diego,
Department of Biology,
La Jolla,
California 92037, USA.

J.F.Feldman — State University of New York at Albany,
Department of Biological Sciences,
Albany,
New York 12203, USA.

M.Haberey — State University of New York at Albany,
Department of Biological Sciences,
Albany,
New York 12203, USA.

J.W.Hastings — Harvard University,
Biological Laboratories,
Cambridge,
Massachusetts 02138, USA.

T.Iino — University of Tokyo,
Laboratory of Genetics,
Faculty of Science,
Hongo,
Tokyo, Japan.

H.Koffler
Purdue University,
Department of Biological Sciences,
Lafayette,
Indianna 47907, USA.

T.M.Konijn
Universiteitscentrum de Uithof,
Hubrecht Laboratory,
Utrecht,
The Netherlands.

Ching Kung
University of California,
Department of Biological Sciences,
Santa Barbara,
California 93106, USA.

J.P.Mascarenhas
State University of New York at Albany,
Department of Biological Sciences,
Albany,
New York 12203, USA.

E.M.McGroarty
Purdue University,
Department of Biological Sciences,
Lafayette,
Indiana 47907, USA.

R.L.Miller
Temple University,
Department of Biology,
Philadelphia,
Pennsylvania 19122, USA.

J.R.Mitchen
Purdue University,
Department of Biological Sciences,
Lafayette,
Indiana 47907, USA.

Y.Naitoh
University of California,
Department of Zoology,
Los Angeles
California 90024, USA.

W.Nultsch
University of Marburg,
Department of Botany,
Marburg,
Germany.

D.Osborn
Michigan State University,
Department of Biophysics,
East Lansing,
Michigan 48823, USA.

M.L.Sargent	University of Illinois, Botany Department, Urbana, Illinois 61801,USA
P.Satir	University of California, Department of Physiology-Anatomy, Berkeley, California 94720,USA.
M.Simon	University of California at San Diego, La Jolla, California 92037,USA.
R.W.Smith	Purdue University, Department of Biological Sciences, Lafayette, Indiana 47907,USA.
S.B.Stevens	State University of New York at Albany, Department of Biological Sciences, Albany, New York 12203,USA.
K.Tokuyasu	University of California at San Diego, Department of Biology, La Jolla, California 92037,USA.
G.Tollin	The University of Arizona, Department of Chemistry, Tucson, Arizona 85721,USA.
D.C.Wood	University of Pittsburgh, Department of Psychology, Pittsburgh, Pennsylvania 15213,USA.
D.O.Woodward	Stanford University, Department of Biological Sciences, Stanford, California 94305,USA.

PREFACE

Organisms are constantly being bombarded by stimuli in their environment (and also by internal stimuli), and a common way of responding is by movement. This is an aspect of irritability, or excitability, or behaviour. Response to stimuli by movement is found in all organisms: it represents one of the universalities of biology. Yet at the molecular level it is one of the least understood of biological phenomena.

Micro-organisms are no exception. If motile, they respond to stimuli by active movement (taxis); if sessile, they respond by growth movements (tropisms). Responses by movement are known among micro-organisms to such stimuli as chemicals, electric current, gravity, light, temperature, touch, and vibrations.

The behaviour of micro-organisms is an exciting subject, first of all for its own sake, but in addition because it may reveal facts and concepts that are applicable to understanding behaviour in more complicated organisms (even us) and because it may help to understand the movement of cells and tissues during differentiation and development of higher plants and animals.

In 1906 H.S.Jennings published his masterful book, "Behavior of the Lower Organisms" (reprinted 1962 by Indiana University Press, Bloomington, Indiana, USA.). Since that time no book has appeared on that subject. When Dr. Josè Ruiz-Herrera invited me on behalf of the 10th International Congress of Microbiology to organise a symposium on the behaviour of microorganisms for that Congress, I was thrilled, because it was clear that this could represent the first opportunity since 1906 to bring together under one cover the progress in this area. So here it is.

This book represents the proceedings of a four-day symposium, "The Behaviour of Micro-organisms", held as part of the 10th International Congress of Microbiology in Mexico City, August 9 to 15, 1970.

I have tried to cover the behaviour of micro-organisms in the broadest form possible - from bacteria to moulds, algae, protozoa, sperm, and pollen, from motile organisms to non-motile ones, from responses to short stimuli to habituation (or "learning"), and biological clocks are also represented.

Although I tried hard to include all current work in this area, nevertheless some very deserving specialists did not get invited, or could not accept invitations. The bibliography below includes references to the work of some of these people, and also to the work of the following individuals (with area indicated in parentheses) who were actually on the program but for one reason

A*

or another could not attend or could not produce a manuscript: Dr.E.Cerde-Olmedo (phototropism and sensory integration in Phycomyces), Dr.I.R.Gibbons (biochemistry of cilia, eucaryotic flagella, and sperm tails), Dr.J.Rosenbaum (biochemistry of flagella of Chlamydomonas), and Dr.B.A.D.Stocker (genetics of bacterial flagella).

The primary purpose of the bibliography, however, is to list reviews on the behaviour of micro-organisms, In addition, it refers to a few very recent articles of special importance. Attention should also be called to a number of excellent films on the behaviour of micro-organisms, produced and sold by Institut für Wissenchaftlichen Film, Nonnenstieg 72. Gottingen 34, Germany.

While I am responsible for choosing the contributors to this symposium, I would like to emphasize that I did not edit these papers, either for style or scientific content, so I will assume no responsibility for the language, organiation, or science; this responsibility lies with the individual contributor. Each contributor has proofread his own section and in many cases has brought the contents up to the 1972 level.

I would like to thank our Mexican hosts for their great hospitality, financial support, and other help. In particular, thanks go to Dr. Luis F.Bojalil., secretary general of the Congress, Dr. Josè Ruiz-Herrera, secretary in charge of the sections of General Microbiology and Microbial Biochemistry, and Dr. Adolfo Pèrez-Miravete, coordinator of publications.

Julius Adler
Departments of Biochemistry and Genetics
University of Wisconsin
Madison,Wisconsin,USA.

MOSTLY REVIEWS; A FEW IMPORTANT RECENT PAPERS; AND SOME TOPICS NOT COVERED IN THE TEXT

General

Allen, R. D. and Kamiya, N., editors (1964). Primitive Motile Systems in Cell Biology. Academic Press. London.

Ball, N.G. (1969). Tropic, nastic, and tactic responses. pp 119-228 in vol VA, Plant Physiology, edited by F.C. Stewart. Academic Press. London.

Burge, R.E. and Holwill, M.E. (1965). Hydrodynamic aspects of microbial movement. pp. 250-269 in Function and Structure in Micro-organisms. Fifteenth Symposium of the Society for General Micro-biology. Cambridge University Press. Cambridge, England.

Carlile, M.J. (1966). The orientation of zoospores and germ-tubes. Colston Papers, 18, 175-187. Butterworth's Scientific Publications, London.

Dryl, S.,editor (1970). Symposium on physiology of motor responses in Protozoa. Acta Protozoologica 7, 292-383.

Gibbons, I.R. (1968). The biochemistry of motility. A.Rev. Biochem. 37,521-546.

Halldal, P., editor (1970). Photobiology of Microogranisms. Wiley-Interscience. London. Especially chapter 8-13.

Jahn,T.L. and Bovee, E.C. (1964). Protoplasmic movements and locomotion in Protozoa. pp. 62-129 in Biochemistry and Physiology of Protozoa, vol. III, edited by S.H. Hunter. Academic Press. London.

Jahn, T.L. and Bovee,E.C. (1965). Movement and locomotion of mirco-organisms. A.Rev. Microbiol. 19, 21-58.

Jahn, T.L. and Bovee, E.C. (1967). Motile behavior of Protozoa. pp. 41-200 in Research in Protozoology, vol. I, edited by T-T. Chen. Pergamon Press. London.

Newton, B.A. and Kerridge, D. (1965). Flagellar and ciliary movement in micro-organisms. pp. 220-249 in Function and Structure in Micro-organisms. Fifteenth Symposium of the Society for General Microbiology. Cambridge University Press. Cambridge, England.

Ruhland, W., editor (1959, 1962). Physiology of movements. Encyclopedia of Plant Physiology. (Handbunch der Pflanzenphysiologie.) Vol. XVII, Parts 1 and 2. Springer-Verlag. Berlin. (Truly encyclopedic, covers all aspects of movements in plants, including bacteria, algae, and fungi. Total 1809 pages. Mostly in German, partly in English.)

Chemotaxis in Bacteria

Berg, H.C. (1971). How to track bacteria. Rev. Sci. Instr. 42, 868-871.

Berg, H.C. and Brown, D.A. (1972). Chemotaxis in Escherichia coli: Analysis by three-dimensional tracking. Submitted to Nature.

Dahlquist, F.W., Lovely, P., and Koshland, D.E. Jr. (1972). Quantitative analysis of bacterial migration in chemotaxis. Nature New Biology 236, 120-123.

Weibull, C. (1960). Movement. pp. 153-205 in The Bacteria, vol. I, edited by I.C. Gunsalus and R.Y. Stanier. Academic Press. London.

Chemotaxis in Fungi

Barksdale, A.W. (1969). Sexual hormones of Achyla and other fungi Science 166, 831-837

Hickman, C.J. and Ho, H.H. (1966). Behaviour of zoospores in plant-pathogenic Phycomycetes. A. Rev. Phytopathology 4, 195-220

Machlis, L. (1969). Zoospore chemotaxis in the watermole Allomyces. Physiol. Plant. 22, 126-139

Machlis, L. (1969). Fertilization-induced chemotaxis in the zygotes of the watermold Allomyces. Physiol. Plant. 22, 392-400.

Machlis, L., Nutting, W.H., and Rapoport, H. (1968). The Structure of Sirenin. J. Am. Chem. Soc. 90, 1674-1676. (Sex attractant in watermold.)

Machlis, L. and Rawitscher-Kungel, E. (1963). Mechanisms of gametic approach in plants. Int. Rev. of Cyto. 15, 97-138.

Chemotaxis in Leukocytes

Becker, E.L. (1969). Enzymatic mechanisms in complement-dependent chemotaxis. Fedn. Proc. Fedn. Am. Socs. Exp. Biol. 28, 1704-1709.

Harris, H. (1960). Mobilization of defensive cells in inflammatory tissue. Bact. Rev. 24, 3-14.

Ramsey, W.S. and Grant, L. (1973). Chemotaxis. Chapter 5 in The Inflammatory Process, vol. I, edited by B. Zweifach, L. Grant, and R.T. McCluskey. Academic Press. London. (Chemotaxis in all organisms, but particularly in leukocytes.)

Sorkin, E., Borel, J.F., and Stecher, V.J. (1970). Chemotaxis of mononuclear and polymorphonuclear phagocytes. Chapter 25, pp. 397-421, in Monocuclear Phagocytes, edited by R. van Furth. F.A. Davis Co. Philadelphia.

Chemotropism

Bonner, J.T. (1971). Aggregation and differentiation in the cellular slime molds. A. Rev. Microbiol. 25, 75-92

Delbrück, M. (1972). Signal transducers: terra incognita of molecular biology. Angew. Chem. 11, 1-6

Rosen, W.G. (1962). Cellular chemotropism and chemotaxis. Q.Rev. Biol. 37, 242-259.

Phototaxis and Other Light Responses in Bacteria

Clayton, R.K. (1964). Phototaxis in microorganisms. pp 51-77 in Photobiology, edited by A.C. Giese. Academic Press. New York.

Oesterhelt, D. and Stoeckenius, W. (1971). Rhodopsin-like protein from the purple membrane of Halobacterium halobium. Nature New Biology 233, 149-152. Blaurock, A.E. and Stoeckenius, W. (1971). Structure of the purple membrane. ibid pp 152-154

Phototaxis in Algae and Protozoa

Halldal, P. (1964). Phototaxis in Protozoa. pp. 277-296 in Biochemistry and Physiology of Protozoa, vol. III, edited by S.H. Hunter. Academic Press. London.

Haupt, W. (1966). Phototaxis in algae. Int. Rev. Cytol. 19, 267-299

Jahn, T.L. and Bovee, E.C. (1968). Locomotive and motile responses of Euglena. pp. 45-108 in The Biology of Euglena, vol. I, edited by D.E. Buetow. Academic Press. London

Tollin, G. (1969). Energy transductions in algal phototaxis. pp. 417-446 in vol. III, Current Topics in Bioenergetics, edited by D.R. Sanadi. Academic Press. London.

Phototropism

Bergman, K., Burke, P.V., Cerdá-Olmedo, E., David, C.N., Delbrück M., Foster, K.W., Goodell, E.W., Heisenberg, M., Meissner, G., Zalokar, M., Dennison, D.S., and Shropshire, W., Jr. (1969). Phycomyces, Bact. Rev. 33, 99-157.

Carlile, M.J. (1965). The photobiology of fungi. A.Rev. Pl. Physiol. 16, 175-202.

Page, R.M. (1968). Phototropism in fungi. pp 65-90 in vol. III Photophysiology, edited by A.C. Giese. Academic Press. London.

Thimann, K.V. (1967), Phototropism. Chapter I, pp. 1-29, in Comprehensive Biochemistry, vol. 27, edited by M. Florkin and E.H. Stotz. Elsevier Publishing Co. Amsterdam.

Behavior and Movement of Ciliated and Flagellated Protozoa

Eckert, R. (1972). Bioelectric control of ciliary activity. Science 176, 473-481.

Kinosita, H. and Murakami, A. (1967). Control of Ciliary Motion. Physiol. Rev. 47, 53-82.

Naitoh, Y. and Kaneko, H. (1972). Reactivated Triton-extracted models of Paramecium: modification of ciliary movement by calcium ions. Science 176, 523-524.

Párducz, B. (1967). Ciliary movement and coordination in ciliates. Int. Rev. Cyto. 21, 91-128.

Pitelka, D.R. and Child, F.M. (1964). The locomotor apparatus of ciliates and flagellates: relations between structure and function. pp. 131-198 in Biochemistry and Physiology of Protozoa, vol. III, edited by S.A. Hunter. Academic Press. London.

Behavior and Movement of Amoebae

Allen, R.D. (1972). Biophysical aspects of pseudopod formation and retraction, in Biology of the Amoeba, edited by K. Jeon. Academic Press. in press.

Wolpert, L. (1965). Cytoplasmic streaming and ameboid movement. pp. 270-294. In Function and Structure in Micro-organisms. Fifteenth Symposium of the Society for General Micro-biology. Cambridge University Press. Cambridge, England.

Flagella and Motility of Bacteria

Doetsch, R.N. (1971). Functional aspects of bacterial flagellar motility. Crit. Rev. Microbiol. 1, 73-103.

Doetsch, R.N. and Hageage, G.J. (1968). Motility in procaryotic organisms; problems, points of view, and perspectives. Biol. Rev. 43, 317-362.

Iino, T. (1969). Genetics and chemistry of bacterial flagella, Bact. Rev. 33, 454-475.

Joys, T.M. (1968). The structure of flagella and the genetic control of flagellation in Eubacteriales. A review. Antonie van Leeuwenhock J. Microbiol. Serol, 34, 205-225

Kerridge, D. (1961). The effect of environment on the formation of bacterial flagella. pp. 41-68 in Microbial Reactions to Environment, Eleventh Symposium of the Society for General Microbiology, Cambridge University Press. Cambridge, England.

Silverman, M.R. and Simon, M.I. (1972). Flagellar assembley mutants in Escherichia Coli. J.Bacterial. in press. (Polyhook mutants).

Cilia, Eucaryotic Flagella, Sperm Tails, and Other Microtubules

Adelman, M.R., Borisy, G.G., Shelanski, M.L., Weisenberg, R.C., and Taylor, E.W. (1968). Cytoplasmic filaments and tubules. Fedn. Proc. Fedn. Am. Soc. Exp. Biol. 27, 1186-1193.

Bishop, D.W., editor (1962). Spermatozoan Motility. American Association for the Advancement of Science. Washington, D.C. Publication No. 72

Brokaw, C.J. (1971). Bend propagation by a sliding filament model for flagella. J. Exp. Biol. 55, 289-304.

Gibbons, B.H. and Gibbons, I.R. (1972). Flagellar movement and adenosine triphosphatase activity in sea-urchin sperm extracted with Triton X-100. J. Cell. Biol. 54, 75-97.

Porter, K.R. (1966). Cytoplasmic microtubules and their function. pp. 308-345 in Principles of Biomolecular Organization, CIBA Foundation Symposium. Little, Brown and Co., Boston.

Sleigh, M.A., editor (1973). Cilia and Flagella. Academic Press. London. (Contains reviews by various experts on structure, function, and chemistry of cilia and eucaryotic flagella,)

Summers, K.E. and Gibbons, I.R. (1971). Adenosine triphosphate-induced sliding of tubules in trypsin-treated flagella of sea-urchin sperm. Proc. Nat. Acad. Sci. USA. 68, 3092-3096.

Whitman, G.B., Carlson, K., Berliner, J., and Rosenbaum, J. (1972). Chlamydomonas flagella. I. Isolation and electrophoretic analysis of microtubules, membrances, mastigomenes, and matrix fraction.

J. Cell Biol. September. II. Distribution of tubulins 1 and 2 in the outer doublet microtubules. ibid.

"Learning"

Corning, W.C. and Ratner, S.C. (1967). Chemistry of Learning, Invertebrate Research. Especially article by P.B. Applewhite and H.J. Morowitz. pp. 329-340. Plenum Press. New York.

McConnell, J.V. (1966). Comparative physiology: learning in invertebrates. A. Rev. Physiol. 28, 107-136. (Especially pp. 111-113.

Thorpe, W.H. and Davenport, D., editors (1964). Learning and associated phenomena in invertebrates. Animal Behavior, Supplement No. 1. Especially articles by D.D. Jensen (pp. 9-20) and B. Gelber (pp. 21-29), Bailliere, Tindall, and Cassell, Ltd. London.

Ungar, G., editor (1970). Molecular Mechanisms in Memory and Learning. (Especially pp. 72-75). Plenum Press. London

Biological Clocks

Aschoff, J., editor (1965). Circadian Clocks. North Holland Publ. Co.

Brown, F.A., Hastings, J.W., and Palmer, J. (1970). The Biological Clock. Academic Press, New York.

CONTENTS

CHEMOTAXIS AND CHEMOTROPISM

CHEMOTAXIS IN *ESCHERICHIA COLI*

J. Adler
University of Wisconsin,
Departments of Biochemistry and Genetics,
Madison,
Wisconsin 53706, U.S.A.

1. Introduction

Motile bacteria are attracted to a variety of chemicals – a phenomenon called chemotaxis (for a review, see Weibull, 1960). Although chemotaxis by bacteria has been recognized since the end of the nineteenth century, thanks to the pioneering work of Engelmann, Pfeffer, and other biologists, the mechanisms involved are still almost entirely unknown. How do bacteria detect the attractants? How is this sensed information translated into action; that is, how are the flagella directed?

To learn about the detection mechanism that bacteria use in chemotaxis, it is important first to know *what* is being detected. One possibility is that the attractants themselves are detected. In that case, extensive metabolism of the attractants would not be necessary for chemotaxis. There is another possibility: the attractants themselves are not detected but, instead, some metabolite of the attractants is detected (for example, the pyruvate inside the cell); or the energy produced from the attractants, perhaps in the form of adenosine triphosphate, is detected. In these cases, metabolism of the attractants would be necessary for chemotaxis. The idea that bacteria sense the energy produced from the attractants has, in fact, gained wide acceptance for explaining chemotaxis (and also phototaxis) (Clayton, 1964; Links, 1955).

To try to determine which of these possibilities is correct, experiments were carried out with *Escherichia coli* bacteria, which had previously been demonstrated to exhibit chemotaxis toward various organic nutrients (Adler, 1966). The results show that extensive metabolism of the attractants is not required, or sufficient, for chemotaxis. Instead, the attractants themselves are detected.

The systems that bacteria use to detect chemicals without metabolizing them are here called "chemoreceptors". Efforts to identify the chemoreceptors are described.

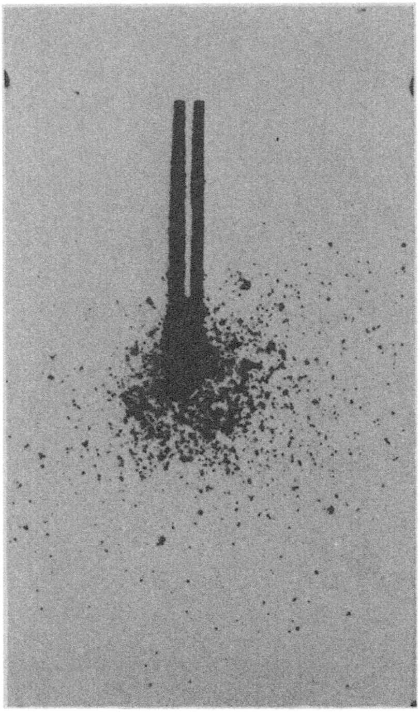

Figure 1. Photomicrograph showing attraction of Escherichia coli bacteria to aspartate. The capillary tube (diameter, ~25 microns) contained aspartate at a concentration of 2×10^{-3} M. (Photomicrograph by Scott W. Ramsey; dark-field photography.)

2. A Quantitative Method for Studying Chemotaxis

In the 1880's Pfeffer (Pfeffer, 1884, 1888) demonstrated chemotaxis by exposing a suspension of motile bacteria to a solution of an attractant in a capillary tube and then observing microscopically that the bacteria accumulated first at the mouth of the capillary (Figure 1) and later inside. A modification of this method, which permits quantitative study of chemotaxis, is here described briefly; a full account will be given elsewhere. (Adler, 1972).

Wild-type Escherichia coli K12, strain W3110, was used, except where otherwise indicated. A capillary tube containing a solution of attractant was pushed into a suspension of bacteria on a slide. After incubation at 30°C for 60 minutes, the capillary was taken out of the bacterial suspension and washed to remove bacteria adhering to the outside. The number of bacteria inside the capillary was then measured by plating the contents of the capillary and counting colonies the next day. The standard deviation is 9 per cent.

A typical result for glucose at various concentrations is shown in Figure 2. (All sugars mentioned, including fucose, have the D- configuration, and all amino acids mentioned have the L- configuration.) From such a dose-response curve – or, better, from a double log plot – one can estimate a threshold concentration for accumulation inside the capillary, in this case about 4×10^{-7} M.

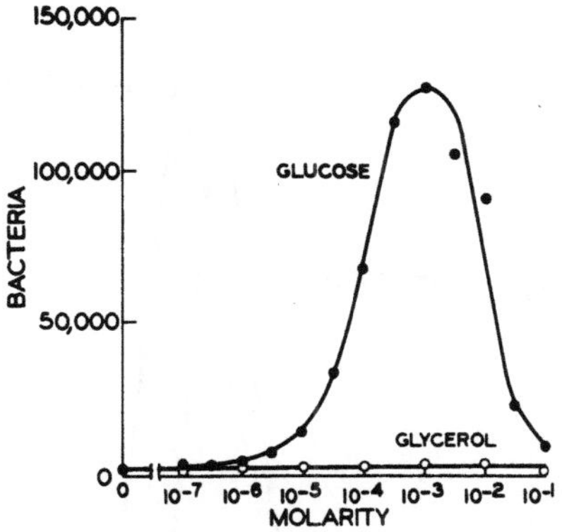

Figure 2. Graph showing chemotaxis toward glucose (solid circles) but not toward glycerol (open circles). Wild-type (strain W3110) bacteria were used, and the experiment lasted 1 hour.

(The threshold is actually lower than this, since the glucose is being used up.) At the highest concentrations, so much attractant diffuses out that the bacteria which have accumulated outside the capillary do not enter in the time allowed. The peak concentration varies with time of incubation, rate of use of the attractant, and other factors.

Results similar to that shown for glucose in Figure 2 were obtained for other attractants – for example, galactose, ribose, aspartate, and serine.

3. Evidence that the Attractants Themselves are Detected

The following five approaches lead to the conclusion that chemotaxis is not a consequence of the metabolism of the attractants but, rather, that the attractants themselves are detected. A more complete documentation of the data can be found elsewhere (Adler, 1969).

(a) Some Chemicals that are Extensively Metabolized Fail to Attract Bacteria.

This result makes it clear that metabolism of a chemical and energy production from it are not sufficient to make a chemical an attractant.

Among a number of chemicals that are readily metabolized and yield energy, as judged by the ability of Escherichia coli to grow on them in the absence of any other carbon and energy source, there are some that fail to attract the bacteria or that attract them very weakly. This includes galactonate, gluconate, glucuronate, glycerol, α-ketoglutarate, succinate, fumarate, malate, and pyruvate. The case of glycerol is shown in more detail in Figure 2. The inability of glycerol to attract bacteria had already been shown by Pfeffer (Pfeffer, 1884, 1888). The failure of some of these chemicals to attract bacteria was not attributable to an inhibition of chemotaxis.

Among the chemicals that are extensively metabolized but fail to attract bacteria (or attract them very weakly) are some that are the first products in

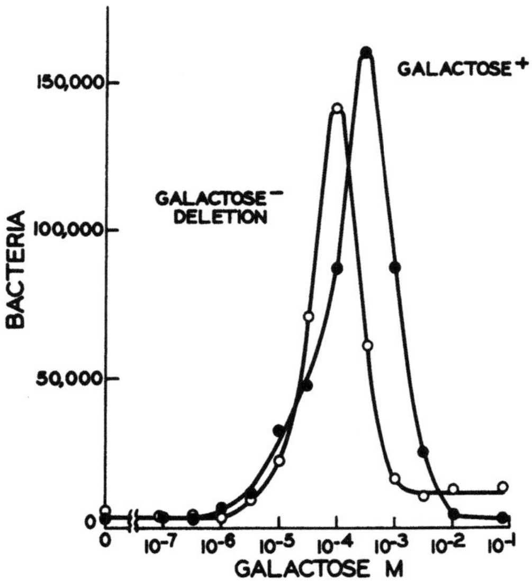

Figure 3. Graph showing chemotaxis toward galactose by a wild-type strain, W3110 (solid circles), and by galactose⁻ mutant, SU 742 (open circles) which has the genes for the three enzymes of galactose metabolism deleted. The incubation time was 1 hour.

the metabolism of the attractants aspartate and serine. First products should also attract, if bacteria detect metabolites of the attractants, or energy produced from the attractants.

Pyruvate, oxalacetate, malate, fumarate, and succinate are, of course, also intermediates in the metabolism of glucose, galactose, and ribose, which are good attractants.

(b) Some Chemicals that are Essentially Nonmetabolizable Attract Bacteria

It has now been found that mutant bacteria that have lost the ability to metabolize an attractant are still attracted to it, and that bacteria are attracted to largely nonmetabolizable analogues of attractants.

(i) Mutant Bacteria that have Lost the Ability to Metabolize a Chemical are Attracted to It. Mutants which lack three enzymatic activities essential for the metabolism of galactose (galactokinase, galactose-1-phosphate uridyltransferase, and uridine diphosphogalactose-4-epimerase) are strongly attracted to galactose, as compared to wild-type bacteria (Figure 3). Evidence has been presented (Adler, 1969) that these mutants are 99.5 per cent or more blocked in their metabolism of galactose, relative to a wild-type strain.

A mutant defective in its ability to metabolize glucose because of mutations in the genes for phosphoglucose isomerase and glucose-6-phosphate dehydrogenase was attracted to glucose as strongly as its wild-type parent (Adler, 1969). The mutant was 97 per cent blocked in its metabolism of glucose, relative to the wild-type parent.

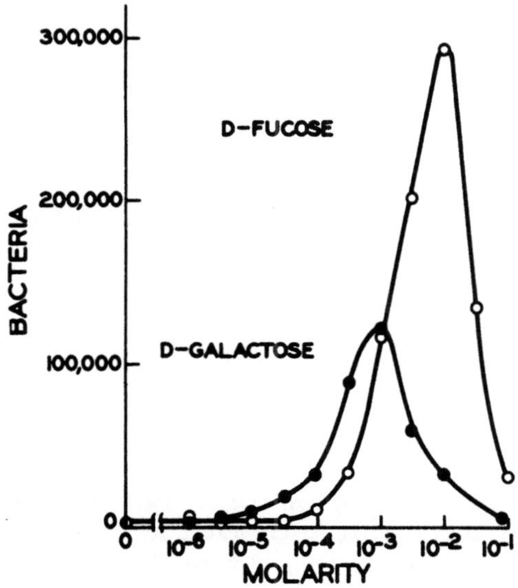

Figure 4. Graph showing chemotaxis toward D-fucose (open circles) and D-galactose (solid circles). Wild-type bacteria (W3110) were used, and the experiment lasted 1 hour.

(ii) Some Essentially Nonmetabolizable Analogues of Metabolizable Chemicals Attract Bacteria. D-Fucose (6-deoxy-D-galactose) is a galactose analogue that is not a source of carbon and energy for growth (Buttin, 1963). Nevertheless the bacteria are attracted to it. In Figure 4 the responses of bacteria to D-fucose and D-galactose are compared. It may be seen that D-fucose is an effective attractant, though its threshold concentration for chemotaxis is higher than that of D-galactose, as might be expected for an analogue. The D-fucose had been purified to remove metabolizable impurities such as galactose or glucose. (L-Fucose, while an excellent source of carbon and energy for growth, is inert as an attractant.)

The evidence that D-fucose is metabolized at 1 per cent or less of the rate at which D-galactose metabolism occurs has been presented elsewhere (Adler, 1969).

Three glucose analogues which were known to be non-metabolizable are also attractants: 2-deoxyglucose, α-methyl glucoside, and L-sorbose. The three analogues were purified before use in order to remove glucose or other contaminants.

c) Chemicals Attract Bacteria Even in the Presence of a Metabolizable Chemical

If bacteria detect metabolites of an attractant, or energy produced from it, then the addition of a metabolizable chemical should stop chemotaxis by flooding the cells with metabolites and energy. This was not found to be the

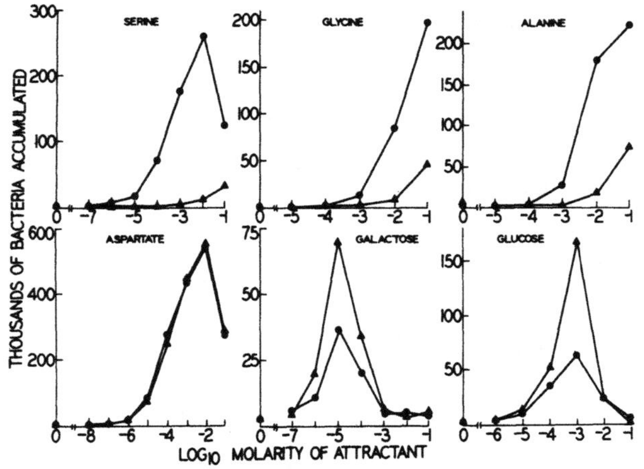

Figure 5. Graph comparing chemotaxis by the serine receptor mutant, AW518 (triangles), and its parent, AW405 (circles). (From Hazelbauer et al., 1969). The experiment lasted 45 min.

case for either metabolizable or nonmetabolizable attractants (Adler, 1969). Thus the presence of the metabolizable chemicals pyruvate or succinate in the bacterial suspension and in the capillary did not block chemotaxis toward galactose, glucose, aspartate, or serine. Even the chemicals that are not metabolized – fucose, or galactose in the case of the galactose$^-$ mutant, or glucose in the case of the glucose$^-$ mutant – attracted bacteria perfectly well in the presence of pyruvate or succinate. Nor did glucose block chemotaxis toward aspartate or serine.

(d) Attractants that are Closely Related in Structure Compete with Each Other but not with Structurally Unrelated Compounds

This finding supports the conclusion that it is the attractants themselves that are detected, and that there exists a variety of specific receptors.

In these experiments one attractant at its peak concentration is put into the capillary tube, and another attractant at a concentration of 0.01 M is put into both the capillary and the bacterial suspension. If the two attractants use the same chemoreceptor, the response should be inhibited; if they do not, the response should not be affected. (Inhibition could result from other causes too, but failure to obtain inhibition is strong evidence that the attractants use different receptors.) Experiments of this nature were first carried out in the late nineteenth century (Rothert, 1901). Some of our results follow; a more detailed report will be presented elsewhere (Mesibov and Adler, 1972; Adler, Hazelbauer and Dahl, 1972).

Chemotaxis toward fucose was completely inhibited by the presence of galactose, and in the reciprocal experiment there was nearly complete inhibition. This suggests that fucose and galactose use the same chemoreceptor (the "galactose receptor").

Glucose completely eliminated taxis toward galactose, but in the reciprocal experiment the inhibition was only about 60 to 70 per cent, no matter

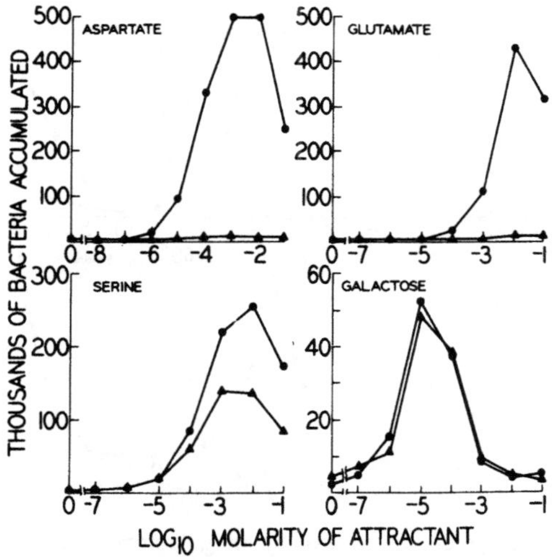

Figure 6. Graph comparing chemotaxis by the aspartate receptor mutant, AW539 (triangles), and its parent, AW 405 (circles). (Mesibov and Adler, 1972.) The experiment lasted 45 min.

how high the concentration of galactose was. This suggests that the receptor which detects galactose also detects glucose but that, in addition, there is another receptor that detects glucose but not galactose (the "glucose receptor").

Similar experiments show that fructose, maltose, mannitol, and ribose are each detected by a specific chemoreceptor.

Glucose did not block taxis toward serine or aspartate, and neither did galactose, fucose, or ribose. In the receiprocal experiments, aspartate failed to inhibit taxis toward any of the sugars. (Serine slightly inhibits chemotaxis toward all other attractants, and this inhibition remains unexplained.) These results show that the receptors which detect the sugars are different from those which detect the amino acids.

Aspartate did not inhibit taxis toward serine so evidently there are separate receptors for detecting these two amino acids (the "aspartate receptor" and the "serine receptor"). On the other hand, aspartate completely inhibited taxis toward glutamate, and complete inhibition was found in the reciprocal experiment, so it appears that aspartate and glutamate use the same receptor.

The various chemicals that are not attractants or that attract very weakly all failed to inhibit chemotaxis toward the attractants.

(e) There are mutants which fail to Carry Out Chemotaxis to Certain Attractants but are still able to Metabolize them

If there are chemoreceptors in bacteria and if they are specific, there should be mutants that are defective in their response to some attractants but

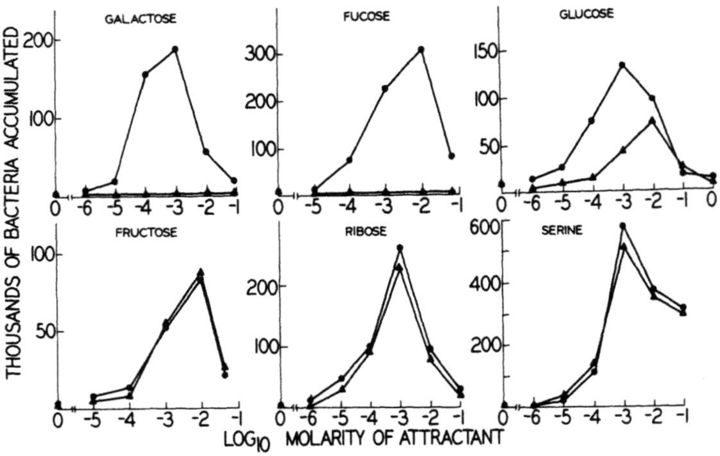

Figure 7. Graph comparing chemotaxis by the galactose receptor mutant, AW520 (triangles), and its chemotaxis revertant, AW521 (circles). (From Hazelbauer et al., 1969). The experiment lasted 1 hour.

not to others, because of a defect in a single receptor. Such mutants of Escherichia coli have now been found (Hazelbauer et al., 1969; Mesibov and Adler, 1972).

One mutant, defective in the "serine receptor", (Figure 5) fails to be attracted to serine, except for a very weak response at the highest concentrations, and shows much-reduced taxis toward glycine, alanine, and cysteine. (These residual responses result from the "aspartate receptor".) The mutant is attracted normally to aspartate and glutamate, and (better than normally) to the various sugars. It oxidizes and takes up L-serine at the same rate that its parent does.

Another mutant, lacking the "aspartate receptor", (Figure 6) shows no chemotaxis toward aspartate and glutamate, nearly normal taxis toward serine, alanine, glycine, and cysteine, and normal taxis toward the various sugars. The rate of oxidation and uptake of aspartate is the same for the mutant and its parent.

A third mutant, missing the "galactose receptor", (Figure 7) is not attracted to galactose and fucose and is attracted to glucose at a higher-than-normal threshold (3×10^{-5} M instead of 4×10^{-7} M). (This residual response to glucose results from the "glucose receptor".) It is attracted normally to maltose, mannitol, fructose, ribose, serine, and aspartate. Metabolism of galactose is normal in the galactose receptor mutants. In some of the mutants there is a defect in the uptake of galactose, which will be discussed below.

The existence of these mutants argues for specific receptors and provides additional support for the idea that detection of the attractants is independent of their metabolism.

4. How Many Chemoreceptors?

To determine how many kinds of chemoreceptors there are, three approaches are being used. The first is to ask whether a given attractant is

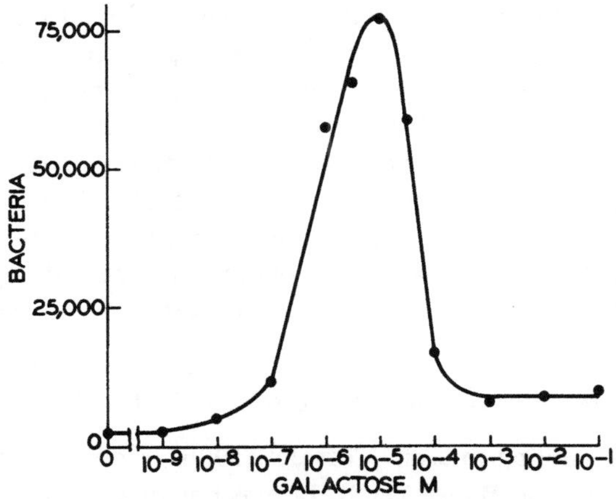

Figure 8. Graph showing chemotaxis toward galactose by a mutant, 20SOK⁻, defective in the uptake of galactose and also lacking galactokinase. The experiment lasted for 1 hour.

still effective when another attractant is present. The second is to try to isolate mutants defective in individual receptors. A third approach is to study the inducibility of specific taxes (presumably the inducibility of specific receptors). For example, taxis toward galactose and fucose is inducible by galactose.

The conclusion from results obtained so far (Adler, 1969; Adler, Hazelbauer and Dahl, 1972; Mesibov and Adler, 1972) is that there are at least the eight chemoreceptors shown in Table 1. Oxygen is known to be an attractant for E. coli (Adler, 1966), so there could be a receptor for it, but this question has not been investigated so far. A survey of possible other attractants or of repellents has not been completed.

It is conceivable that, besides chemoreceptors, at least some bacteria might have receptors specialized to detect light, gravity, or temperature, since all these stimuli are known to elicit tactic responses in some bacteria (Weibull, 1960).

5. What is the Nature of the Chemoreceptors?

One possibility is that the chemoreceptors are the first enzymes in the metabolism of the chemicals. This possibility has been excluded in the case of galactose, because mutants that lack galactokinase still respond perfectly well. Another possibility is that the chemoreceptors are the permeases.

What role, if any, is played in chemotaxis by permeases and other components essential for transport of substances into the cell? To find out, mutants defective with respect to transport have been investigated from the standpoint of chemotaxis.

Figure 8 shows good attraction to galactose by an Escherichia coli mutant, 20SOK⁻, that is defective in the uptake of galactose (Buttin, 1963; Rotman et al., 1968) to the extent of a 99.5 per cent block (Adler, 1969) owing to the absence of both galactose permease and β-methyl galactoside permease activity (Rotman et al., 1968), and that, in addition, is unable to grown on, or to metabolize, galactose, as a result of a mutation in the gene for galactokinase. The threshold concentration for taxis toward galactose appears to be even lower (about 2×10^{-9} M) for the mutant than for strains that are wild-type with respect to galactose transport (compare Figure 8 with Figure 3); actually the thresholds are probably the same for the mutant and the wild-type bacteria, but the latter consume the galactose and in this way destroy the gradient.

Thus transport is not required for chemotaxis, and the chemoreceptors therefore appear to be located somewhere on the "outside" of the cell.

The galactose binding protein (Anraku, 1968), a component needed for the transport of galactose (Boos, 1969), is present in 20SOK$^-$ (Hazelbauer and Adler, 1971); it must be missing an additional component needed for galactose transport. We (Hazelbauer and Adler, 1969) have now found that the galactose binding protein is also needed for galactose taxis, and that this is the component of the galactose receptor that recognizes galactose, glucose, and a number of structurally related chemicals. The evidence (Hazelbauer and Adler, 1969) follows:

(a) The specificity of the galactose binding protein is the same as the specificity of the galactose receptor.

(b) Most of the galactose taxis mutants are defective in the transport of galactose, as mentioned above, and these all have very low levels of galactose binding protein.

(c) Galactose taxis can be eliminated by a mild osmotic shock which releases the galactose binding protein from the cells, and then galactose taxis can be restored by the addition of pure galactose binding protein. Addition of galactose binding protein from a mutant that is attracted to galactose only at high concentrations results in restoration of taxis only at high concentrations.

(d) The galactose chemoreceptor is saturated at concentrations above 10^{-6} M, and so is the galactose binding protein.

There must be one or more additional components of the galactose chemoreceptor, since at least one of the galactose taxis mutants has normal galactose binding protein (Hazelbauer and Adler, 1971). We are trying to find out what this additional component(s) is.

The role of the binding protein and the relationship between transport and taxis are summarized as follows:

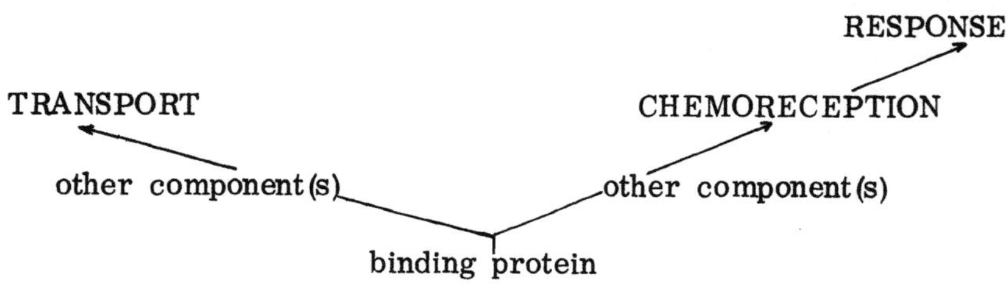

We have also found osmotically shockable binding proteins for maltose and ribose that appear to serve the corresponding chemoreceptors (Hazelbauer and Adler, 1971). For the remaing chemoreceptors (see Table 1) the binding proteins must be more firmly bound to the cell envelope, since the shock fluid did not contain them.

TABLE 1. Partial list of chemoreceptors in Escherichia coli

Attractant	Chemoreceptor name	Threshold† molarity
	Fructose receptor	
D-Fructose		1×10^{-5}
	Galactose receptor	
D-Galactose		4×10^{-7}
D-Glucose		4×10^{-7}
D-Fucose		3×10^{-5}
	Glucose receptor	
D-Glucose		3×10^{-5}
	Maltose receptor	
Maltose		3×10^{-6}
	Mannitol receptor	
D-Mannitol		7×10^{-6}
	Ribose receptor	
D-Ribose		3×10^{-7}
	Aspartate receptor	
L-Aspartate		6×10^{-8}
L-Glutamate		5×10^{-6}
	Serine receptor	
L-Serine		3×10^{-7}
L-Cysteine		5×10^{-6}
L-Alanine		7×10^{-5}
Glycine		3×10^{-5}

†The threshold values are lower in mutants unable to take up or metabolize a chemical.

A two-enzyme system (the "phosphotransferase system") which catalyzes the phosphorylation of glucose and certain other sugars is required for the transport of these chemicals (Roseman, 1969). Enzyme I catalyzes the phosphorylation of a heat-stable protein by phosphoenolpyruvate; enzyme II then catalyzes the transfer of phosphate from the heat-stable protein to the sugar, and there are specific enzyme II's for different sugars. Three mutants of Escherichia coli that lack enzyme I activity and a mutant defective in the heat-stable protein all showed normal chemotaxis toward glucose (Adler, 1969). An E. coli mutant defective in the enzyme II activity that phosphorylates glucose and α-methyl glucoside was attracted normally to these chemicals (Adler, 1969). Thus neither enzyme I, nor the heat-stable protein, nor enzyme II activity is required for this chemotaxis. However, these two sugars are detected by both the galactose and glucose receptors. Since galactose taxis was also normal in these mutants, the phosphotransferase system is not required by the galactose receptor but it remains possible that it is required by the glucose receptor. We are currently determining if the phosphotransferase system, or a part of it, plays a role in the functioning of the glucose, fructose, and mannitol receptors; all three chemicals are transported via this system (Roseman, 1969).

The permeases and related binding proteins are by themselves not sufficient for chemotaxis: many chemicals for which transport mechanisms and binding proteins exist fail to attract bacteria. Examples are the following amino acids for which active transport is known in Escherichia coli (Piperno, 1966): L-glutamine, L-histidine, L-isoleucine, L-leucine, L-methionine, L-phenylalanine, L-tryptophan, L-tyrosine, and L-valine.

6. How do Chemoreceptors Work?

As to the mechanism of chemoreceptors in bacteria, this still remains unknown. Boos has shown that the galactose binding protein undergoes a conformational change when it binds galactose (Boos et al., 1972). Somehow this change may be "felt" by the additional component(s). Then this information is transmitted to the flagella, either by a diffusible substance or by a conformational change of macromolecules perhaps in the cell membrane. The latter mechanism could involve something like a receptor potential or an action potential. In the protozoa such changes in potential have been observed prior to the reversal of cilia or to emission of light (Eckert, 1965a and b; Kinosita and Murakami, 1967; Naitoh, 1966; Naitoh and Eckert, 1969). The change might be propagated along the membrane so as to reach all the flagella. In fact, the base of the flagellum is in close association with the cell membrane (van Iterson et al., 1966; also DePamphilis, this volume). The flagella could then respond by changing their orientation in some way. See H. C. Berg (1972, submitted to Nature) for a study of how individual Escherichia coli behave in a chemical gradient.

We have isolated and reported on 40 mutants which are generally nonchemotactic, i.e., they fail to carry out chemotaxis toward any of the attractants (Figure 9) – amino acids, sugars, or oxygen – though the bacteria are perfectly motile (Armstrong et al., 1967). Since it is unlikely that a single mutation would lead to a loss of all the kinds of chemoreceptors, these mutants are probably defective at some stage beyond the receptors, as shown diagrammatically in Figure 10. The defect could be in a transmitting system through which information from all the receptors is channeled to the

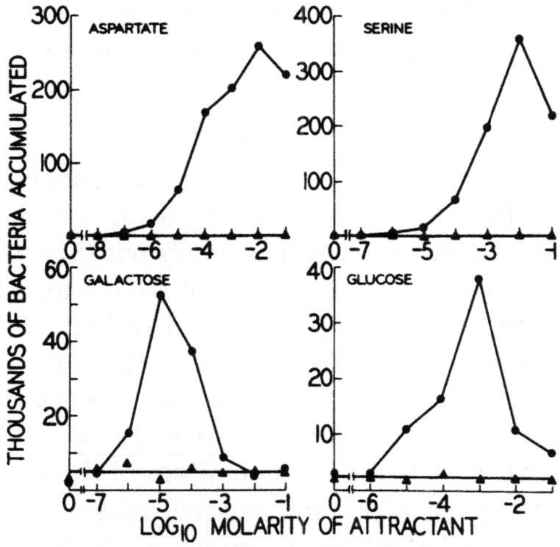

Figure 9. Graph comparing chemotaxis by the generally non-chemotactic mutant, M353 (triangles), and its parent AW330 (circles). The experiment lasted 1 hour.

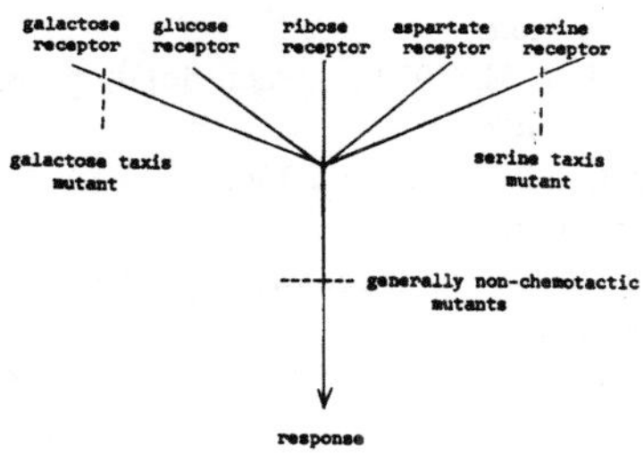

Figure 10. The scheme for chemotaxis suggested in this article, showing location of defects in the various mutants. Only 5 of the 8 chemoreceptors are indicated.

flagella, or in the responding mechanism itself. Genetic analyses of the mutants have shown that three genes are involved (Armstrong and Adler, 1969a and b). Further studies of these mutants may lead to an understanding of the way in which the chemoreceptors direct the flagella.

The availability of behavioral mutants of bacteria – for example, mutants of the types reported here – together with the existence of a great body of knowledge about the genetics and biochemistry of Escherichia coli, should make the bacterial system a favorable one for studying simple forms of behavior and perhaps even some primitive kinds of "learning". From such studies might emerge a set of facts and concepts that can be applied to investigations of more complex phenomena in higher organisms.

7. Summary

Extensive metabolism of chemicals is neither required, nor sufficient, for attraction of bacteria to the chemicals. Instead, the bacteria detect the attractants themselves. The systems that carry out this detection are called "chemoreceptors". There are mutants that fail to be attracted to one particular chemical or to a group of closely related chemicals but still metabolize these chemicals normally. These mutants are regarded as being defective in specific chemoreceptors. Data obtained so far indicate that there are at least eight different chemoreceptors in Escherichia coli. The chemoreceptors are not the enzymes that catalyze the metabolism of the attractants; nor are they certain parts of the permeases and related transport systems, and uptake itself is not required or sufficient for chemotaxis. In the case of the galactose receptor, the galactose binding protein is the component that recognizes the attractants detected by that chemoreceptor.

REFERENCES

Adler, J. (1966). Science 153, 708.
Adler, J. (1969). Science 166, 1588.
Adler, J. (1972). J. Gen. Microbiol. in press.
Adler, J., Hazelbauer, G. L., and Dahl, M. M. (1972). J. Bacteriol. in press.
Anraku, Y. (1968). J. Biol. Chem. 243, 3123.
Armstrong, J. B. and Adler, J. (1969a). J. Bacteriol. 97, 156.
Armstrong, J. B. and Adler, J. (1969b). Genetics 61, 61.
Armstrong, J. B., Adler, J., and Dahl, M. (1967). J. Bacteriol. 93, 390.
Boos, W. (1969). European J. Biochem. 10, 66.
Boos, W., Gordon, A. S., Hall, R. E., and Price, H. D. (1972). J. Biol. Chem. 247, 917.
Buttin, G. (1963). J. Mol. Biol. 7, 164.
Clayton, R. K. (1964). In Photophysiology, ed. by A. C. Giese, vol. 2, p. 51, New York: Academic Press.
Eckert, R. (1965a). Science 147, 1140.
Eckert, R. (1965b). Science 147, 1142.
Hazelbauer, G. L. and Adler, J. (1971). Nature New Biology 230, 101.
Hazelbauer, G. L., Mesibov, R. E., and Adler, J. (1969). Proc. Nat. Acad. Sci. U. S. 64, 1300.
Iterson, W. van, Hoeniger, J. F. M., and van Zanten, E. N. (1966). J. Cell Biol. 31, 585.
Kinosita, H. and Murakami, A. (1967). Physiol. Rev. 47, 53.
Links, J. (1955). Thesis, University of Leiden. (in Dutch; summary in English).
Mesibov, R. and Adler, J. (1972). J. Bacterial. in press.
Naitoh, Y. (1966). Science 154, 660.
Naitoh, Y. and Eckert, R. (1969). Science 164, 693.
Pfeffer, W. (1884). Untersuch. Botan. Inst. Tubingen 1, 363.
Pfeffer, W. (1888). Untersuch. Botan. Inst. Tubingen 2, 582.
Piperno, J. R. W. (1966). Thesis, University of Michigan.
Rothert, W. (1901). Flora, 88, 371.
Rotman, B., Ganesan, A. K., and Guzman, R. (1968). J. Mol. Biol. 36, 247.
Roseman, S. (1969). J. Gen. Physiol. 54, 138.
Weibull, C. (1960). In The Bacteria, ed. by I. C. Gunsalus and R. Y. Stanier, vol. 1, p. 153. New York: Academic Press.

ACKNOWLEDGEMENTS

The research discussed was supported by a grant from the U.S. National Institutes of Health. I thank Margaret Dahl for having carried out many of the experiments described here, and G. L. Hazelbauer and R. E. Mesibov for major contributions.

Much of this paper is reproduced from an article published in Science (Adler, 1969) by permission of the American Association for the Advancement of Science (copyright 1969).

CHEMOTAXIS IN CILIATE PROTOZOA

S. Dryl

M. Nencki Institute of Experimental Biology,
Department of Cell Biology,
Polish Academy of Sciences,
3 Pasteur Street,
Warsaw 22, Poland.

1. INTRODUCTION

The free-living ciliate protozoa are cosmopolitan organisms which can be easily found in streams, rivers, lakes, ponds, and bodies of stagnant water from various parts of the world. It is evident that they can live and reproduce under variable conditions of external environment thanks to highly developed capacity of motor response towards chemical, mechanical, photic, thermal, electric, and gravitional stimuli. The relatively high rate of swimming of the organism and the perception of chemical stimuli ahead of it provide additional advantages for finding favorable living conditions and for avoiding noxious effects in the surrounding medium.

The term "chemotaxis" was used for the first time by Pfeffer (1883, 1884, 1888) in his studies on chemo-attractive and chemo-repellent factors for the fern sperms. The positive chemotaxis of Paramecium towards oxygen was observed first by Verworn (1889) and Loeb and Hardesty (1895), while Loeb and Budget (1897) noticed negative chemotactic response towards acids and alkaline substances. It was stressed by Massart (1889) that the ciliate protozoa are sensitive to changes of osmotic tension in the external medium and not to its chemical composition. He even suggested the use of the term "tonotaxis" instead of "chemotaxis" but this view was ruled out by Jennings (1897) who brought strong evidence that the ciliate protozoa show true chemotactic response towards appropriate stimuli and osmotic pressure does not play any significant role in this respect.

Jennings (1897, 1899 a, 1900, 1906) has shown that the chemotactic response in the ciliate protozoa is achieved by means of so-called "avoiding reaction" (AR) which in the case of negative response appears at the boundary of the medium being tested while in the case of positive chemotaxis the animal swims without reaction to medium containing the positive chemotactic stimulus,

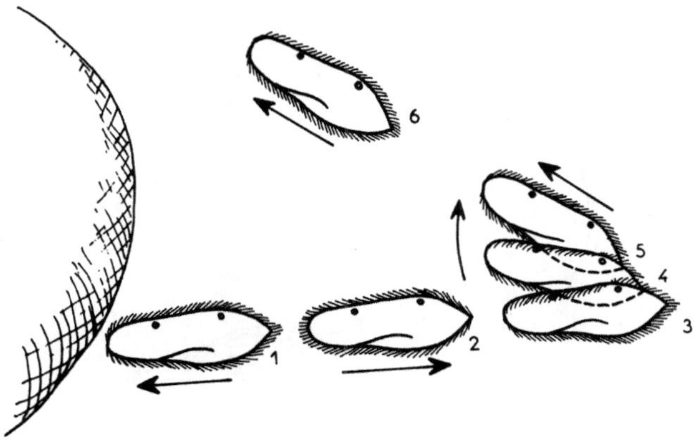

Figure 1. Avoiding reaction of Paramecium towards external stimulus (schematic). (1-3) short-lasting ciliary reversal. (3-5) Aboral turning, pivoting, or circling. (6) swimming in the new direction. (After Jennings, 1906).

showing AR on the boundary of the primary medium. In the case of Paramecium the fully expressed AR is characterized by short-lasting backward movement followed by turning to the aboral side of the body and forward movement in the new direction.

As concerns the theoretical approach to the problem of motor response in protozoa it should be pointed out that after the early naive period of anthropomorphism, the behavior of unicellular organisms proved to be a very useful tool for experimental studies on motor response to various external stimuli, with special attention paid to reactions described as tropisms, taxes, and kineses.

Loeb (1890, 1912, 1918) suggested that the overwhelming majority of animals possess the bilateral anatomical symmetry which is also expressed by function of their sense organs and locomotor apparatus. The animal stimulated in the same way from both sides of its plane of symmetry moves in a straight line towards the stimulus (positive tropism) or away from the stimulus (negative reaction). However, if the intensity of stimulation on one side of the body is increased or decreased, the asymmetry of physiological processes in the peripheral and central nervous system and in corresponding effectors (muscle, glands, etc.) will be manifested by a change of direction of movement until a new symmetry of body position is reached and consequently the animal will move again along the straight line towards or away from the stimulus. According to Loeb the locomotion of the animal consists of forced movements as a result of action of external stimuli on symmetrical components of nervous or locomotory systems.

One of the earliest serious objections against Loeb's theory of tropisms was raised by Jennings (1897, 1900, 1904 a, 1906) who showed that as a rule the unicellular organisms respond to external stimuli and that this response is carried out by the organism as a whole unit and not by local reaction of locomotory cell organelles on the cell surface only. Taking into account AR as a

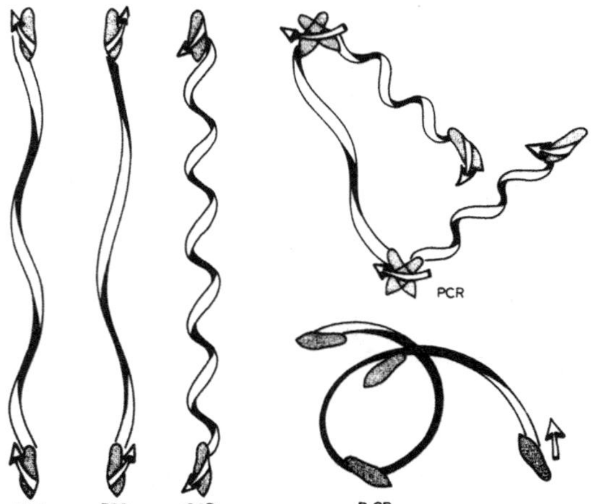

Figure 2. Schematic presentation of various kinds of response in Paramecium caudatum. FLS = normal, forward left-spiraling movement. FRS = forward right-spiraling movement. CCR = continuous ciliary reversal. PCR = periodic ciliary reversal. (After Kuznicki 1966).

basic motor response of the organism to external stimuli Jennings (1904 b, 1906) described the behavior of paramecia and other ciliate protozoa by means of Morgan's principle of "trial and error". Later on Mast (1911, 1913, 1914, 1915) and Alverdes (1922 a, 1922 b, 1922 c) were strongly opposing the rigidity of the mechanistic concept of Loeb's theory on the basis of their own observations on the behavior of protozoa under normal and experimental conditions.

Kühn (1919) in his classification system of elementary reactions included some ideas of Loeb and his opponents, dividing the reactions to external stimuli into so-called phobo-taxes and topo-taxes. According to his view all reactions of protozoa based on AR should belong to the group of phobo-taxes while all oriented reactions to the source of stimulation (e.g., light) should be classified as topo-taxes.

More detailed classification of elementary reactions was proposed by Frankel and Gunn (1961) who divided the reactions of animals to external stimuli into three large groups: kineses, taxes, and tranverse orientations. According to this classification the kinetic phenomena of protozoa described as "chemo-taxis" should belong to the group of "klino-kineses" in which frequency or amount of turning per unit time depends on the intensity of stimulation. However, many authors, even recently (Dryl 1961 a, Rosen 1962, Jahn and Bovee 1968, Dryl and Grebecki 1966), still use the traditional term "chemotaxis" to describe the non-directed movements of protozoa towards external chemical stimuli.

2. Mechanism of Chemotaxis

Depending upon the species of animals under study, the normal progressive locomotion of the ciliate protozoa is based on the action of various locomotor

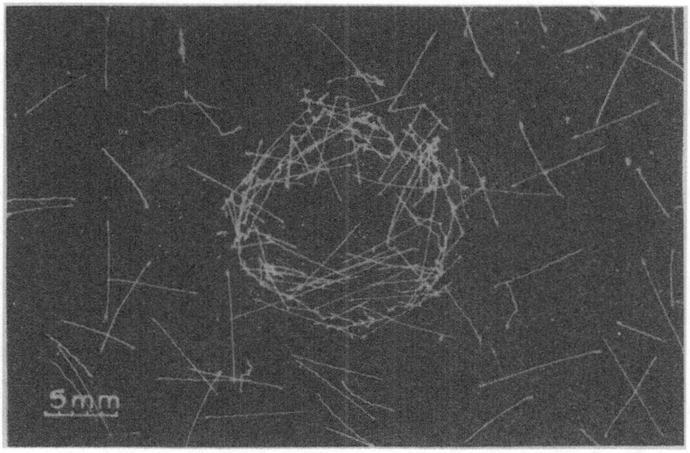

Figure 3. Positive chemotactic response of Paramecium caudatum towards optimum pH range 5.2-6.4 T; pH of surrounding medium 7.8. A number of avoiding reactions visible on the boundary between two solutions. Recording of movement carried out by Dryl's time-exposure macrophotographic technique. Scale = 5 mm. Exposure time = 5 seconds. (Dryl, 1963).

cell organelles like cilia, AZM (Adoral Zone Membranelles), cirri, and contraction of myonemes. As a rule the animal moves along the spiraling line when swimming freely in the liquid medium or along circles and arcs when swimming close to the substrate. This normal pattern of forward locomotion undergoes a sudden change of direction if the organism meets on its way an external stimulus of sufficient intensity to affect the function of the locomotor apparatus. It is worth mentioning in this connection that at present we distinguish in Paramecium at least four patterns of ciliary reversal responses which are classified as follows:

1. Avoiding reaction (AR), which was described in detail by Jennings (1899 a, b, 1904 b, 1906) and in the fully developed form is expressed by the following phases: a) short-lasting reversal of ciliary beat which forces the animal to swim backwards; b) pivoting, circling, and turning to the aboral side of body, and finally; c) forward movement in the new direction (Figure 1). In the case of weak stimulus AR may be limited to the aboral turning or forward swimming along curved line.

2. Periodic ciliary reversal (PCR), which is characterized by a short-lasting reversal of ciliary beat (backward movement) followed by turning to the aboral side and a short-lasting period of the normal forward motion, each phase of movement occuring alternately one after another at intervals of 0.5-1 sec. on average. This response appears in typical form in Paramecium during exposure to the appropriate concentrations of Ba^{2+} and Ca^{2+} in external medium (Dryl 1961 c).

3. Partial ciliary reversal (PaCR), which appears as a circling backward movement with part of the cilia beating in normal and another part in

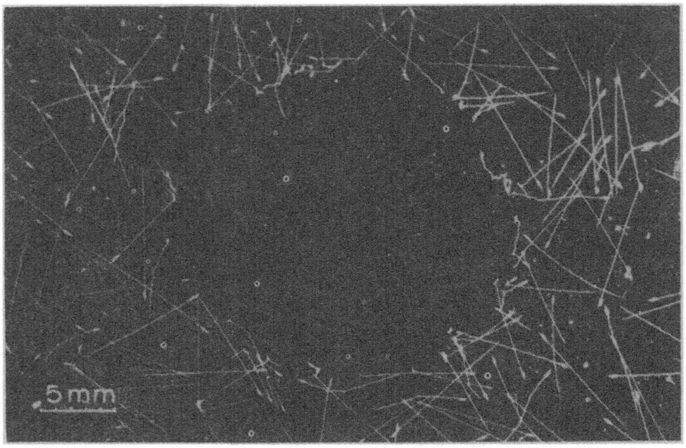

Figure 4. Negative chemotactic response of Paramecium caudatum towards 2.10^{-2} M solution of $MgCl_2$. Recording of movement carried out by Dryl's time-exposure macrophotographic technique. Scale = 5 mm. Exposure time = 5 seconds. (Dryl, original).

reversed direction. This kind of ciliary response was demonstrated by Parducz (1959) and Grebecki (1965 a) in Paramecium and in Stylonychia by Dryl (1969) and Machemer (1965).

4. Continuous ciliary reversal (CCR) expressed by long-lasting backward movement along spiraling line with anticlockwise rotation of body around its longitudinal axis (Figure 2).

Jennings has described AR as the only motor reaction which appears in response to chemotactic stimuli in external medium. However, Alverdes (1922 a, c) pointed out that Jennings' definition of AR does not include all motor responses of Paramecium at the boundary of applied external stimuli. According to him the animal may react by means of adoral instead of aboral turning in response to mechanical stimulus or chemical agents and it may swim along arcs or can react with reversal of ciliary beat within a limited area of pellicle in response to local stimuli. In extensive studies on coordination of ciliary movement and mechanism of AR in Paramecium, Parducz (1956, 1959, 1967) also cast doubt upon the validity of Jenning's view and brought evidence that a numberof other reactions than those described by Jennings may appear as a result of external stimulation of Paramecium. Dryl (1952, 1961 a, 1963) was able to demonstrate that Paramecium may show PaCR instead of AR response towards some chemical agents (low concentrations of barium chloride or hight concentrations of potassium chloride) and in similar way Bujwid-Cwik and Dryl (unpublished) noticed that under certain experimental conditions Paramecium aurelia may show PCR instead of AR as a boundary reaction to weak concentrations of quinine and some other chemical agents. In both cases the pseudo-positive chemotactic aggregations of animals appeared at the boundary of tested solutions in consequence of inhibition of progressive movement while typical AR response was observed at higher concentrations of substances under study.

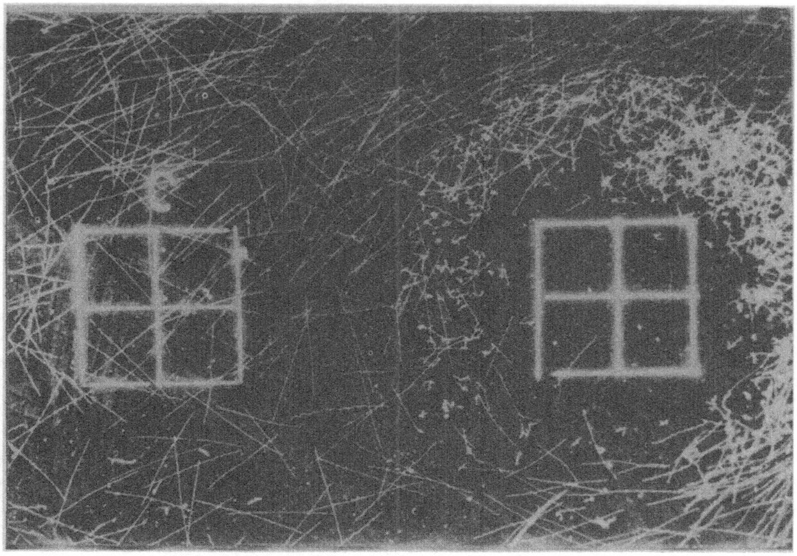

Figure 5. Negative chemotactic response of Paramecium aurellia towards mixed solution containing KCl and $CaCl_2$ in equal concentration of 16×10^{-3} M. The primary medium (C) contained 16×10^{-3} M $CaCl_2$ only. PCR response visible as boundary reactions between primary and tested medium. Recording of movement carried out by Dryl's time-exposure macrophotographic technique. The length of margin of small square = 5 mm. Time of exposure = 3 seconds (Bujwid-Cwik and Dryl, original).

The PCR responses in ciliates are reminiscent of random turnings observed in planaria Dendrocoelum lacteum (Ulyott 1936; Gunn, Kennedy and Pielou 1937) and according to classification by Frankel and Gunn (1967) they should be considered as a typical example of klinokinesis in which the rate of random turnings of animals depends on the intensity of stimulation.

As a rule the negative chemotactic response in Paramecium is accompanied by decrease of swimming rate (Dryl, 1961 b) and this fact cannot be neglected in evaluation of chemotactic response to given stimulus. It is clear therefore that quantitative analysis of chemotactic response of paramecia and other ciliates is always difficult because of possible "contamination" by such chemokinetic factors like: slackening of forward movement of animals within tested solution or occurence of PaCR or PCR as boundary reactions. Fortunately the new time exposure macrophotographic technique for recording the movement of protozoa (Dryl, 1958, 1963) and quantitative method for studying the chemotactic response in ciliate protozoa (Dryl, 1959 a) provide a more or less objective picture of chemotactic reaction under given experimental conditions. A typical positive chemotactic response of Paramecium towards solution showing a pH range within limits of chemotactic optimum (pH = 5.4-6.4) is shown in Figure 3, while negative chemotactic response towards higher concentration of $MgCl_2$ (2.90^{-2} M) is demonstrated in Figure 4. In both cases AR responses are recorded in form of zig-zag lines at the boundary between

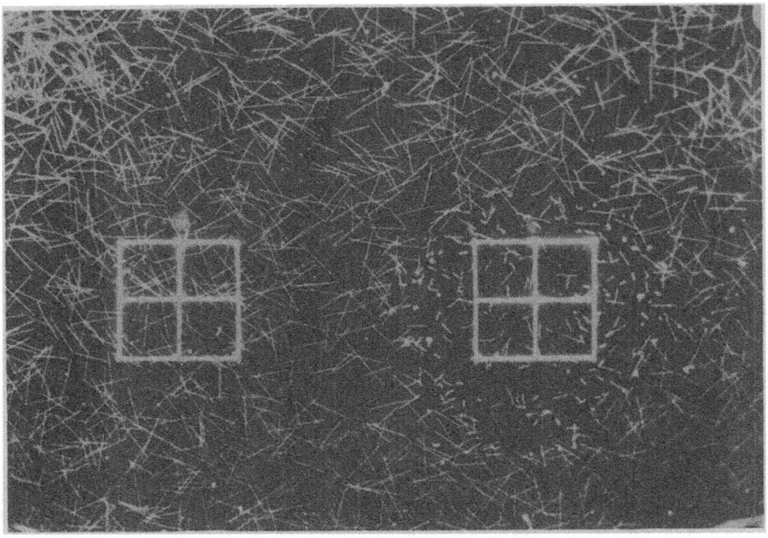

Figure 6. Negative chemotactic response of Paramecium caudatum towards solution containing NaCl in concentration 16×10^{-3} M. The slackening of movement of paramecia is visible within tested medium on the right. Recording of movement carried out by Dryl's time-exposure macrophotographic technique. The length of margin of large square = 5 mm. Time of exposure = 3 seconds. (Dryl, original).

initial medium and tested solution. The recorded PCR responses on the boundary of negative chemotactic solution are shown in Figure 5, while slackening of forward movement within tested solution can be easy recognized in Figure 6.

From a physiological point of view AR or any other boundary reaction (PCR or PaCR) should be considered as a first step of increased excitability of the protozoan cell since it is well known that ciliary reversal is correlated with depolarization of cell membrane (Kinosita, 1954; Yamaguchi, 1960 a, b; Kinosita, Dryl, and Naitoh, 1964 a, b, c) and there is a clear analogy between observed cathodal ciliary reversal in protozoa (Ludloff, 1895; Kinosita, 1936; Jahn, 1961) and cat-electronus of nerve and muscle cells which reflects an increase of their excitation state.

Jennings (1897) noticed that paramecia may show CCR in response to high concentrations of potassium chloride in external medium, while Mast and Nadler (1926) and Oliphant (1938, 1942) showed that monovalent cations induce CCR whereas bivalent or trivalent ones are indifferent in this respect.

The dependence of potassium-induced CCR in Paramecium caudatum on the presence of calcium in external medium was first emphasized by Kamada (1938, 1940). Kamada and Kinosita (1940) noticed antagonism between external K^{1+} and Ca^{2+} in their effects on the excitation state of Paramecium as it was expressed by duration of induced ciliary reversal. Jahn (1962) calculated the data of Kamada and Kinosita and found that the maximal duration of CCR is

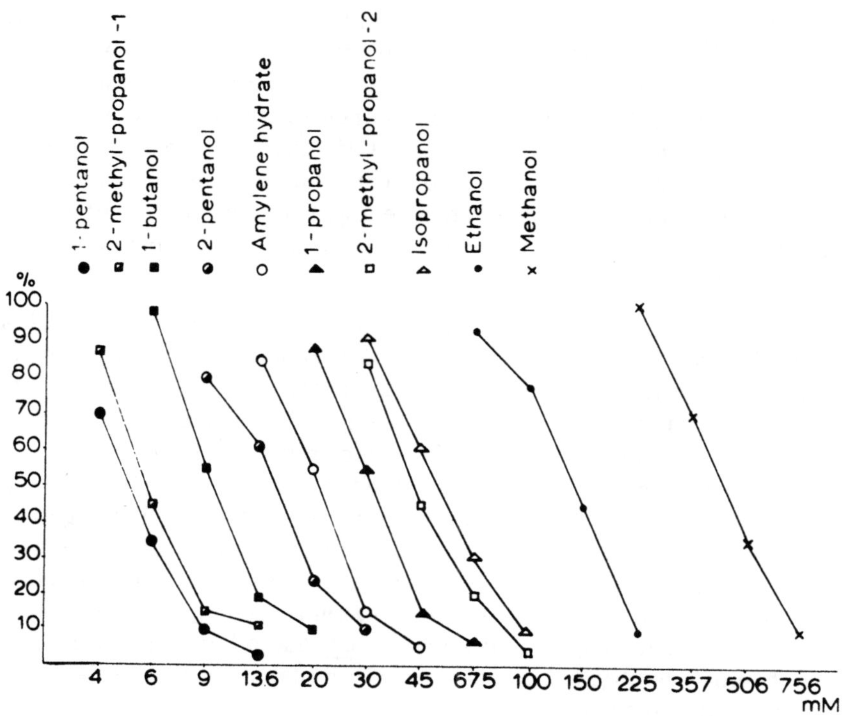

Figure 7. Chemotactic effects of lower alcohols on Paramecium caudatum expressed in percentage of animals entering the area of tested solution of alcohol in relation to the number of animals in the control area devoid of alcohol. (Dryl, 1959 b).

constant when concentration of K^{1+} is proportional to the square root of Ca^{2+} in external medium. This represents the Gibbs–Donnan ratio $[K^{1+}]/\sqrt{[Ca^{2-}]}$ = const. and suggests that ciliary reversal is caused by potassium ions which compete with calcium adsorbed at the cell membrane, releasing Ca^{2+} from their binding sites within a postulated ion exchange system localized at the cell surface. The detailed studies on stimulating effects of external chelating (EDTA), calcium-binding (citrates) or calcium-precipitating (oxalates) agents in Paramecium revealed the following sequence of motor response in dependence on the concentration of substances under study: Normal forward movement → PCR → CCR → PaCR → slow forward movement, which proved to be reversible if recalcification procedure was started early enough so that the animals did not perish (Grebecki, 1964, 1965 b). A similar series of motor responses was noticed by Kuznicki (1966) in Paramecium exposed to a number of other cations at different levels of external calcium. Kuznicki suggested that all the above mentioned cations induce ciliary reversal by competing action on the membrane-bound calcium. This assumption was confirmed by Naitoh and Yasumasu (1968) who were able to show that ^{45}Ca-binding by paramecia was inhibited by the monovalent cations in good agreement with Gibbs –Donnan principle. The authors suggested that calcium ions liberated from the anionic sites of the cell membrane by an exchange reaction with other anions induce ciliary reversal. Naitoh (1968, 1969 a, b) suggested that calcium ions activate the contractile system energized by ATP, necessary for induction of ciliary reversal. In this way the ciliary reversal would be analogous in its mechanism to contraction of muscle cells. The recent studies by Naitoh and Eckert (1968) brought evidence that cationic permeability depends on the level of saturation of the anionic binding sites with Ca^{2+} and an increase of the cation conductance is associated with decrease of bound calcium. It looks as though calcium binding mechanism may play an essential role both in the permeability of cell membrane and in ciliary response, coupling in this way excitation and contractile systems in Paramecium.

It should be emphasized that recent studies of Stentor coeruleus indicate that negative chemotactic response of this ciliate to quinine solutions depends on Gibbs–Donnan equilibrium of potassium and calcium ions in external medium (Pietrowicz-Kosmynka, 1970). The susceptibility of Stentor towards quinine decreased parallel to increase of value of ratio $[K^{1+}]/\sqrt{[Ca^{2+}]}$ and chemotactic response was completely abolished at values higher than 1.5. It was found also recently by Bujwid-Cwik and Dryl (unpublished) that negative chemotactic response of Paramecium aurelia towards various cations (K^{1+}, Na^{1+}, Mg^{2+}) decreases parallel to increase of concentration of Ca^{2+} in external medium, showing good agreement with Gibbs–Donnan principle. These results suggest that chemotactic response in Paramecium and other ciliates is based on the same basic physiological mechanism which plays essential role in other motor responses of protozoa.

It was suggested by the author elsewhere (Dryl, 1970) that in terms of physiology of the cell membrane Paramecium – and perhaps other ciliates – possess the chemosensitive input and the electrosensitive conductile components localized within the cell membrane, while transmission of impulse from the cell surface to locomotor organelles (cilia, cirri, myonemes) may correspond to the output component of the general scheme postulated by Grundfest (1957, 1959) for all kinds of excitable cells. Such organization of components within cell is reminiscent of the "primary type" invertebrate sense organs (Grundfest, 1964) where the sensory message is received in the reception portion of the cell and after formation of the graded generator potential is encoded in form of single or multiple all-or-none spikes which appear in the conductile portion of the same cell.

If we assume in accordance with Parker (1919), Grundfest (1964), and Duncan (1967) that the simple receptor–effector system of the cell (devoid of conductile portion) is the most primitive one in the animal kingdom, then we should consider the three-component system in Paramecium as a more advanced step in the evolution of excitability at the cellular level.

As regards the localization of chemoreceptive area within pellicle, Jennings and Jamieson (1902) and Horton (1935) demonstrated that fragments of paramecia possess the same capacity of response towards chemical stimuli as non-operated, intact animals. However, Alverdes (1922 b, c) pointed out that the cilia of the anterior region of Paramecium are more sensitive to chemical, thermal, and mechanical stimuli than those from the posterior end of the animal, while other authors (Parducz, 1956; Grebecki, 1965 a) suggested that peristomal cilia might be more sensitive to external stimuli than somatic ones. The existence of anterior–posterior polarization of excitability of the protozoan cell was postulated also for Opalina (Kinosita, 1954), Dileptus (Doroszewski, 1961) and Spirostomum (Seravin 1962, 1963).

3. Chemotactic Response of Ciliate Protozoa to Various Factors in External Environment

In his pioneer studies on chemotaxis in Paramecium aurelia and other ciliate protozoa Jennings (1899) divided the chemical compounds into: chemo-attractive (causing positive chemotactic reaction), chemo-repellent (causing negative chemotaxis), and chemo-indifferent (causing no chemotactic reaction at all) substances. He was not able to find any correlation between the intensity of chemotactic response and noxious effects of tested compounds. According to him the univalent and bivalent cations possess strong negative chemotactic properties, the trivalent cations weaker ones, while weak acids and anions have positive chemotactic properties. In this way solutions of salts derived from univalent and bivalent cations cause negative chemotactic response due to the proponderance of cation over anion, whereas solutions of salts derived from trivalent cations cause positive chemotactic reaction as a result of prevalence of anion over cation in their chemotactic activities. Jennings noticed an increase of negative chemotactic action parallel to decrease of atomic weight of the cation, while Kagan (1939) suggested that intensity of negative chemotactic reaction goes up parallel with an increase of the valency of cations and in a group of cations with equal valency it increases parallel to the magnitude of atomic weight.

The following range of cations was established by Dryl (1952, 1961) in dependence on the threshold values of their negative chemotactic action on Paramecium caudatum: $Ca^{2+} \geq Na^{1+} > Mg^{2+} \geq Li^{1+} > K^{1+} > Ba^{2+}$. This ranking of cations does not indicate any correlation between chemotactic action and the valency of cation or between chemotactic properties and atomic weight among cations with equal valency. A similar range of cations was reported recently by Dryl and Pietrowicz-Kosmynka (1968) in studies on chemotactic response of Stentor coeruleus and this species proved to be even more sensitive to chemotactic action of cations then Paramecium. The recent results achieved in studies on intracellular potential of Paramecium indicated following range of cations: $Ca^{2+} > Na^{1+} > Mg^{2+} > K^{1+} > Ba^{2+}$ in dependence on the magnitude of negative intracellular potential in 2 mM and 20 mM concentrations of corresponding chlorides (Kinosita, Dryl, and Naitoh, 1964). This finding may suggest that negative chemotactic properatires of cations are in some way related to their depolarizing effects on the cell membrane. The data indicating correlation between lower rates of forward movement and depolarization of cell membrane also support this view – if we take into accounts that the slackening of the forward movement is usually associated with negative chemotactic action of cations (Dryl, 1961 a).

Jennings (1899, 1906) indicated that paramecia and other ciliate protozoa respond positively to those chemotactic stimuli which signalize the presence of bacteria or other kinds of food in the external environment. Similar observations were reported by Blattner (1926) for Spirostomum ambiguum. It was suggested by Jennings and Moore (1902) and Moore (1903) that positive response of paramecia to a slightly acid medium has adaptive character, since under normal conditions it brings the animals into an environment abundant in food and bacteria which produce large quantities of carbon dioxide during the process of respiration. In contradiction to Jennings' view Barrat (1905) suggested that positive chemotaxis is only the transient phase of negative chemotaxis and there is no reason to distinguish both kinds of response as separate reactions. However, further studies on this line brought clear evidence that positive and negative chemotaxis exist as separate phenomena although both of them are based on the occurrence of an avoiding reaction as a boundary response between the initial and test solution.

Lozina-Lozinskij (1929 a, b, c) observed in paramecia high rate of food vacuole formation in suspensions of dyes causing positive chemotaxis, when compared with animals exposed to suspensions of dyes inducing negative chemotactic response or no response at all. Lozina-Lozinskij noticed also correlation between the positive chemotactic properties and phagotrophic response of Paramecium towards suspensions of India Ink, Carmine, and B. subtilis. The positive chemotactic response towards food was also reported in Dileptus (Chen, 1950) and Tetrahymena (Corliss, 1960) although no specific food-attractant substance could be distinguished.

The optimum pH range for chemotaxis in Paramecium caudatum was established by Dryl (1952, 1959 a) between 5.4 and 6.4, i.e. the animals gather themselves in solutions showing pH within these limits. The established optimum causes alleviation of the negative chemotactic action of potassium ions and other negative chemotactic factors. These effects of pH may be of great biological importance since they indicate the way in which paramecia under natural conditions may eventually enter the environment containing chemorepellent factors.

Recently Pietrowicz-Kosmynka (1970) found the chemotactic optimum of pH for Stentor coeruleus between 6.9 and 7.7, thus giving evidence of occurrence of significant physiological differences between Paramecium and Stentor in this respect.

In separate series of experiments with ten lower alcohols Dryl (1959 b) found evidence that stronger negative chemotactic response is associated with higher molecular weight of alcohol and normal compounds prove to be more effective in this respect than iso (Figure 7). It should be pointed out in this connection that a similar range of alcohols was reported by authors studying the smell sensitivity of invertebrates (Dethier and Yost, 1952) and vertebrates (Moulton and Eayrs, 1960), which indicates a rather high degree of development of chemical sense in the ciliate protozoa.

As regards other organic compounds of biological importance, paramecia proved to be chemotactically insensitive to urea, glycerol, and d-glucose (Dryl, 1961 a) in spite of the fact that some bacteria (Adler, 1966) manifest positive chemotactic response towards glucose and galactose as to an utilizable energy source in external environment.

Kadlubowski and Rostkowska (1961) reported positive chemotactic response of the parasitic ciliate Balantidium coli towards some protozoocidal agents like: potassium permanganate, cupric sulphate, formaldehyde, phenol, ethanol, atebrin, chinosol, neosalvarsan, aureomycin, and streptomycin, while Rostkowska (1964) noticed positive chemotaxis of Balantidium towards low concentrations of formic, oxalic, lactic, and citric acids and negative response towards solutions of ammonium chloride, magnesium chloride, calcium chloride, sodium sulphate, sodium iodide, sodium cyanide, glucose, and saccharose. It is not clear whether the reported aggregation responses of Balantidium were true chemotactic or only pseudo-chemotactic reactions, since the authors did not give any information about the pattern of movement, character of boundary reactions, and rate of swimming, i.e., those factors which could be responsible for the observed gatherings of protozoa in tested solutions.

We have still scant data as regards the possible role of ACh–AChase system in evoking response and chemical transmission of stimulus in protozoa. The occurrence of ACh was reported in Paramecium (Bayer and Wense, 1936), while AChase was found Tetrahymena (Pastor and Fennel, 1959; Seaman and Houlihan, 1951; Seaman, 1951). Some authors (Muller and Toth, 1959; Seravin, 1963) noticed that low concentrations of ACh and anti AChase agents lengthen K^{1+}/Ca^{2+} – induced CCR while high concentrations shorten this response. Dryl (unpublished) noticed negative chemotactic response towards ACh in Paramecium caudatum, Paramecium aurelia, Stentor coeruleus, and Spirostomum ambiguum, thus giving support to the earlier observations by Seravin (1964 1969) that ACh may evoke ciliary reversal and contraction of myonemes in Spirostomum. There is no doubt that the ACh–AChase system and perhaps some other transmitter substance may play an essential role in the excitability of protozoa, but more experimental data are needed in order to explain the physiological mechanism of their action on the protozoan cell.

4. Sensory Adaptation in Chemotaxis

Adaptation to stimulus usually exerts modifying effects on the motor reactions of protoza, as was revealed by studies on response to light (Mast and Pusch, 1924; Mast, 1932; Mast, 1937), mechanical stimuli (Jennings, 1906; Wawrzynczyk, 1937; Kinastowski, 1963) and temperature (Mendelsohn, 1902).

Oliphant (1938) has shown in Paramecium multimicronucleatum that adaptation to solutions of sodium, lithium, and potassium salts involved inhibition of ciliary reversal at low concentrations or caused shorter duration of this response at higher concentrations. In Opalina adaptation to potassium chloride solutions reduced their sensitivity to chemical and electric stimuli (Okajima, 1954).

As concerns chemotaxis, Dryl (1959 a) indicated that paramecian adapted to medium containing high concentrations of Na^{1+}, Mg^{2+} did not show much change of response to chemical stimuli, whereas 1-24 hours lasting exposure of animals to potassium-rich medium effected the chemotactic response in a very significant way.

Paramecia show a very characteristic sequence of motor response during exposure to potassium-rich medium (concentration of KCl = $4 \cdot 10^{-2}$ M, concentration of $CaCl_2 = 1 \cdot 10^{-3}$ M). At the beginning the animals react with CCR, which after 5-7 minutes transforms to PaCR and finally (after next 2-3 minutes) there appearas the normal pattern of forward movement with highly reduced rate of swimming. It was shown by Dryl (1952, 1959 a) that paramecia treated in this way loose the capacity of motor response to chemical or mechanical stimuli even after being washed for 1-3 minutes in potassium-free medium. The first response to strong chemotactic stimuli reappears after 3 minutes from the beginning of washing procedure while the normal response to chemotactic stimuli is recovered after 15-20 minutes. In spite of the rather lengthy process of recovery of normal response-capacity towards external stimuli, the normal rate of swimming of Paramecium reappears during first 10-15 seconds of washing and this may suggest that there are separate physiological mechanisms involved in these two phenomena.

Adaptation to potassium is non-specific in action since it causes inhibition of response to all kinds of negative and positive chemotactic stimuli. Recently similar inhibiting effects of potassium on chemotactic response were reported for Stentor coeruleus (Pietrowicz-Kosmynka, 1970).

The mechanism by which potassium ions inhibit the chemotactic response in ciliates is unknown although it may be suggested that it is related in some way to postulated action of potassium ions on the behavior of calcium within the cell surface and induced depolarization of cell membrane.

REFERENCES

Adler, J. (1966). Science 153, 708.

Alverdes, F. (1922 a). Studien an Infusorien uber Flimmerbewegung, Lokomotion und Reizbeantwortung. Berlin, p. 130.

Alverdes, F. (1922 b). Zool. Anz. 55, 19.

Alverdes, F (1922 c). Biol. Zbl. 42, 218.

Barrat, J. O. W. (1905). Zschr. Allg. Physiol. 5, 73.

Bayer, G. and Wense, T. (1936). Pfluger's Arch. ges. Physiol. 237, 417.

Blattner, H. (1926). Ehrbg. Arch. f. Protistenk. 53, 253.

Chen. Y. T. (1950). Q. J. microsc. Sci. 91, 297.

Corliss, J. O. (1960). Parasitol. 50, 111.

Dethier, V. A. and Yost, M. T. (1952). J. Gen. Physiol. 35, 823.

Doroszewski, M. (1961). Acta Biol. exp. 21, 15.

Dryl, S. (1952). Acta Biol. exp. 16, 23.

Dryl, S. (1958). Bull. Acad. pol. Sci. Cl, II 6, 429.

Dryl, S. (1959 a). Acta Biol. exp. 19, 53.

Dryl, S. (1959 b). Acta Biol. exp. 19, 95.

Dryl, S. (1961 a). Acta Biol. exp. 21, 75.

Dryl, S. (1961 b). Bull. Acad. pol. Sci. Cl. II 9, 71.

Dryl, S. (1961 c). J. Protozool. 8 (suppl.) Abstr. 55.

Dryl, S. (1963). Anim. Behav. 11, 393.

Dryl, S. (1965). Progress in Protozool., London Abstr. 308.

Dryl, S. (1969). Motor response of Protozoa to external stimuli. Progress in Protozoology, 124-126, Publishing House "Nauka" Leningrad.

Dryl, S. (1970). Acta Protozool. 7, 325.

Dryl, S. and Grebecki, A. (1966). Protoplasma 62, 255.

Dryl, S. and Pietrowicz-Kosmynka, D. (1968). J. Protozool. 15 (suppl.), 112.

Duncan, C. J. (1967). The molecular properties and evolution of excitable cells. International Series of Monographs in pure and applied Biology (Zoology Division) 35, Pergamon Press Ltd.

Fraenkel, G. S. and Gunn, D. L. (1961). The orientation of Animals. Dover Publications, Inc., New York. p. 376.

Grebecki, A. (1964). Acta Protozool. 2, 69.

Grebecki, A. (1965 a). Acta Protozool. 3, 79.

Grebecki, A. (1965 b). Acta Protozool. 3, 275.

Grundfest, H. (1957). Physiol. Rev. 37, 337.

Grundfest, H. (1959). Evolution of conduction in the nervous system. In: Evolution of Nervous Control from Primitive Oraganisms to Man, 43-86. (Bass, A. D. ed.) Amer. Assoc. Adv. Sci., Washington, D. C.

Grundfest, H. (1964). Evolution of electrophysiological varieties among sensory receptor systems. Essays on Physiological Evolution. Pergamonn Press. Oxford – London – Edinburgh – New York – Paris – Frankfurt.

Gunn, D. L., Kennedy, J. S., and Pielou, D. P. (1937). Nature 140, 1064.

Horton, F. M. (1935). J. Exp. Biol. 12, 13.

Jahn, T. (1961). J. Protozool. 8, 369.

Jahn, T. (1962). J. Cell. Comp. Physiol. 60, 217.

Jahn, T. L. and Bovee, E. C. (1968). Mtile Behavior of Protozoa. In: Research in Protozoology. Ed. by Chen, T. T. Vol. I, 47-200.

Jennings, H. S. (1897). J. Physiol. 21, 258.

Jennings, H. S. (1899 a). Am. J. Physiol. 2, 311.

Jennings, H. S. (1899 b). Am. J. Physiol. 2, 355.

Jennings, H. S. (1900). Am. J. Physiol. 3, 229.

Jennings, H. S. (1904 a). Carnegie Inst. Wash. Pub. 16, 89.

Jennings, H.S. (1904 b). Carnegie Inst. Wash. Pub. 16, 235.

Jennings, H. S. (1906). Behavior of the lower Organisms. p. 366, New York.

Jennings, H. S. and Jamieson, C. (1902). Biol. Bull. 3, 225.

Jennings, H. S. and Moore, E. M. (1902). Am. J. Physiol. 6, 233.

Johnson, W. H. (1929). Biol. Bull. 57, 199.

Kadlubowski, R. and Rostkowska, J. (1961). Acta Parasitol. 9, 109.

Kagan, D. (1939). Trav. Soc. Sci. Wilno, 13, 1.

Kamada, T. (1938). Proc. Imp. Acad. Japan 14, 260.

Kamada, T. (1940). Proc. Imp. Acad. Japan 16, 241.

Kamada, T. and Kinosita, H. (1940). Proc. Imp. Acad. Japan 16, 125.

Kinastowski, W. (1963). Acta Protozool. 1, 201.

Kinosita, H. (1936). J. Fac. Sci. Tokyo Univ. 4, 155.

Kinosita, H. (1954). J. Fac. Sci. Tokyo Univ. 7, 1.

Kinosita, H., Dryl, S., and Naitoh, Y. (1964 a). J. Fac. Sci. Tokyo Univ. Sec. IV 10, 291.

Kinosita, H., Dryl, S., and Naitoh, Y. (1964 b). J. Fac. Sci. Tokyo Univ. Sec. IV 10, 303.

Kinosita, H., Dryl, S., and Naitoh, Y. (1964 c). Bull. Acad. Pol. Sci. Cl. II 12, 459.

Kuznicki, L. (1966). Acta Protozool. 4, 241.

Kuhn, A. (1919). Die Orientierung der Tiere im Raum. Jena, 40 figs, p. 71.

Loeb, J. (1890). Der Heliotropismus der Thiere und seine Uebereinstimmung mit dem Heliotropismus der Pflanzen. p. 118. Wurzburg.

Loeb, J. (1912). The mechanistic Conception of Life. Chicago, p. 232.

Loeb, J. (1918). Forced Movements, Tropisms and Animal Conduct. Philadelphia and London, 42 figs, p. 209.

Loeb, J. and Budgett, S. P. (1897). Zur Theorie des Galvanotropismus. Pfluger's Arch. ges. Physiol. 65, 518.

Loeb, J. and Hardesty, J. (1895). Ueber die Lokalisation der Atmung in der Zelle. Pfluger's Arch. ges. Physiol. 61, 583.

Lozina-Lozinsky, L. (1929 a). Compt. rend. soc. biol. 100, 321.

Lozina-Lozinsky, L. (1929 b). Compt. rend. acad. sci. U.R.S.S. Ser. A 17, 403.
Lozina-Lozinsky, L. (1929 c). Bull. Inst. sci. Lesshaft 15, 91.
Ludloff, K. (1895). Pfluger's Arch. ges. Physiol. 59, 525.
Machemer, N. (1965). Arch. Protistenk. 108, 153.
Massart, J. (1889). Archs. Biol. 9, 515.
Mast, S. O. (1911). Light and the Behavior of Organisms. New York and London, 34 figs, p. 410.
Mast, S. O. (1913). Biol. Zbl. 33, 581.
Mast, S. O. (1914). Biol. Zbl. 34, 641.
Mast, S. O. (1915). Arch. Entm. Mech. Org. 41, 251.
Mast, S. O. (1932). Zschr. vergl. Physiol. 17, 644.
Mast, S. O. (1937). Biol. Bull. 73, 126.
Mast, S. O. and Nadler, J. E. (1926). J. Morph. and Physiol. 43, 105.
Mast, S. O. and Pusch (1924). Biol. Bull. 46, 55.
Mendelssohn, M. (1902). J. Physiol. et path. gen. 4, 393.
Moore, A. (1903). Am. J. Physiol. 9, 238.
Moulton, D. G. and Eayrs, J. T. (1960). Quart. J. exp. Psychol. 12, 99.
Muller, M. and Toth, E. (1959). J. Protozool. 6, (suppl.) 28.
Naitoh, Y. (1968). J. cell. comp. Physiol. 51, 85.
Naitoh, Y. (1969 a). J. gen. Physiol. 53, 517.
Naitoh, Y. (1969 b). Science 164, 963.
Naitoh, Y. and Eckert, R. (1968). Z. vergl. Physiol. 61, 427.
Naitoh, Y. and Yasumasu, I. (1968). J. gen. Physiol. 50, 1303.
Okajima, A. (1954). Annot. Zool. Japon. 27, 46.
Oliphant, J. F. (1938). Physiol. Zool. 12, 19.
Oliphant, J. F. (1942). Physiol. Zool. 15, 443.
Parducz, B. (1956). Acta biol. 7, 73.
Parducz, B. (1959). Ann. Hist. Nat. Mus. Nat. Hung. 51, 227.
Parducz, B. (1967). Int. Rev. Cytol. 21, 91.
Parker, G. H. (1919). The elementary Nervous System. Lippincott, Philadelphia and London, 53 figs, p. 292.
Pastor, E. P. and Fennel, R. A. (1959). J. Morphol. 104, 143.
Pfeffer, W. (1883). Ber. dt. bot. Ges. 1, 524.
Pfeffer, W. (1884). Unters. Bot. Inst. Tubingen 1, 363.
Pfeffer, W. (1888). Unters. Bot. Inst. Tubingen 2, 582.
Pietrowicz-Kosmynka, D. (1970). Chemotaksja u Stentor coeruleus. Ph. D. thesis M. Nencki Institute of Exp. Biology. Warsaw, Poland.
Rosen, W. G. (1962). Q. Rev. Biol. 37, 242.
Rostkowska, J. (1964). Acta Protozool. 2, 81.
Seaman, G.R. (1951). Proc. Soc. Exp. Biol. Med. 76, 169.
Seaman, G. R. and Houlihan, R. K. (1951). J. Cell. Comp. Physiol. 37, 309.
Seravin, L. N. (1962). Tsitologia 4, 545.
Seravin, L. N. (1963). Inst. Tsitol. Akad. Nauk. S.S.S.R. 3, 111.
Seravin, L. N. (1964). Tsitologia 6, 516.
Seravin, L. N. (1969). Tsitologia 11, 659.
Ullyott, P. (1936). J. exp. Biol. 13, 253.
Verworn, M. (1889). Psychophysiologische Protistenstudien, Experimentelle Untersuchungen, Jena, p. 219.
Wawrzynczyk, S. (1937). Acta Biol. exp. 11,
Yamaguchi, T. (1960 a). J. Fac. Sci. Tokyo Univ. IV 8, 573.
Yamaguchi, T. (1960 b). J. Fac. Sci. Tokyo Univ. IV 8, 593.

CHEMOTAXIS OF ANIMAL SPERMATOZOA

R. L. Miller
Temple University,
Department of Biology,
Philadelphia,
Pennsylvania 19122, U. S. A.

SUMMARY

Although the gametes of most animals are presumed to meet by chance, several mechanisms exist which serve to enhance the chances of contact.

1. The size of one gamete (egg) is increased as a target.

2. The other gamete (sperm) remains small and is usually highly motile, showing a persistence of direction. For any population, direction is random, however.

The mobility of the gametes, especially the sperm, may be modified in several ways to increase the probability of collision with the egg. All produce undirected behavior in the sperm.

1. "Thigmotaxis" or the tendency of the sperm to swim near surfaces.

2. Agglutination by egg associated substances.

3. Chemically decreasing motility.

4. Physically decreasing motility.

5. Production of aberrant motility.

Mechanism of direct guidance of sperm to eggs include:

1. Oriented egg coatings or micropyles.

2. Chemotaxis.

Directed sperm migration by means of a chemical gradient has been demonstrated in a number of marine hydroides. The sperm behavior during chemotaxis is compared to sperm behavior during undirected responses.

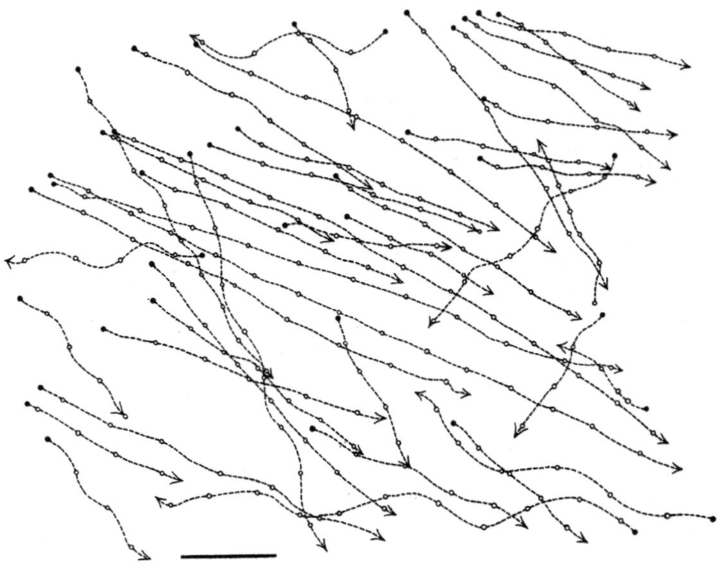

Figure 1. A plot of sperm swimming free of any constraint. The sperm have been released from the upper left. The scale equals 40μ. In this and all other plots, the start of the trail is indicated by the filled circle. The open circles are 10 frames (0.45 seconds) apart. Because of the properties of the optical system, left and right have been reversed in Figures 1 and 2 and 6-9. The species used is Campanularia calceolifera.

1. Introduction

For most organisms fertilization takes place in an aqueous medium. Success is predicated on gamete contact which results ultimately from the locomotion of at least one of the two gametes. The surfaces of both gametes bear adhesive substances specific for the surface of the other cell, which bind the gametes firmly together once collision has occurred. This system has evolved along lines which take advantage of circumstances that increase the probability of collision of randomly moving small objects: (1) one of the two gametes becomes stationary and increases in size, because a larger, immobile target is easier to hit than a small, rapidly moving one; and (2) interaction between randomly dispersed gametes is enhanced if the smaller rapidly swimming cell (sperm) moves in straight lines, turning infrequently, and displays little or no tendency to turn in a particular direction relative to its own path or other objects in its vicinity. This permits a population of these cells to penetrate a large volume of medium with maximum efficiency. Given these conditions, gamete contact may be assumed to occur by chance (Balinsky, 1965) and this is probably so for most animals. However, animals further provide for the meeting of their gametes by attempting to approximate them before or during their release. Simultaneous spawnings, special egg coatings, spawning or mating aggregations, courtship and nesting behaviors, copulation and transport and storage of sperm by the female reproductive tract all serve this purpose in one way or another.

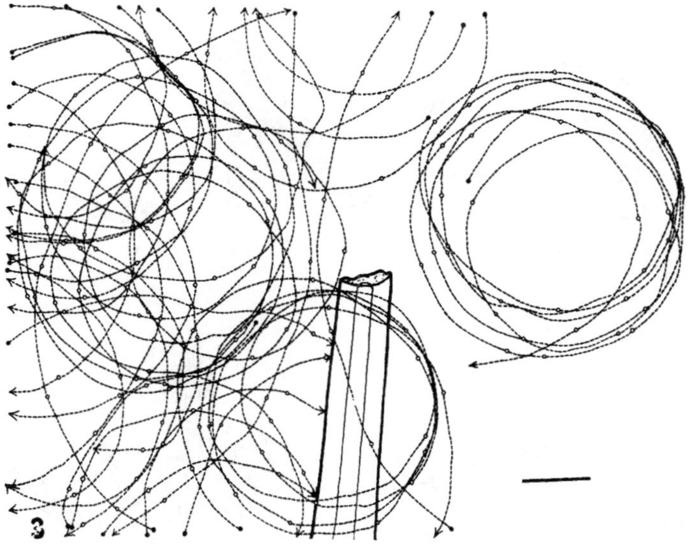

Figure 2. A control preparation where sperm circling on the surface of a microscope slide are exposed to sea water in a pipette. All trails but one in the right half of the plot have been omitted to show the nature of the circling behavior. The scale equals 20 μ. The experimental is shown in Figure 8.

The "chance" system of gamete interactions possesses inherent disadvantages. Since, for any population of sperm, the direction of individual cells is random, and the volume of the medium to be traversed large in comparison to the volume of the eggs, very large numbers of sperm must be produced to ensure contact with most of the eggs. Thus the system will tend to waste sperm. It may also be wasteful of eggs, which might simply be missed by randomly swimming sperm. Paradoxically, problems may arise at the other extreme as eggs can be exposed to excessive amounts of sperm that could lead to polyspermy. Animals have overcome the latter difficulty by developing mechanisms which decrease the number of sperm making contact with the egg. Examples include precipitation and inactivation of excess sperm by agglutination with egg-associated substances, prevention of entry of supernumerary sperm by means of impenetrable egg membranes and restriction of sperm access to one point on the egg surface by means of micropyles. In these ways a balance is struck so that fertilization can take place in the proper manner under a variety of gamete population sizes. It is not likely that all animals will regulate the numbers of sperm approaching the eggs in the same way, though common factors are certainly present in widely diverse groups. Each species adjusts the mechanisms at its disposal to the particular environmental conditions it faces.

A large body of literature (cf. reviews by Machlis and Rawitscher-Kunkel, 1967; Rosen, 1962; Raper, 1952; Wiese, 1969; Zeigler, 1962a, 1962b) exists describing the important role of chemical attractants in bringing the gametes of plants together. Two general chemo-attractive phenomena are

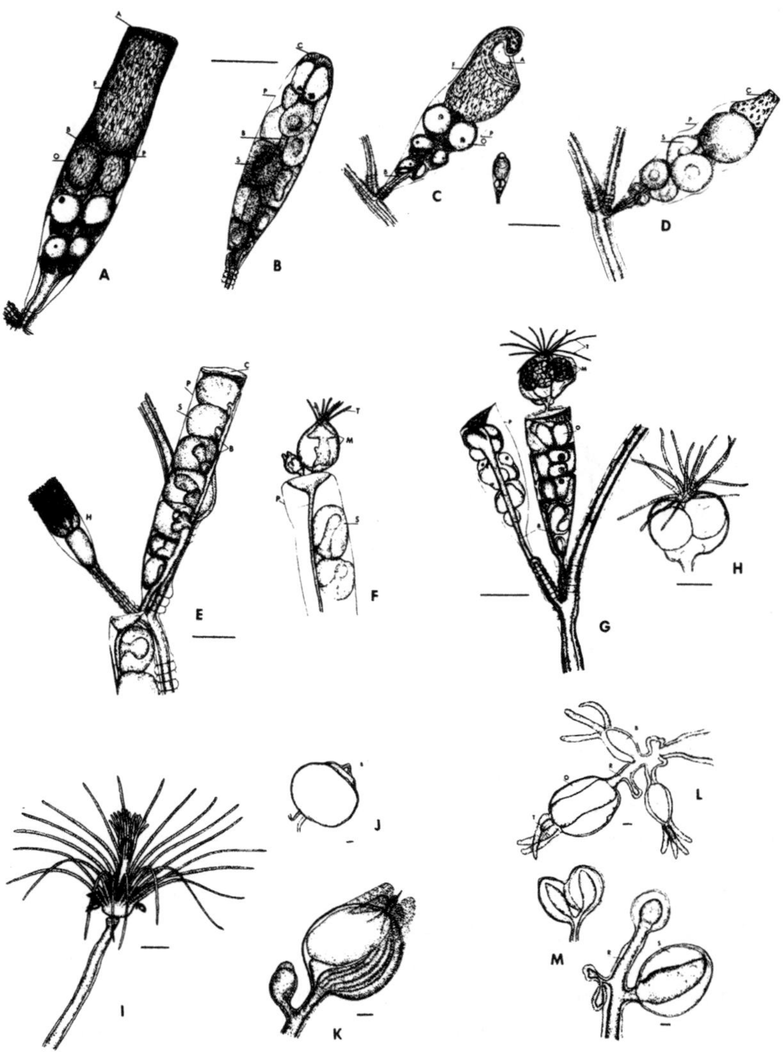

Figure 3. Gonangia and gonophores of some of the hydroids used.

A and B – Female and male, respectively, of Campanularia flexuosa. Scale equals 0.5mm.

C and D – Female and male, respectively, of Campanularia calceolifera, Scale equals 0.5mm.

E and G – Male and female gonangia, respectively, of Gonothyrea loveni. Scale equals 0.3mm.

F and H – Extruded meconidia (gonophores) of E and G. Scale of H equals 0.1mm.

I – Hydranth of Tubularia crocea showing position of gonophores at base of proximal tentacles. Scale equals 1.0mm.

J and K – Male and female gonophores, respectively, of Tubularia crocea. Scale equals 0.01 mm.

L and M – Female and male gonophores, respectively, of Tubularia marina. Scale equals 0.01mm.

Legend: A-aperture of gonangium, B-blastostyle, C-tissue cap of male gonangium of Campanularia, F-funnel tissue of female gonangium of Campanularia, H-hydranth, M-meconidium, O-ovum, P-perisarc, R-raceme, S-sporosac, T-tentacle of gonophore. (From Miller, 1966a, 1970 and unpublished).

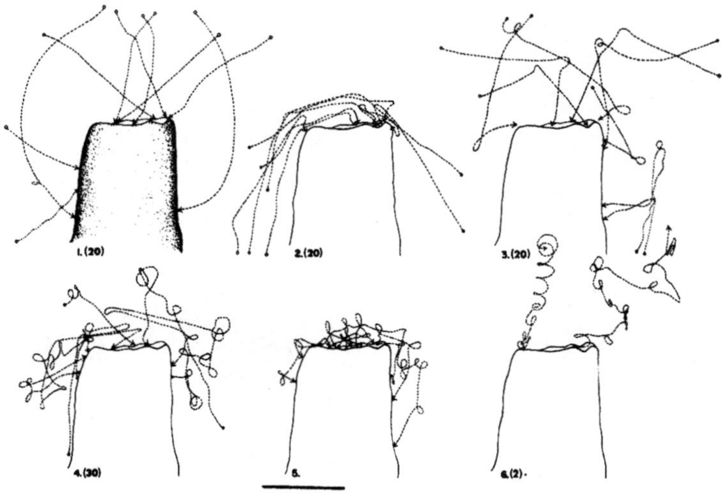

Figure 4. Attraction of C. flexuosa sperm to the aperture of the female gonangium of the same species. The trails have been grouped according to morphological type and the percentage of each type is indicated in parentheses. The scale is 0.4mm. (From Miller, 1966a).

found in plants: (1) chemotaxis, where the motile gamete is free-swimming and makes directed turns in response to a chemical gradient produced by the female gamete (or more often, by cells near it) and (2) chemotropism, where an outgrowing structure, such as a thallus or pollen tube bends in the direction of a chemical gradient produced by another thallus, a gamete, or structure surrounding the gamete.

In view of the diversity of the modes of gametic interactions in animals, and the widespread presence of chemo-attractive phenomena in plants, one is tempted to ask why animals have not utilized this mechanism which almost guarantees the meeting of egg and sperm. Although substances released by eggs and egg related tissues do play some role in keeping animal sperm in the vicinity of the egg (Lillie, 1919) and the sperm's own behavior when confronted with surfaces also acts in this manner (Dewitz, 1886), many of these effects are nonspecific, and some definitely adverse to successful fertilization. They do not involve directed orientation of the sperm to the egg by means of chemical gradients and are considered under the general category of "trap-action" phenomena (Rothschild, 1956).

The presence of chemo-attractive phenomena in plants, and its evident absence in animals, might be partially explained by the fact that in most animals the female gamete does retain some motility, even if only passive. It is usually free of somatic tissue investment, and if not, carries that investment with it. In animals, therefore, the two gametes can be said to move toward each other, whereas in higher plants the male gamete moves toward a totally immobile female gamete.

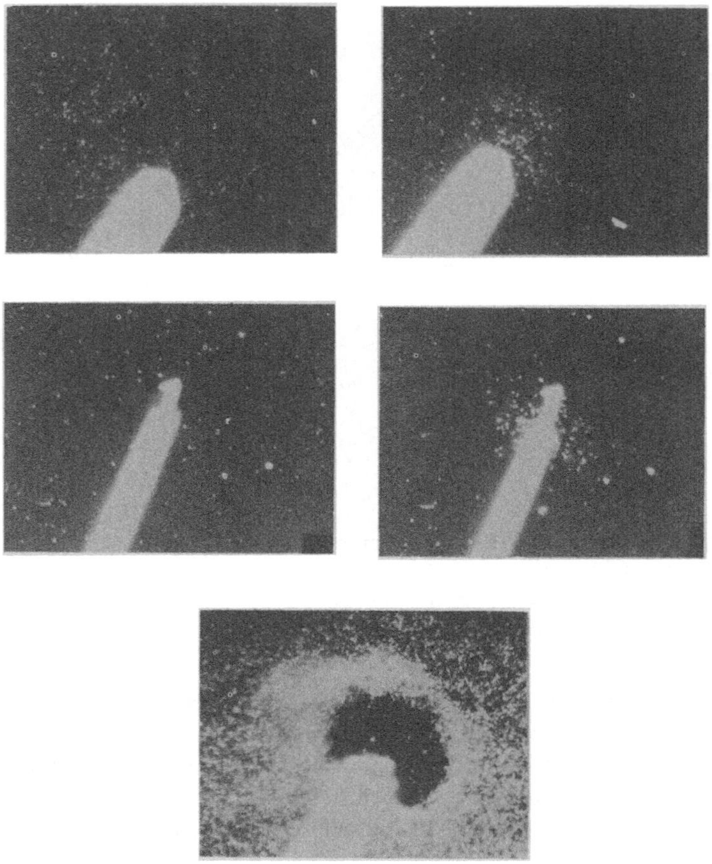

Figure 5. a and b Photographs of blow-out situation equivalent to Figures 2 and 6. a. no material released. b. about one minute after extrusion of active extract. Pipette diameter is 40 μ. c and d Photographs of agar-diffusion situation equivalent to Figures 1 and 8. c. pipette just inserted. d. after 30 seconds. Pipette diameter is 20 μ. e. Control blow-out situation where immobile sperm are pushed aside by sea water ejected from pipette. The clear area gives a rough approximation of the constant concentration zone of attractant existing in front of the pipettes in Figures 6 and 5b. Pipette diameter in 50 μ. (From Miller, 1966a).

2. Existence of Chemotaxis in Animal Sperm

The initial discoveries of Pfeffer (1884) on ferns and mosses, and the type of reasoning just presented, encouraged many investigators to look for chemotaxis during fertilization in animals. Practically all of these workers used Pfeffer's method of introducing egg or tissue extracts into a medium containing swimming sperm by means of a capillary pipette and used the sea urchin or similar form of experimental material. Because Pfeffer's capillary method when used with animal sperm is exceedingly prone to artifact for physical reasons alone (Rothschild, 1956) it is not surprising that many claims for the existence of sperm chemotaxis appeared (Dakin and Fordham, 1924, for example). Furthermore, sperm–sperm interactions were taking place that severely hindered observation of sperm behavior in the gradient. The sea urchin sperm is not ideal for these studies because it moves rapidly, and in crowded

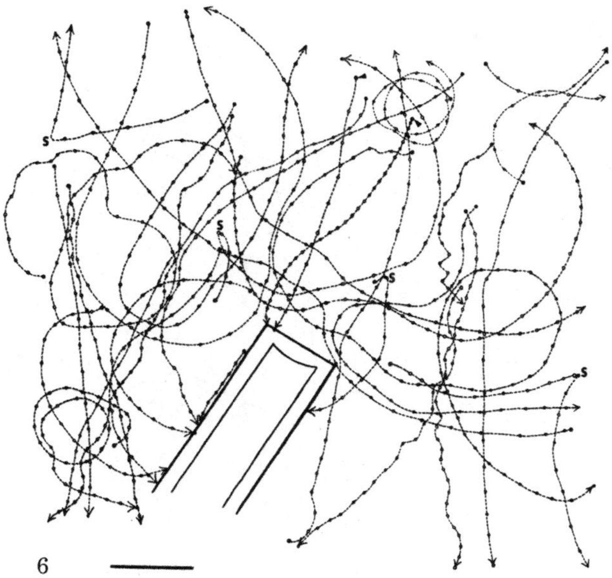

6

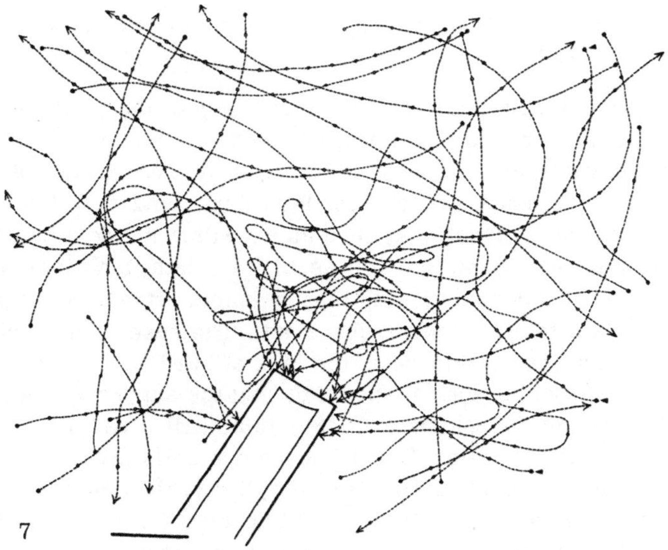

7

Figures 6 and 7. Control and experimental, respectively, where the contents were briefly expelled from the pipette. Points marked S in Figure 6 indicate turns resulting from sperm striking the slice surface. Trials marked with triangles in Figure 7 are those where the sperm deviate as they enter the gradient. The scale equals 40μ. (From Miller, 1966a).

suspension observation of individual behavior is practically impossible. Interpretation was further complicated by a loose definition of chemotaxis which encompassed all aggregations formed by chemical means (Jennings, 1962).

The situation began to clear after the important discoveries of Lillie (1919) on sperm agglutination by secretions emanating from the egg or incorporated in jelly layers surrounding the egg. The "fertilizin" hypothesis provided an explanation for the massive agglutinations of sperm misinterpreted

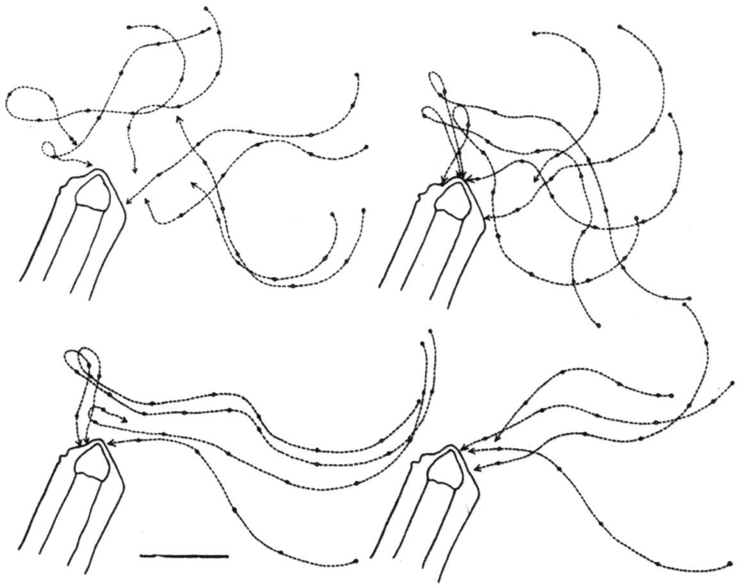

Figure 8. Selected trails from an experimental preparation equivalent to Figure 7, but where the sperm are circling on a surface rather than swimming straight. This plot demonstrates well the ability of some sperm to orientate when entering the gradient. The scale equals 40 μ.

as chemotaxis by workers using the capillary method, though some of their observations still require explanation (Lillie, 1919). Lillie's work was shortly followed by two devastating critiques of the methods and results of earlier workers on sperm chemotaxis by E.B. Wilson (1924) and T.H. Morgan (1927). Using simple physical explanations, such as crowding inside a capillary and random direction of movement, as well as Lillie's data, both men disproved all previous reports by demonstrating that chemical attraction did not have to be invoked to explain the phenomena observed. The ease with which they were able to do this gives some evidence of the lack of hard data on the actual behavior (direction of locomotion) of sperm during the supposed chemotaxis. Results of later workers (Dickmann, 1963) can be criticized on similar grounds. It was further claimed by Weiss (1961) that sperm cells did not possess, by reason of their small size and structural simplicity, the sensory and locomotory capabilities required for as complex a behavioral reaction as taxis movement. The weight of negative evidence was strong enough to produce denials of its existence in every major review between 1925 and 1966 (cf. Miller, 1966a, for literature survey). Work has continued actively on the surface components responsible for gamete adhesion (Metz, 1967), and some of these have effects on sperm motility, if not directionality (Tyler, 1949).

In approaching the study of animal sperm chemotaxis the major question concerns the criteria used to determine the nature of the sperm behavior. The problem is to find a testable definition of chemotaxis which permits elimination of all other phenomena previously included under this category, and which provides critical tests of the suspected chemotactic behavior. Fraenkel and Gunn (1961) in their book <u>The Orientation of Animals</u> define a taxis as a

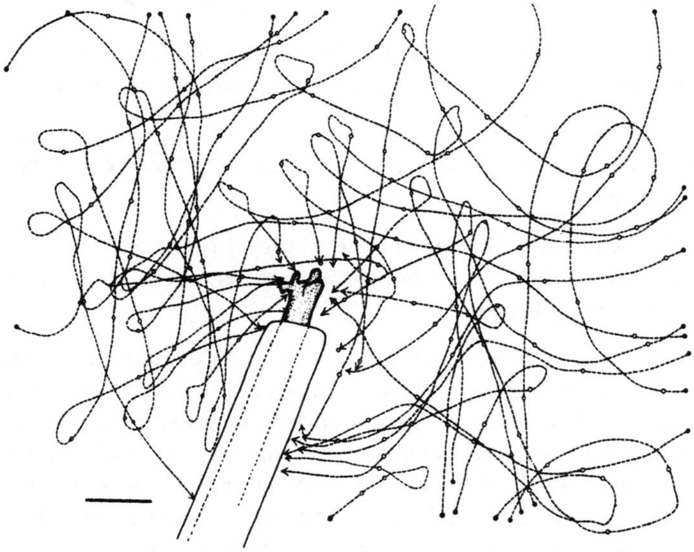

Figure 9. Experimental case whose control is Figure 1. The small mass at the pipette tip is agar inpregnated with extract from Campanularia calceolifera female gonangia. The scale equals 20 μ.

directed movement toward the source of some stimulus, relying on consecutive or simultaneous testing of the gradient to determine direction and implying the presence of one movable or two separate but immobile receptors. The organism's body axis lies in line with the gradient. Several types of taxis movements are subsumed under this general definition. Contrasting with these behaviors are undirected movements, or kineses, in which locomotion is random in direction and no orientation of the axis of the body in relation to the stimulus occurs. Two major types are recognized:

(a) ortho-kinesis – "speed or frequency of locomotion dependent on intensity of stimulation."

(b) klino-kinesis – "frequency or amount of turning per unit time dependent on intensity of stimulation. Adaptation, etc., required for aggregation."

Since demonstration of chemotaxis in sperm requires only that a taxis type of behavior be a component of the total reaction to the chemical gradient, the problem is to determine if the reaction observed satisfies the definition of the most simple taxis movement – klinotaxis. Using Fraenkel and Gunn's summary (1961, pp. 134-5) of the properties of klinotaxis and klinokinesis we find that:

1. Both require a gradient of intensity.

2. Both require a single intensity receptor.

3. Orientation and direction of locomotion of the organism with respect to the gradient is:

(a) random in klinokinesis.
(b) direct and in line with the gradient in klinotaxis.

4. Turning with respect to increasing stimulus intensity:

(a) increases in frequency in klinokinesis, barring adaptation.
(b) occurs by adjustment of regular deviations of the body or part of it in klinotaxis.

5. When presented with two sources of equal intensity, 90° apart, an organism displaying:

(a) klinokinesis will react to the whole of the gradient.
(b) klinotaxis will orient between the two sources, curving into one only when close to both.

The usual types of experiments performed on organisms to determine the mode of orientation are the two-source experiment, elimination of the receptor, and determination of rate of change of direction as related to stimulus intensity. For various technical reasons, none of these experiments has as yet been performed on sperm. It is possible, however, to look at the direction of locomotion with respect to a gradient or source of stimulus and the relationship between turning frequency and stimulus intensity, in the light of the requirements of the Fraenkel and Gunn definition.

3. Animal Sperm Motility and Turning Behavior

Animal sperm move by means of a single propulsive unit – a rearward directed flagellum. Periodic symmetric or asymmetric waves pass from the base to the tip of the flagellum and the resulting forces exerted on the medium propel the sperm forward. The plane of beat bears a definite relationship to the axis of the fibers composing the flagellum (Satir, 1965a, 1965b) and to the axis of the head (Lindahl and Drevius, 1964), which is flattened (Gray, 1955). The wave envelope is nearly planar in invertebrate sperm. Asymmetries in the planar beat cause the sperm both to rotate in a direction opposite to the direction of the asymmetric beat component (Gray, 1955) and to yaw to one side, producing a helical path whose axis is a straight line. The pitch of the helix increases as the forward speed increases. Paths of healthy sperm will therefore be nearly straight lines (Figure 1). Deviation is, however, not necessarily uniform on all sides of the straight-line axis because of the asymmetry of the beat about its axis of propagation (Gray, 1955). Overall, the individual sperm does make regular lateral deviations of its entire body in relation to a stationary object in its environment. The rotation of the sperm coincides with its position on the spiral path, so that to an observer on one side of the path, the sperm at its closest approach during each swing around the path axis presents the same part of the head.

Turning of the sperm such that the direction of the straight-line path is altered is relatively infrequent and appears to be due to indeterminate factors under normal conditions. Turning may be induced by a variety of stimuli, however, the simplest of which is the interaction of the sperm with a surface. There are several possibilities, but if one presumes a non-sticky smooth surface, the behaviors may be narrowed to three. In the first case, the sperm simply impinge on the surface and reflect off at some angle, continuing the path in a new direction. In the second case, the sperm evidence a "thigmotaxis" (Dewitz, 1886) and will interact with the surface such that they swim close to, and parallel with, the surface, but still remain swimming in straight lines (Miller and Brokaw, 1970). This behavior is responsible for the rapid elimination of free-swimming sperm in a narrow volume of medium between two smooth surfaces (Rothschild, 1963). This case leads to a third, where the sperm make contact with the surface such that the cell glides over it and is prevented from rolling. The plane of flagellar beat is also parallel to the surface, but the tendency to yaw in one direction remains and the sperm acts as though it is trying to swim in a spiral path through the surface (cf. Gray, 1955, for a complete analysis). The spiral becomes flattened against the surface, and the cell swims in large open circles, each circle representing one complete turn on the original helix (Figure 2). Circling behavior in sperm has been noted on non-sticky egg surfaces (which are usually smooth) (Dewitz 1886). The behavior is a "trap", in that the sperm are so constrained that they cannot break free of the surface and will circle ineffectually until they run out of energy reserves. The behavior is advantageous, since it tends to keep sperm on the egg surface; but it is a distinct disadvantage in that it tends to remove sperm by adsorbing them to available surfaces, effectively rendering them incapable of fertilizing.

4. Factors Inducing Sperm Aggregation

Besides the "thigmotaxis" described, aggregations of sperm may be obtained by any one or more of several means. On the basis of random movement with a constant low frequency of turning, totally reflecting surfaces and unlimited time, every sperm in a suspension must pass through a pre-selected area. If this area is treated with some chemical agent that slows the cells down, causes aberrant motility (such as spinning or tight circling), traps them in mucus, causes them to stick to each other (agglutination) or prevents their escape from the affected area (avoidance behavior), then an aggregation will build up. These aggregations can be distinguished from a taxis behavior by noting the behavior of the sperm as they enter the affected area.

Egg water (fertilizin) agglutinated sperm produce an aggregation which consists of clumps of agglutinated cells, many of these clumps being evenly dispersed within the affected area (Tyler, 1940) or arranged in a circular band in a boundary around a clear area into which no sperm penetrate (Lillie, 1919). Since egg water agglutination in sea urchins and other invertebrates is often reversible, sperm will penetrate into the clear area eventually, and the clumps will finally disperse. If egg water is added to the suspension again, no aggregations will occur (Tyler, 1941) so the sperm cannot be reagglutinated. They are, however, incapable of fertilizing eggs (Tyler, 1959).

Sperm slowed by chemical agents also aggregate uniformly, but turn little if at all and if not rendered totally immobile will increase their swimming speed as they leave the aggregation. The amount of aggregation will be directly related to the amount of time the sperm spend in the area where the slowing takes place. This behavior is equivalent to orthokinesis (Fraenkel and

Gunn, 1961). Sperm made to undergo tight circling or spinning using solutions of heavy metals or organic compounds do so uniformly within the aggregate zone, or in a ring as in the case of agglutinating sperm. No directionality of movement is seen other than a slow precession of the circular paths, and sperm showing this behavior are considered to be damaged cells. The behavior is equivalent to a simple klinokinesis.

The aggregative behavior of sperm in mucus or egg jellies is complicated by the increased viscosities of the medium. Direct effects include suppression of the beat in the posterior half of the flagellum with extreme slowing of forward progression (Brokaw, 1966; Miller, 1970). Observations of movements close to eggs under these circumstances have been made by Buller (1903), who found that sea urchin sperm penetrating egg jellies were indifferent to the position of the egg, and by Miller (unpublished observations) in the hydroid Cordylophora, who observed sperm penetrating the jelly-like gonophore wall. Directed migration may exist in Gonothyrea (Miller, 1970), however. Directed penetration has been observed in the lamprey (Kille, 1962) and the bitterling (Suzuki, 1961a, 1961b), possibly in the herring, Clupea (Yanagimachi, 1957; Yanagimachi and Kanoh, 1953) and the fly (Henking, 1888). In the four latter cases, the eggs bear a micropyle, which is the only path by which the sperm can penetrate to the eggs and the orientation of the sperm appears to be determined by structured components of the egg surface.

None of these aggregating mechanisms necessarily requires the presence of a chemical gradient. Assuming a gradient situation, two general cases may be considered: where the sperm respond to a specific concentration difference only, displaying a boundary reaction either when entering or leaving the gradient and where the sperm respond to the changing stimulus intensity continuously. Several workers have studied the behavior of microorganisms in gradients of various substances, mostly using the method of Pfeffer or modifications of it. The classical case of Paramecium becoming trapped in dilute acid is well known (Jennings, 1962). The organism does not deviate when passing into the gradient, and does not orientate to the center of the gradient once inside. On reaching an area in the gradient where the concentration of aggregating substance decreases, the organism experiences a physiologically effective concentration difference and turns away from the area. The direction taken after the turn is random in relation to the gradient axis, however, so that although the organisms can aggregate by this method, they do not show orientation to the gradient source per se. They reach the gradient area by chance, enter it without deviation toward the stimulus source, but cannot leave and thus become trapped. This reaction is called klinokinesis by Fraenkel and Gunn (1961).

Clearly, klinokinesis is distinguishable from klino-taxis, even if the organism only deviates as it leaves or enters the gradient. If the organism moves in a path straight toward the stimulus source after turning then we have evidence for klino-taxis. If the organism does not orient in line with the gradient as it moves within the aggregation zone, the reaction is klinokinesis. Once attraction has occurred, the organisms cannot leave the attractive area, no matter what the method of aggregation, since both behaviors cause the organism to turn back into the attractive zone. Organisms which turn continuously as the gradient strength increases must show adaptation in order to avoid uncontrolled spinning behavior at higher concentrations. Turning modulated to the gradient strength seems far too complex a behavior for microorganisms and is often not displayed in higher forms known to be capable of it (Fraenkel and Gunn, 1961). Usually the gradient source, once perceived by the organism, is approached directly if a taxis is occurring.

5. Observations of Sperm Aggregations in Hydroids

Some intriguing reports of sperm activation and aggregation around the micropyle of eggs of certain fishes (Yanagimachi, 1957; Suzuki, 1961a, 1961b) and a report of sperm aggregations at the surface of the egg of a medusan only at the position of the germinal vesicle (Dan, 1950) led to a reinvestigation of the possibility that sperm chemotaxis did occur in some animals (Miller and Nelson, 1962). Assuming some consistency in morphological patterns and their functions, the resemblance of reproductive structures by hydroids to plants made it appear that this group of plant-like animals might display the phenomenon.

Organisms used in this work currently include Campanularia flexuosa, Campanularia calceolifera. Tubularia crocea, Tubularia marina, Tubularia larynx, Gonothyrea loveni, and Clava leptostyla. These hydroids all produce sexual structures which are modified, sessile medusa (Figure 3). The gametes ripen within them, and are shed when ripe in the case of the males, or maintained in situ during embryogenesis in the case of the females. Since fertilization is internal and the sperm's access to the egg blocked by the gonangium, some mechanisms must exist for bringing sperm close to the egg and keeping them there. This is especially important for sessile organisms living in areas of current and wave action. The evidence is clear (Miller, 1966a) that aggregations of highly motile sperm build up at areas of the gonangium or gonophore where access to the egg is likely. Extracts of the gonangia will produce similar aggregations (Miller, 1966a, 1966b). The question is whether the sperm behavior leading to the development of aggregations resembles either a klinokinetic or klinotactic behavior.

Demonstration of species specificities during attraction of hydroid sperm serves to eliminate physical trap actions of various kinds (Miller, 1966a). Table 1 displays the current state of the sperm-gonangium and sperm-extract interactions among the genera and species so far investigated. The complicated nature of the specificities is demonstrated by the presence of almost complete specificity between species within one genera (Campanularia), total lack of specificity between species within another (Tubularia), complete cross-reactivity between species in two genera (Campanularia and Gonothyrea) and partial specificity across suborders (C. flexuosa vs. Tubularia). Orthokinetic behavior is eliminated by observing the speed of sperm approaching the source of the stimulus. As demonstrated in Miller (1966a), sperm velocity increases as they approach the stimulus source.

TABLE 1

	Female Gonangia or Extracts						
Sperm	C. flexuosa	C. calceolifera	G. loveni	T. crocea	T. larynx	T. marina	C. leptostyla
C. f.	+(±)	±(-)	-(-)	+(-)	+(-)	?(-)	?(-)
C. c.	-(-)	+(+)	-(-)	-(-)	?(-)	-(-)	?(-)
G. l.	-(-)	+(+)	+(±)	-(-)	?(-)	-(-)	?(?)
T. c.	-(-)	-(-)	-(-)	+(+)	+(+)	+(+)	?(?)
T. l.	-(?)	-(?)	?(?)	+(+)	+(+)	?(?)	?(±)
T. m.	-(-)	-(-)	-(-)	+(+)	?(?)	+(+)	?(?)
C. l.	-(?)	-(?)	-(?)	?(?)	?(-)	?(?)	-(-)

Note: These tests were run as described in Miller, 1966a. The signs are as follows: +) a positive reaction; -) no reaction; ±) a weak reaction; and ?) test not performed. The sign before the parenthesis indicates the result of the test of sperm vs. the living female sexual structure; that within the parenthesis indicates the result of the test of sperm vs. an alcoholic extract of the female gonangia or gonophores.

Sperm swimming in the vincinity of a female gonangium or a pipette containing extract of the female gonangia may be followed by plotting the sperm movements photographed on motion picture film (16 mm) and projected frame by frame (Miller, 1966a). Both direction and speed may be determined from these plots. A plot of sperm aggregating at the gonangium tip in C. flexuosa is shown in Figure 4. Similar turns have been segregated according to type and percentages of the total have been calculated. At least 40 per cent of the sperm make non-random turns taking them closer to the aperture of the female gonangium. Since the aperture is so large in contrast to the size of the sperm, precise determination of the directionality of the path after the turn in relation to the stimulus source is not possible. This can be more easily done using pipettes as stimulus sources, expecially if they are true diffusion sources.

Pipettes containing extract have been used which produce non-uniform and uniform diffusion cases. In the former, the attractive substance diluted in sea water is actively expelled from the pipette for an instant producing an area of constant high concentration just in front of the pipette. Diffusion then takes place from the edges of this zone. In the latter case, the pipettes are prepared by permitting active sea water to diffuse into agar-filled micropipettes. This produces a concentration gradient whose source is the pipette opening itself. Aggregations produced by these two types of stimulus sources and their controls are shown in Figure 5, a-d, and the plots of representative trails shown in Figure 6, 7 and 2, 9, respectively. In the case of the blow-out stimulus source (Figure 7 and Figure 5, a and b), the aggregation is rather open, occurring in an area around the pipette about equivalent to that shown in Figure 5e. Analysis of the tracks (Figure 7) shows that the sperm may turn as they enter the gradient (Figure 8), but they always turn when attempting to leave (Figures 7 and 8). It is worth noting that the sperm in these preparations are swimming against the slide surface, and are thus constrained to move in open circles. This makes deviations toward the pipette tip as the sperm enter the gradient all the more significant. Once inside the gradient the sperm swim straight across the area in front of the pipettte where the concentration difference is presumed to be minimal because of the blow-out situation. On reaching the boundary, the sperm turn back into the zone of uniform concentration, but appear better orientated to the pipettte. Unfortunately, the strength and form of the gradient cannot be measured in this case, for lack of concentration data and because of turbulence at the pipette opening

Although it is evident that the sperm in the above situation are following non-random paths after entering the gradient, a more striking demonstration of non-random behavior and precision of orientation is possible using agar-diffusion sources (Figures 9, and 5c and d). In this case the sperm make straight paths to the center of the pipette opening from all directions (Figure 9) and will form tight aggregations around sources less than 10μ in diameter. For most of the paths observed, the aggregating sperm turn when leaving the area of attraction. The turns are always made to the left (Miller, 1966a), a consequence of the fact that the sperm are circling counter-clockwise against the surface of the slide. The sperm are artificially contrained from making a three-dimensional turn under these conditions and evidently cannot turn in the other direction. Although these turning behaviors could be used to argue for a klinokinesis-type of orientation, the evident non-random orientation to the stimulus source after the turn is made is coincident with klinotaxis. Further statistical analysis is under way in an effort to prove the point more firmly.

6. Propectus

One question remains to be answered. It concerns the possible mechanisms regulating the sperm behavior during chemotaxis. I have already pointed out that the normal path of the sperm in three-dimensional space is required for klinotactic behavior. The form of the path of circling sperm produces the same result. Because of beat asymmetry, the sperm are constrained to rotate in one direction (Gray, 1955) and can be assumed to be more likely to turn in this direction when responding to the chemotactant. This accounts for the prevalence of one kind of turn in sperm swimming on glass surfaces. Although deviation toward the source is possible by adjustment during approach (Figure 8), most, on perceiving the gradient, turn toward a decreasing concentration to determine the approximate direction of the source and align their path axis in that direction. Thus, the amount of turn, though restricted to the direction of the yaw component, is related, presumably, to the stimulus concentration difference perceived by the sperm. It is the apparently precise regulation of the amount of turning, especially in those sperm turning in response to increasing concentrations, which at least implies the existence of a receptor mechanism that can rapidly detect very small changes in concentration. The detection is then somehow translated into an asymmetry superimposed on the normal flagellar beat (Miller and Brokaw, 1970).

REFERENCES

Balinsky, B. I. (1965). An Introduction to Embryologv. 2nd Edition, Philadelphia, Saunders.
Buller, A. H. R. (1903). Q. J. Micr. Sci. 46, 145.
Brokaw, C. J. (1966). J. Exp. Biol. 45, 115.
Dakin, W. J. and Fordham, M. G. C. (1924). J. Exp. Biol. 1, 103.
Dan, J. C. (1950). Biol. Bull. 99, 412.
Dewitz, J. (1886). Arch. ges. Physiol. 38, 358.
Dickmann, Z. (1963). J. Exp. Biol. 40, 1-5.
Fraenkel, G. S. and Gunn, D.L.(1961). The Orientation of Animals. New York, Dover.
Gray, J. (1955). J. Exp. Biol. 32, 802.
Henking, H. (1888). Zeitschr. f. wiss. Zool. 46, 289.
Jennings. H. S. (1962). Behavior of the Lower Organisms. Bloomington, Indiana University Press.
Kille, R. A. (1962). Exp. Cell. Res. 20, 12-17.
Lillie, F. R. (1919). Problems of Fertilization. Chicago. University of Chicago Press.
Lindahl, P. E. and Drevius, L. O. (1964). Exp. Cell. Res. 36, 632.
Machlis, L. and Rawitscher-Kunkel, E. (1967). Fertilization. New York, Academic Press, 1, 177.
Metz, C. B. (1967). Fertilization. New York, Academic Press, 1, 163.
Miller, R. L. (1966a). J. Exp. Zool. 162, 23.
Miller, R. L. (1966b). Am. Zool. 6, 509.
Miller, R. L. (1970). J. Exp. Zool. 175, 493.
Miller, R. L. and Brokaw, C. J. (1970). J. Exp. Biol. 52, 699.

Miller, R. L. and Nelson, L. (1962). Biol. Bull. 123, 477.
Morgan, T. H. (1927). Experimental Embryology. New York, Columbia University Press.
Pfeffer, W. (1884). Untersuch. a. d. Botanische Inst. zu Tubingen 1, 363.
Raper. J. R. (1952). Bot. Rev. 18, 447.
Rosen, W. G. (1962). Q. Rev. Biol. 37, 42.
Rothschild, L. (1956). Fertilization. London, Methuen and Co.
Rothschild, L. (1963). Nature 198, 1221.
Satir, P. (1965a). J. Cell. Biol. 26, 805.
Satir, P. (1965b). Protoplasmatol. 3E, 1.
Suzuki, R. (1961a). Annot. Zool. Japon. 34, 18.
Suzuki, R. (1961b). Annot. Zool. Japon. 34, 24.
Tyler, A. (1940). Biol. Bull. 78, 159.
Tyler, A. (1941). Biol. Bull. 81, 190.
Tyler, A. (1949). Am. Natur. 83, 105.
Tyler, A. (1959). Exp. Cell. Res., Suppl. 7, 183.
Weiss, P. (1961). Exp. Cell. Res. Suppl. 8, 260.
Wiese, L. (1969). Fertilization. New York, Academic Press, 2, 135.
Wilson, E. B. (1924). The Cell in Development and Heredity. New York, Macmillan.
Yanagimachi, R. (1957). Annot. Zool. Japon. 30, 114.
Yanagimachi, R. and Kanoh, Y. (1953). J. Fac. Sci., Hokkaido Univ., Ser. 6, Zool. 11, 487.
Zeigler, H. (1962a). Handbuch der Pflanzenphysiologie 17/2, 396.
Zeigler, H. (1962b). Handbuch der Pflanzenphysiologie 17/2, 484.

CHEMOTAXIS AND AGGREGATION IN SLIME MOLDS

T.M. Konijn
Universiteitscentrum de Uithof,
Hubrecht Laboratory,
Utrecht,
The Netherlands.

Two factors are of prime importance for cell aggregation in the slime molds: chemotaxis and adhesion. The latter is least understood. New light has been shed on chemotaxis by recent observations on attraction of myxamoebae of the cellular slime molds.

Attractants may effect both chemotaxis and adhesion. Attraction and adhesion of cells have in common that both of them are specific. Since cells of different species may be attracted to a common center and sort out later to differentiate into separate species, adhesion at the multicellular stage is more specific than the chemotactic response at the unicellular stage.

Chemotaxis plays a key role at two stages in the life cycle of the cellular slime molds: at the vegetative and at the aggregative phase. Myxamoebae feed on bacteria. Bacteria are not only the food source but also secrete substances that attract amoebae. Cells multiply as long as bacteria are present. Starving amoebae undergo morphological, physiological, and biochemical changes, which prepare them for the social aggregative phase.

The aggregation is also mediated by a chemotactic compound. This attractant secreted by the amoebae in an aggregate establishes a diffusion gradient which the single amoebae nearby will orient.

The aggregate of the species we will be mainly concerned with, Dictyostelium discoideum, develops into a slug shaped free-moving body of cells and finally differentiates into a simple fruiting structure, consisting of spores supported by vacuolated stalk cells.

Although it was assumed that the aggregation phase was mediated by chemotaxis, there was no evidence for this supposition until Runyon (1942) was able to show that aggregations occurring on one side of a dialyzing membrane would coincide with aggregations formed on the other side.

Proof came from Bonner (1947) who demonstrated that aggregating centers placed in a slowly moving stream of water were capable of attracting amoebae only downstream from them. He termed the attractant "acrasin".

A qualitative assay to test for acrasin was developed by Shaffer (1956). The attracting agent was unstable unless it was dialyzed or extraction was carried out in methanol (Shaffer, 1956) or hydrochloric acid (Sussman, Lee, and Kerr, 1956). The inactivation apparently was due to a non-dialyzable enzyme.

R. R. Sussman et al. (1958), using the Shaffer assay, suggested that the chemotactic agent consisted of three components, different ratios being used as a mechanism of species specificity.

The identification of the attractant in D. discoideum was carried out with a quantitative assay, which has been developed in Professor Kenneth B. Raper's laboratory at the University of Wisconsin (Konijn, 1961).

1. Microbiological Assay for Attractants of Myxamoebae

The small population assay that will be described, requires a hydrophobic agar surface of a specific rigidity.

After agar has been washed frequently with deionized water, dissolved by boiling and has been allowed to gelate, the agar surface is hydrophobic (Ennis and Sussman, 1958).

The lack of salts causes a harmful hypotonicity to cells placed on such an agar surface (Konijn and Raper, 1961). When salts are added back before gelation of the washed agar, the agar surface remains hydrophobic but becomes a more suitable medium to hold the myxamoebae (Konijn and Raper, 1961). Populations of myxamoebae can be grown in situ with bacteria on such an agar, or pregrown amoebae can be placed on it as small droplets of a cell suspension. The amoebae do not cross the boundaries of the droplets in which they are placed on the agar, in contrast to their behavior on a normal hydrophilic agar or on a hydrophobic agar surface of too low rigidity.

An essential condition for the small population bioassay is that the hydrophobic agar surface is sufficiently rigid to keep the cells within the boundaries of the droplet, yet weak enough to allow the cells to cross the margins of the drop when attracted by an external stimulus. The attractant outside the drop can be another population with aggregating myxamoebae (Figure 1), a bacterial population, or an extract containing chemotactic compounds.

The chemotactic agent for the aggregation of amoebae of <u>D. discoideum</u> is adenosine 3',5'-monophosphate (cyclic AMP) (Konijn et al., 1967). Its activity was expressed as a clear attraction at cyclic AMP concentrations of 10^{-5} to 10^{-6} M (Figure 2). At higher cyclic AMP concentrations (10^{-3} to 10^{-4} M) in the attracting drops the amoebae in the responding populations crossed the boundaries of the drop at all sides (Figure 3). Phosphodiesterase, the inactivating enzyme of cyclic AMP (Chang, 1968) could be responsible for this crawling of amoebae

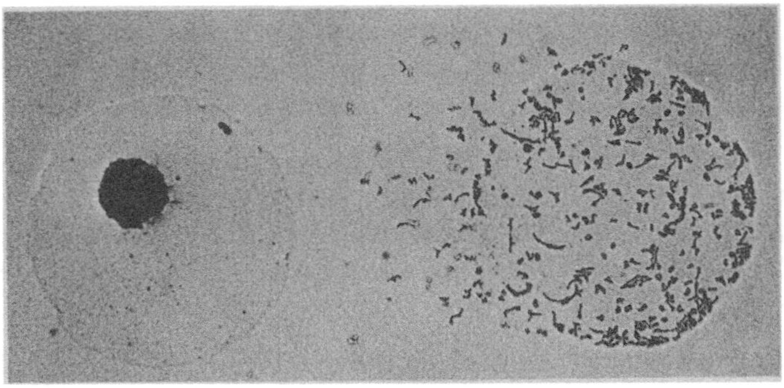

Figure 1. Chemotaxis in Dictyostellium discoideum. The aggregation in the drop on the left attracts myxamoebae outside the boundary of the drop on the right. Cells inside the drop move on the agar surface. Cells outside the drop crawl through the agar. (From Konijn, 1970). ×60.

in all directions, away from the original amoeboid population (Konijn, 1969). At this concentration cyclic AMP which normally initiates the social phase prevents aggregation. At high concentrations of cyclic AMP aggregates are dispersed completely, even when nearly all streams have entered the aggregate (Konijn, 1969).

Above a concentration of 10^{-2} to 10^{-3} M amoebae clump together in small groups of cells (Figure 4); apparently the receptor mechanism of the amoebae becomes overloaded. These clumps of cells move seemingly at random over the surface inside the drop.

All these different reactions can occur when extracts are tested for the presence of cyclic AMP. The assay becomes more quantitative by measuring the distance over which the attracting drop can induce myxamoebae in the responding drop to cross its boundary (Konijn, 1970).

Another way to quantify this method is the dilution of an active extract until not all but only a certain percentage of the responding populations react positively. The response to extracts with weak activity is amplified by placing the extract 3-5 times at 5 min intervals near the sensitive myxamoebae. At very low concentrations of cyclic AMP, 10^{-8} to 10^{-9} M, amoebae are not attracted outside the responding drop but become pressed against the margin. Such a response is considered positive if at least twice as many cells are pressed against the margin closest to the attracting drop than on the opposite side (Figure 5). Since the volume of the attracting drops is 0.1 μl, less than 10^{-12} g of cyclic AMP can induce a positive response as shown in Figure 5.

When 10^{-12} g of cyclic AMP diffuses into the agar at a distance of 300 μ from the responding drop the number of cyclic AMP molecules that activate the individual cells has to be extremely small.

The cyclic AMP content in an extract can be estimated by diluting a commercial cyclic AMP solution to a known concentration at which a similar percentage of positively responding populations will be observed as evoked by

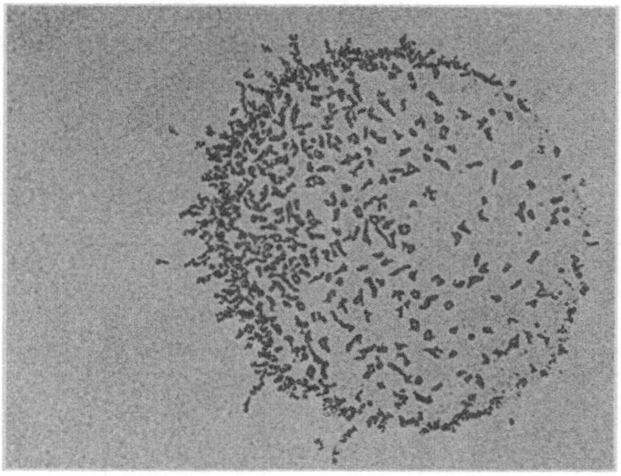

Figure 2. Drops (0.1 μl) containing 3 × 10^{-8} g cyclic AMP were deposited three times at 5 min intervals to the left of the responding drop. ×80.

the extract. Two-fold differences in cyclic AMP concentrations are shown this way (Konijn, 1970).

The myxamoebae of D. discoideum react specifically to cyclic AMP. Other cyclic nucleotides or analogues of cyclic AMP are less active (Konijn et al., 1969). Purification of the extract, which is tested for its cyclic AMP content, by column and paper chromatography, makes it possible to confirm that the observed activity is due to cyclic AMP and not to analogues of it or other cyclic nucleotides.

The presence of cyclic AMP has been demonstrated in higher organisms where it may function as a "second messenger" in hormone action (Sutherland et al., 1965). Cyclic AMP is also present in bacteria where it may play a role in the regulation of enzyme synthesis and catabolite repression (Perlman and Pastan, 1968; De Crombrugghe et al., 1969; Monard et al., 1969).

The high sensitivity and specificity of this technique made it a suitable assay to demonstrate the presence of cyclic AMP in various bacteria, yeasts, spleen, liver, kidney, and heart, and in milk and urine. Purification of the extracts showed that cyclic AMP was the chemotactic agent. Purification was not required to assay the extracts because also the activity in crude extracts could be assessed. A typical example of cyclic AMP determination on urine is shown in Table 1. The concentration that was found was similar to cyclic AMP concentrations recorded in the literature (Butcher and Sutherland, 1962).

The small population assay has been used in a variety of projects; e.g. to obtain conclusive evidence that cyclic AMP is involved in the physiological melanophore reaction in Xenopus laevis (Van de Veerdonk and Konijn, 1970) and to show that effect of parathyroid extract on the cyclic AMP content of embryonic mouse calvaria (Herrmann-Erlee and Konijn, 1970).

TABLE 1. Comparison of the Chemotactic Response Induced by Different Concentrations of Urine and Cyclic 3',5'-AMP. The Drops with Attractant were Placed Three Times with Five-Minute Intervals Near (Less than 0.45 mm) the Responding Drops. Observation Took Place Five Minutes after the Last Deposition. (From Konijn, 1970)

	Urine		3',5'-AMP		Urine	
	dil. ×500		0.01 μM		dil. ×2000	
	total positive	percent positive	total positive	percent positive	total positive	percent positive
test 1	25	83	32	73	14	48
test 2	22	88	25	73	20	59
test 3	18	60	22	47	7	23

2. Effect of the Environment on Aggregation

Raper (1940) discovered that higher temperature, lower humidity and light shortened the period of time before aggregation starts. As long as the cells which secrete acrasin and the cells which respond to it are both occupying the same population there is no apparent way to study the influence of the environment on these two cell groups. Therefore myxamoebae were put in two separate populations, from which one was deposited earlier than the other on a hydrophobic agar surface of a specific rigidity. The responding populations were generally placed at distances of 100 to 1500 μ from the attracting populations. Cell attraction over this measured distance was marked positive if myxamoebae moved outside the margins of the responding drop to the attracting drop (Figure 1).

Sensitive cells of D. discoideum responded mainly between the beginning and the completion of aggregation in the attracting drop, although some secretion of acrasin by amoebae still in the preaggregative phase was shown (Konijn, 1965; Bonner et al., 1969). At lower temperatures the amoebae were attracted more strongly than at higher temperatures. Cells, which were incubated at 13° were attracted over double the distance than when incubation took place at 28.5° (Konijn, 1965). The stronger attraction at low temperatures was not due to an increased sensitivity of the responding cells to chemotactic agents (Konijn, 1969). No information is available on the effect of temperature on the enzymes adenyl cyclase and phosphodiesterase, which respectively activate the production and destruction of cyclic AMP.

Another environmental factor, light, reduced the chemotactic effect of aggregating myxamoebae (Konijn and Raper, 1966). The territory size of aggregations and consequently the sorocarps of D. discoideum are smaller when formed in light than in darkness. A possible explanation for the smaller aggregates in light could be the attraction of sensitive myxamoebae over shorter distances. Light affects the acrasin secreting cells in the aggregate and not the responding populations which react similarly in light and darkness if an artificial attracting source has been used (Konijn, 1969).

The acrasin secretion by different sized aggregates was determined by changing the cell density in the attracting populations. Whether 500 or 5000 cells occupied the attracting drop (0.6 mm diameter), the chemotactic response that was induced by the different sized aggregates was the same (Konijn, 1968). The independence of the chemotactic response was not limited to D. discoideum but also responding populations of P. pallidum reacted independently of the number of cells in the attracting drop.

3. Propagation of the Chemotactic Stimulus

The attraction over distances of 1600 μ exceeds by far the orienting effect of aggregates found earlier by Bonner (1947) and Sussman and Lee (1955). A response was marked positive if cells crossed the boundary of the drop which meant pentrating into the agar. However, a positive response may be observed before the cells creep into the agar outside the responding drop (Figure 5). The actual sphere of attraction, therefore, extends over a larger area than measured earlier (Konijn, 1965, 1968).

A significant consequence of this attraction over a distance of more than 160 times the diameter of an amoeba is that all amoebae in a aggregation territory could be attracted by the aggregate. Such a direct effect of a center could be an alternative for the relayed system of attraction as proposed by Shaffer (1958, 1962). If aggregation depends on a relay system, pulses of acrasin, secreted by a center, diffuse to neighboring amoebae and induce these cells to move to the center. The activated cells themselves release acrasin to the more centrifugally situated cells, which will be activated. A concentrated zone of acrasin diffuses outward and, in this way, large aggregates with streams extending over more than one cm could be formed. Large aggregates have been observed if amoebae were grown in situ (Shaffer, 1958) or at high cell density (Gerisch, 1965, 1968). When amoebae were grown in situ their food source, the bacteria, were present in large numbers. Since attractants and other compounds are secreted by the bacteria these products may have influenced the later developing aggregates and consequently aggregation territories. Amoebae in such large aggregation territories are attracted not only by the center but also by the long streams, which secrete acrasin equally well as the center (Shaffer, 1962).

Gerisch (1965), who had removed his cells from a liquid culture, transferred the myxamoebae to a glass surface. The aggregates, which covered large territories, originated from sheets of cells in which the myxamoebae stuck to each other. Additional to chemotaxis, adhesive forces may also have influenced the territory sizes of these large aggregates.

Amoebae that were washed before deposition and whose population density was such that all amoebae were free before aggregation covered a smaller area with a radius of 0.65 to 0.8 mm during aggregation (Bonner and Hoffman, 1963; Konijn and Raper, 1966; Sussman and Sussman, 1969). The size of such a territory may be sufficiently small to be controlled by the pulses of acrasin that are secreted by the developing aggregate.

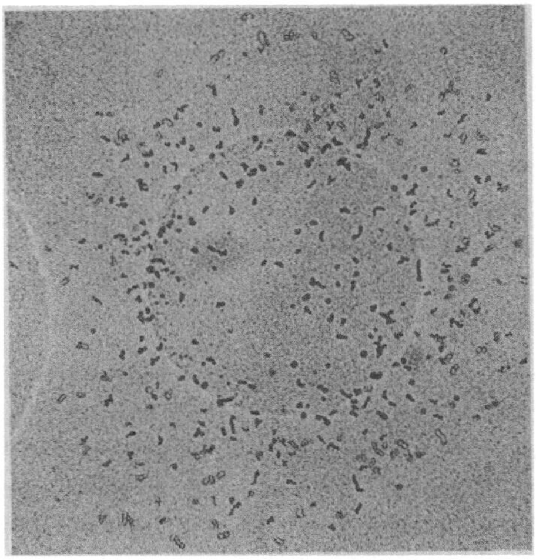

Figure 3. As Figure 2. Drops contain 3×10^{-6} g cyclic AMP. (From Konijn, 1970). ×60.

If an aggregate has to control a whole territory, without a relay of the attractant, its area should be marked at a rather early stage of aggregation, when only a few cells occupy the center; otherwise other cells in its territory will start their own aggregates. A small group of cells, indeed, secretes acrasin maximally and a ten-fold increase in the number of amoebae in the center does not raise the production of acrasin (Konijn, 1968). Apparently with more amoebae in the aggregate the acrasin production per cell is reduced.

If the amoebae at the periphery of an aggregation territory are attracted to the center directly the velocity of the inward movement should be lower than that of amoebae close to the center.

The velocity of the inward movement of amoebae, however, is constant during aggregation (Gerisch, 1965, 1968). This constant speed, again, was measured at high cell densities where even cells at the periphery touched each other. Probably such a sheet of cells may be compared with a stream of an aggregate. Streams of aggregates have the same chemotactic effect as centers (Shaffer, 1962). Therefore these sheets of cells with similar characteristics as streams may transfer pulses differently from free amoebae.

A limitation of the relay system is its unlimited propagation. When all aggregates start at the same time competition among the various centers could confine the propagation of the relay to their own areas. Environmental conditions, such as light, may cause a large variation in the time at which aggregation starts. Large populations of D. discoideum aggregate optimally after an initial dark period of 6 to 8 hr, followed by light (Konijn and Raper, 1965). After a short initial dark period a very few aggregates are formed early and rest of the amoebae may come together one or more hours later. The early aggregations do not extend their sphere of attraction over large areas of uncommitted cells (Konijn and Raper, 1966) as would be expected if the stimulus were relayed to peripheral cells. Their size is even smaller

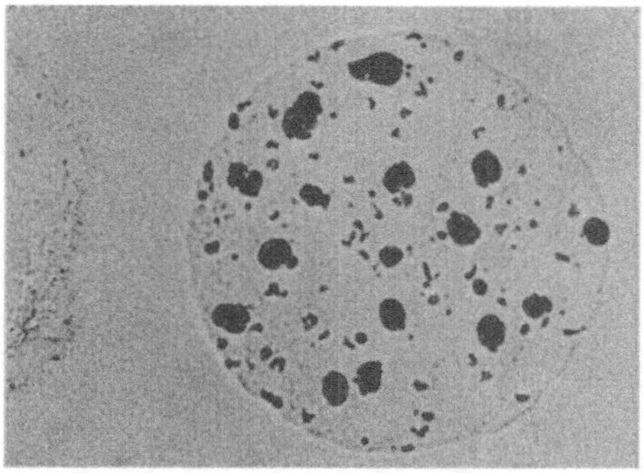

Figure 4. As Figure 2. Drops contain 3×10^{-3} g cyclic AMP. ×80.

than when all aggregates appear at the same time. The extension of the aggregation was not obstructed by a sudden change in cell density or a different physiological age of the myxamoebae.

Probably the process of aggregation is too complicated to be explained exclusively by either a relay or a direct stimulation from the developing aggregate. A thorough study by time lapse photography and a better knowledge about the adenyl cyclase and phosphodiesterase activity may help clarify the intricacies of cell aggregation.

4. Chemotaxis in Dictyostelium and Polysphondylium

Cyclic AMP is synthesized in at least two genera of the cellular slime molds. It has been isolated from Polysphondylium pallidum (Konijn et al., 1968) and identified as the acrasin, synthesized by amoebae of D. discoideum (Konijn, Chang, and Bonner, 1969). Barkley (1969), using the same purification techniques, isolated and identified cyclic AMP as the attractant in D. discoideum by starting out with dialyzed products of the amoebae. In addition to its chemotactic effect cyclic AMP increases the adhesiveness of cells (Konijn et al., 1968).

The species of Dictyostelium that are attracted by cyclic AMP are: D. discoideum (Konijn et al., 1967), D. mucoroides, D. purpureum (Konijn et al., 1968) and D. rosareum. Myxamoebae of these species are attracted when drops of a cyclic AMP solution of 10^{-6} to 10^{-8} M are placed close to the amoebae. At higher concentrations of cyclic AMP the cells cross the boundaries of the drops at all sides. If the assumption that this is a consequence of the inactivation of cyclic AMP by phosphodiesterase is correct (Konijn, 1969) the centrifugal movement of amoebae in all directions would indicate that all these species produce phosphodiesterase. Incubation of myxamoebae with 10^{-5} M cyclic AMP results in a minimal activity of phosphodiesterase. Higher and lower concentrations than 10^{-5} M increase the phosphodiesterase activity (in collaboration with G. Speziali).

The smaller species, D. minutum, D. lacteum, D. aureum, D. polycephalum, and D. vinaceo-fuscum, (all generously provided by Professor Kenneth B. Raper) are not attracted by cyclic AMP; even after frequent application of

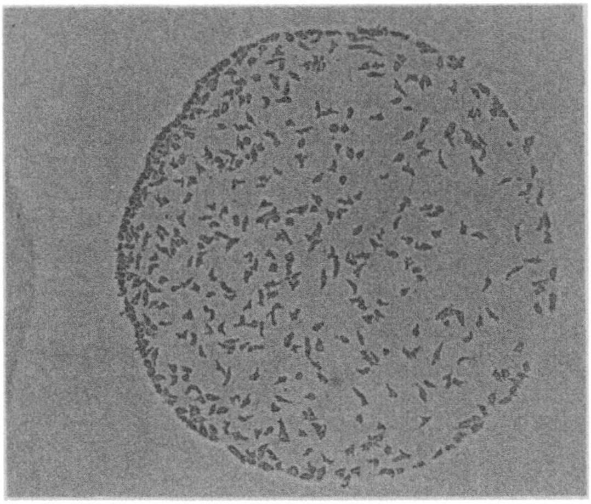

Figure 5. Population of myxamoebae on washed non-nutrient agar of low rigidity. Drops (0.1 μl) containing 3×10^{-13} g cyclic AMP were deposited three times at 5 min intervals to the left of the responding drop. (From Konijn, 1970). ×95.

the cyclic nucleotide. The attractants for these species, which are still under investigation, seem to be widespread in nature. Biological materials that attract nearly all these species are: bacteria, milk, urine, and liver homogenate. The attractants are dializable and their molecular size is in the same range as that of cyclic AMP.

The main attractant(s) of the genus Polysphondylium is also, like cyclic AMP, a small molecule which is present in bacteria, urine, and milk. It is unlikely that cyclic AMP itself is the attractant, since it does not have a chemotactic effect at concentrations of 10^{-2} M to 10^{-8} M, nor with frequent (8-16) applications at intervals of 5, 2, or 1 min. Only at high concentrations of cyclic AMP (10^{-2} M) in the attracting drops are the finished aggregates of Polysphondylium flattened and more aggregates (4-10) are formed in the amoebae populations then normal (1-3).

The active bacterial product which attracts P. pallidum was not inactivated by purified phosphodiesterase (kindly provided by Dr. R.W. Butcher). A crude enzyme extract of amoebae decreased the activity of the bacterial attractant.

A complication during purification of the Polysphondylium active bacterial fractions was the reduction in activity with increasing purity of the extracts.

The possibility that D. discoideum may secrete a cofactor which is necessary for Polysphodylium to be activated by cyclic AMP was studied in a mixture of D. discoideum with P. pallidum or P. violaceum. Amoebae were mixed in various ratios. No positive effect of the extracellular metabolites secreted by D. discoideum on amoebae of P. violaceum was noticeable. The chemotactic response of D. discoideum was reduced in these mixed populations when cyclic AMP was applied nearly. Despite some cell divisions that should have taken place the total number of cells dwindled to 1/4 or 1/3 of the original population and debris of cellular fragments was spread all over the drop. A time lapse film of a mixed population of D. discoidum and P. pallidum (1:1) revealed that, instead of cooperating, the amoebae of D. discoideum attacked the smaller P. pallidum amoebae and after most P. pallidum amoebae were destroyed, amoebae of D. discoideum started to engulf other cells of their own species.

Since the attractants of Polysphondylium and the small Dictyostelium species had certain characteristics such as molecular weight in common with cyclic AMP, the effect of other cyclic nucleotides and analogues of cyclic AMP was examined. Some cyclic nucleotides show some minor attraction, e.g. thymidine 3',5'-monophosphate, if applied near amoebae of D. lacteum. On the other hand an extract of homogenized axolotl embryos contained a strong chemotactic agent for amoebae of P. pallidum.

There are indications that the species which do not react to cyclic AMP are sensitive to specific attractant(s) that act at very low concentrations. Small populations (ca 1000 cells) of D. aureum and P. violaceum attract amoebae in responding drops that are 1500 μ away. The chemotactic agent secreted by D. vinaceo-fuscum activates cells over a distance up to 2200 μ. If the attractant diffuses over the agar surface and into the agar the concentration of it, by the time it reaches an amoeba in the responding population, must be extremely low.

Size alone does not determine whether a species will be attracted by cyclic AMP. A small mutant of D. mucoroides (generously supplied by Dr. Erik Bille-Hansen) with sorocarps of similar size as D. minutum, was attracted by cyclic AMP, whereas D. minutum does not respond to cyclic AMP.

Sensitivity to cyclic AMP often coincides with clear pulsations during aggregation. Amoebae of D. purpureum, D. mucoroides, D. discoideum, and D. rosareum, which are all sensitive to cyclic AMP, move inward to the center of the aggregate in rhythmic waves. Most large Dictyostelium species pulsate at 5 min intervals. The rhythmic waves in D. rosareum appear at intervals of 20 min. Recently Robertson and Cohen discovered pulsations in Polysphondylium at intervals of 80 sec.

It is obvious from time lapse films that a longer interval coincides with a stronger pulse. Early aggregates of D. rosareum may disintegrate completely before they come together again with the next pulsation and several amoebae in advanced aggregates become free again between pulsations.

Clear pulsations is not a prerequisite for attraction by cyclic AMP in D. discoideum. Strain 66 of this species (kindly supplied by Dr. G. Gerisch) does not show clear pulsations (Gerisch et al., 1966) but is sensitive to cyclic AMP.

A third characteristic often found in species that are insensitive to cyclic AMP is the presence of founder cells. Certain cells in a population may round off and attract other cells that are nearby. These founder cells, first described by Shaffer, are shown to be active in P. violaceum (Shaffer, 1961), P. pallidum (Francis, 1965) and D. minutum (Gerisch, 1964), which are species that are not sensitive to cyclic AMP. No evidence is available yet about founder cells in species that are sensitive to cyclic AMP.

5. Chemotaxis in the Myxomycetes

The true slime molds differ from the cellular slime molds in several respects: myxamoebae of the true slime molds can develop into flagellated swarm cells, cells may fuse and form a multinucleated true plasmodium and amoebae as well as the plasmodium of the true slime molds feed by phagocytosis

The presence of mating types in this group simplifies the small population assay. Mating types that are missing their complementary mating strains do not form a plasmodium and allow testing of these cells over long periods of time whereas the cellular slime molds are optimally attracted over a short period immediately before aggregation. A disadvantage of the myxamoebae of the Myxomycetes is that they cannot be stored overnight at a low temperature to improve the test conditions (Konijn et al., 1968) because all cells encyst in the cold.

Myxamoebae of Didymium irridis and Physarum pusillum were attracted by live bacteria and bacterial extracts; the chemotactic activity was proportional to the bacterial concentration (Konijn and Koevenig, 1970). Also fragments of plasmodia were attracted by the bacteria. The fragments of the plasmodia crossed the boundaries of the drops in which they were deposited and crawled over the hydrophobic agar surface to the bacterial population to engulf them.

Gel filtration indicated that the molecular weight of the main attractant(s) was near that of cyclic AMP but cyclic AMP itself (10^{-2} to 10^{-8} M) did not attract myxamoebae and plasmodia even when the cyclic nucleotide was applied 8 times.

Further purification of the bacterial extract resulted in a reduced chemotactic response of the myxamoebae (Konijn and Koevenig, 1970).

The true slime molds were less specific in their chemotactic response than the cellular slime mold D. discoideum. Mixtures of amino acids (each 0.1 M) at pH 7.0 attracted myxamoebae; especially when L-tryptophan was present. It is not known yet whether this sensitivity to amino acids depends on chemo-receptors, as shown by Adler (1969) in bacteria, or is only based on a chemotaxis to nutrients.

6. Chemotaxis of Myxamoebae to Bacteria

Arndt (1937) observed the tendency of amoebae to move to bacteria. Renewed interest for chemotaxis started in the early sixties when Samuel (1961) showed the attraction of D. mucoroides amoebae to a dab of E. coli. Bacteria attracted amoebae of D. discoideum over large distances, without intervening amoebae, and the attraction was studied with the small population assay (Konijn, 1961).

A dialyzed bacterial water extract was chromatographed on Whatman No. 1 paper in butyl alcohol–acetic acid–water (4:1:5). The wash-water of paper strips of one cm each was tested with the assay, the active fractions were pooled, concentrated, and by paper electrophoresis at pH 3.9 it was shown that the charge of the active molecule was negative. The active fractions deposited close to sensitive amoebae delayed aggregation, disturbed aggregation patterns in drops where amoebae were coming together, and attracted cells outside the boundaries of the small populations.

A large increase in activity was possible by using a concentrated bacterial water extract, which was collected by growing E. coli on large trays, washing off the bacteria and centrifuging them (Konijn et al., 1969). The concentrated supernatant was fractionated by gel-filtration, paper chromatography and paper electrophoresis at pH 3.9. After each fractionation the fractions were tested with the assay and the active fractions collected, concentrated, and further purified.

The purified product had an UV absorption spectrum, which strongly suggested that the attracting compound was a derivative of adenine (Konijn et al., 1967). The above-mentioned characteristics and the presence of the attracting compound in bacteria and urine, both known to contain cyclic AMP, led to the testing of commercial adenosine 3',5'-monophosphate (cyclic AMP), which was active at amounts of 0.01 ng (Konijn et al., 1967). Further purification of the highly purified active bacterial extract on a DEAE A-25 Sephadex column and with active charcoal resulted in a product that migrated identically as cyclic AMP in three different solvents (Konijn et al., 1969).

Secretion of cyclic AMP by bacteria was less dependent on the environmental conditions than its secretion by amoebae. The chemotactic activity of bacteria or bacterial extracts was not reduced by light or higher temperature. Whereas the attraction by aggregating amoebae was largely independent of the size of the aggregate, bacterial populations were more attractive at higher cell density than at low density. At high densities E. coli attracted cells of amoebae populations that were deposited as far as 5 mm from the bacteria (Konijn, 1969). Bacterial drops near amoebae delayed aggregation in the responding drop or inhibited aggregation completely.

All species of Dictyostelium and Polyspondylium were attracted by E. coli and other gram-negative and gram-postive bacteria (Konijn, 1969). There may be some difference in the chemotactic activity, even within the same bacterial species. The attraction sphere of E. coli, B/r, extends over a larger distance than that of E. coli, 281.

Since cyclic AMP is the only natural attractant isolated from E. coli, and no other chemotactic agents are found that are active at such low concentrations, it is suggested that all bacteria secrete cyclic AMP which would function as an effective food-seeking mechanism for myxamoebae.

Recently Bonner et al. (1970) indicated that a second chemotactic factor may be of great importance during the vegetative phase of the myxamoebae. This chemotactic agent is a large non-dialyzable molecule, present in bacterial extracts and demonstrated in an assay (Bonner et al., 1966) where an active compound is mixed with the agar before gelation. A square of Cellophane covered with amoebae is transferred to the agar and the distance over which cells moved away from the Cellophane square in a certain period of time is used as a criterion for the activity of the compound added to the agar.

This second chemotactic compound is not active in the small population assay. Bonner et al. (1970) found that this compound does not diffuse through agar, whereas the diffusion of large molecules as haemocyanin with a molecular weight of 6,600,000 are scarcely affected in a 0.5 per cent agar-gel and only slightly in a 1 per cent agar-gel (Polsen, 1958). Several acid and basic dyes, tested on a hydrophobic agar surface, diffused through the agar, independent of the charge of the molecule.

The further purification of this second chemotactic system is of great importance since, should it not only serve in nutrition but also activate the amoeboid membrane, it could indicate the presence of different chemo-receptors.

CONCLUSIONS

By using a microbiological assay it was possible to show that cyclic AMP is the main, if not the only attractant during aggregation of myxamoebae. At low concentrations cyclic AMP initiates the social phase but at higher concentrations it prevents the coming together of myxamoebae. Concentrated solutions of cyclic AMP disperse aggregates, even in an advanced stage.

The specific response to cyclic AMP allows the use of myxamoebae in a bio-assay to measure the levels of this nucleotide in extracts of various biological materials.

Myxamoebae are attracted more strongly at low temperatures or in darkness than at high temperatures or in light. The chemotactic response is largely independent of the number of cells in the aggregate.

The chemotactic activity of cyclic AMP is limited to the large *Dictyostelium* species. Chemotaxis in the true slime molds may be mediated by more than one attractant.

Gram-positive and gram-negative bacteria, and also milk and urine, attract myxamoebae of the genera *Dictyostelium* and *Polysphondylium*. Since species which are not sensitive to cyclic AMP are attracted by cyclic AMP sources as bacteria, milk, and urine, it is tempting to speculate that the unknown attractants for *Polysphondylium* and the small *Dictyostelium* species may be, as cyclic AMP, functional in higher organisms.

REFERENCES

Adler, J. (1969). Science 166, 1588.

Arndt, A. (1937). Wilhelm Roux Arch. EntwMech. Org. 136, 681.

Barkley, D. S. (1969). Science 165, 1133.

Bonner, J. T. (1947). J. Exp. Zool. 106, 1.

Bonner, J. T., Barkley, D. S., Hall, E. M., Konijn, T. M., Mason, J. W., O'Keefe, III, G., and Wolfe, P. B. (1969). Devl Biol. 20, 72.

Bonner, J. T., Hall, E. M., Sachsenmaier, W., and Walker, B. K. (1970). J. Bact. 102, 682.

Bonner, J. T. and Hoffman, M. E. (1963). J. Embryol. Exp. Morph. 11, 571.
Bonner, J. T., Kelso, A. P., and Gillmor, R. G. (1966). Biol. Bull. 130, 28.
Butcher, R. W. and Sutherland, E. W. (1962). J. Biol. Chem. 237, 1244.
Chang, Y. Y. (1968). Science 160, 57.
De Crombrugghe, B., Perlman, R. L., Varmus, H. E., and Pastan, I. (1969). J. Biol. Chem. 244, 5828.
Ennis, H. L. and Sussman, M. (1958). Proc. Nat. Acad. Sci. U.S.A. 44, 401.
Francis, D. W. (1965). Devl. Biol. 12, 329.
Gerisch, G. (1964). Wilhelm Roux Arch. EntwMech. Org. 155, 342.
Gerisch, G. (1965). Wilhelm Roux Arch. EntwMech. Org. 156, 127.
Gerisch, G. (1968). Curr. Topics Devl Biol. 3, 157.
Gerisch, G., Normann, I., and Beug, H. (1966). Naturwissenschaften 53, 618.
Herrmann-Erlee, M. P. M. and Konijn, T. M. (1970). Nature 227, 177.
Konijn, T. M. (1961). Ph.D. Thesis. University of Wisconsin. Madison, Wisconsin.
Konijn, T. M. (1965). Devl Biol. 12, 487.
Konijn, T. M. (1968). Biol. Bull. 134, 298.
Konijn, T. M. (1969). J. Bact. 99, 503.
Konijn, T. M. (1970). Experientia 26, 367.
Konijn, T. M., Barkley, D. S., Chang, Y. Y., and Bonner, J. T. (1968). Am. Nat. 102, 225.
Konijn, T. M., Chang, Y. Y., and Bonner, J. T. (1969). Nature 224, 1211.
Konijn, T. M. and Koevening, J. (1971). Mycologia 63, 901.
Konijn. T. M. and Raper, K. B. (1961). Devl Biol. 3, 725.
Konijn, T. M. and Raper, K. B. (1965). Biol. Bull. 128, 392.
Konijn, T. M. and Raper, K. B. (1966). Biol. Bull. 131, 446.
Konijn, T. M., van de Meene, J. G. C., Bonner, J. T., and Barkley, D. S. (1967). Proc. Nat. Acad. Sci. U.S.A. 58, 1152.
Konijn, T. M., van de Meene, J. G. C., Chang, Y. Y., Barkley, D. S., and Bonner, J. T. (1969). J. Bact. 99, 510.
Monard, D., Janecek, J., and Rickenberg, H. V. (1969). Biochem. Biophys. Res. Commun. 35, 584.
Perlman, R. L. and Pastan, I. (1968). J. Biol. Chem. 243, 5420.
Polsen, A. (1958). Biochim. biophys. Acta 29, 426.
Raper, K. B. (1940). J. Elisha Mitchell Scient. Soc. 56, 241.
Robertson, A. and Cohen, M. H. Manuscript in preparation.
Runyon, E. H. (1942). Collecting Net 17, 88.
Samuel, E. W. (1961). Devl Biol. 3, 317.
Shaffer, B. M. (1956). J. Exp. Biol. 33, 645.
Shaffer, B. M. (1958). Q. J. Microsc. Sci. 99, 103.
Shaffer, B. M. (1961). J. Exp. Biol. 38, 833.
Shaffer, B. M. (1962). Adv. Morphogen. 2, 109.
Sussman, M. and Lee, F. (1955). Proc. Nat. Acad. Sci. U.S.A. 41, 70.
Sussman, M., Lee, F., and Kerr, N. S. (1956). Science 123, 1171.
Sussman, M. and Sussman, R. R. (1969). Symp. Soc. Gen. Microbiol. 19, 403.
Sussman, R. R., Sussman, M., and Fu, F. L. (1958). Bact. Proc. 32.
Sutherland, E. W., Øye, I., and Butcher, R. W. (1965). Recent Progr. Horm. Res. 21, 623.
van de Veerdonk, F. C. G. and Konijn, T. M. (1970). Acta endocr., Copenh. 64, 364.

POLLEN TUBE CHEMOTROPISM

J.P. Mascarenhas
State University of New York at Albany,
Department of Biological Sciences,
Albany,
New York 12203, U.S.A.

The pollen tube of flowering plants may grow through as much as 50 cm of the stylar tissue, enter the micropyle of an ovule and then discharge from its tip two non-motile sperm cells in the immediate vicinity of an unfertilized egg. This review is concerned with the factors that direct the pollen tube to the egg.

The series of events that occur in the process will first be briefly reviewed. After meiosis, the developing pollen grain enlarges and its walls thicken greatly. Its nucleus then divides mitotically forming a vegetative and a generative cell. Depending on the plant species, the generative cell may divide forming two sperm cells either before pollen maturation is complete or during the growth of the pollen tube in the pistil. The pollen grain which thus may be bi- or tri-nucleate when it is released from the anther, is carried by wind, insects or other agents to the stigma of the pistil, the female part of the flower (Figure 1). Conditions on the pistil are favorable for the germination of the pollen grain which then germinates by extruding a tube, the pollen tube, through a germ pore. The pollen tube grows in between the cells of the stigma and down into the style. Most pollen tubes grow very rapidly, some achieving rates greater than 35 mm an hour. Styles can be extremely variable in length. In some species the style is practically non-existent, whereas in others, e.g., corn, it may attain a length of about 50 cm.

An outstanding feature of the organization of the pistil is that the stigma is connected with the interior of the ovary by a tissue, the stigmatoid tissue (Esau, 1953), consisting of cells that are secretory (Rosen, 1971). Styles may be hollow, solid, or a combination of the two. In hollow styles, e.g., lily, the stigmatoid tissue lines the stylar canal. In most angiosperms the styles are solid. The stigmatoid tissue is present, nevertheless, usually in the form of strands of considerably elongated cells staining deeply with cytoplasmic stains. Stigmatoid tissue occurs on the placenta within the ovary, and in some species

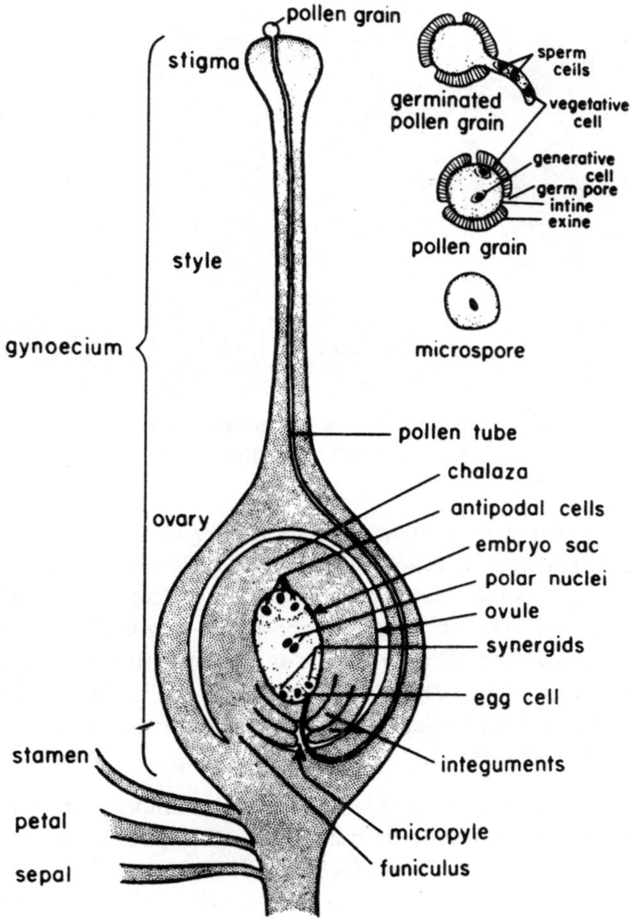

Figure 1. Diagrammatic longitudinal section of a flower, showing the pathway of the pollen-tube to the egg.

on parts of the ovule as well (Esau, 1953). In solid styles the pollen tube usually passes through the stigmatoid tissue by intercellular growth. Upon reaching the ovarian cavity, the pollen tube follows the stigmatoid tissue lining the ovary wall and the placenta, and eventually comes in contact with an ovule. The ovary may contain from one to several hundred ovules depending on the species, attached to various parts of the lining of the ovary wall. The tube enters the ovule in a very specific manner. In most plants it enters through the micropyle. In some plants the pollen tube enters the ovule through the chalazal end. Even in such cases, the tube usually continues its growth over the surface of the embryo sac and penetrates it only after arriving near the end containing the egg cell. The tube penetrates the wall of the embryo sac, bursts open, discharges its contents, and fertilization occurs. For a more detailed description of the events preceding fertilization in flowering plants the reader is referred to the monograph by Maheshwari (1950).

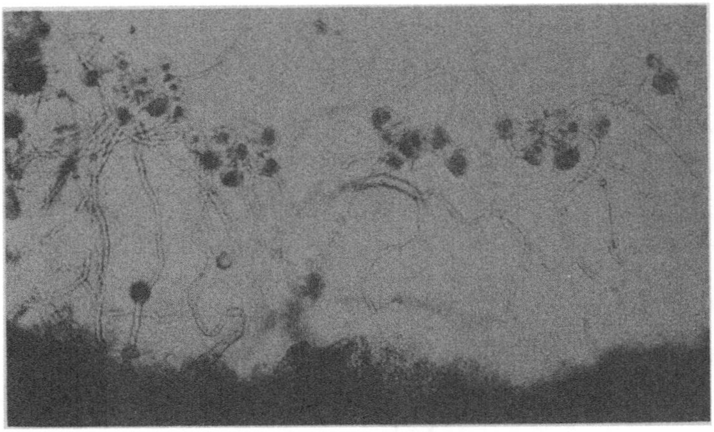

Figure 2. The chemotropic growth of pollen tubes of Antirrhinum majus to ovules (bottom of picture).

Why does the pollen tube grow through the style and enter the embryo sac always in so specific a manner? Is it chemically directed, or is the anatomy of the pistil tissues such that just by elongating it automatically arrives at the micropyle? The structure of the pistil might play an important part; however, this review will only consider the chemically controlled directional growth of pollen tubes. Different aspects of pollen tube chemotropism have been covered in several recent reviews (Mascarenhas and Machlis, 1962a; Rosen, 1962, 1968, (1971).

Molisch in 1889 in Germany was the first to demonstrate that pistil tissues contained some substance or substances that could control the direction of growth of pollen tubes. When freshly cut styles of Narcissus tazetta (daffodil) were placed on a sugar gelatin drop, pollen tubes growing in the vicinity were very strongly attracted towards the stigma and cut surface of the style. Figure 2 shows the type of test used by Molisch and most workers since. As the pollen and ovules or other test material are placed on the surface of the agar medium this test has been called the "surface" test. The "surface" test is not a very reliable test, although when there is a positive reaction it is very dramatic. The relative merits of the different assay procedures used for measuring chemotropism can be found in Mascarenhas and Machlis, (1962a), and Rosen (1964).

Since Molisch, several other workers have demonstrated this type of chemotropism in a wide variety of plants. The results of all the work reported in the literature were tabulated (Mascarenhas and Machlis, 1962a) and it was found that out of 105 plant species tested, chemotropism of pollen tubes to pistil tissues was observed in 57 species or 54 per cent of the plants. This is probably an underestimate, as several factors, such as the unreliability of the "surface"-test, release of inhibitors of pollen tube growth when tissues are damaged, use of pistil parts at the wrong stage of maturity, etc., could give negative results. Welk, Millington, and Rosen (1965) have found that in two species of lily the presence of chemotropic activity in the pistil progresses basipetally as a wave commencing at the stigma 3 to 5 days before the anthers of the flower release their pollen and appearing at the ovules 1 to 2 days later. It is thus important to select pistil tissue at the right stage of development if any chemotropic activity is to be demonstrated.

Pollen from many plants is able to respond chemotropically to vegetative tissue and to pistil tissues from related and unrelated plant species (see review by Mascarenhas and Machlis, 1962a). Hence, the chemotropic factor(s) seems to be widely dispersed among plants and/or there are several factors to which pollen tubes can react chemotropically.

The first attempt to isolate the chemotropic factor was made by Tsao (1949). She found that it was reasonably water soluble, stable to boiling for 10 min, stable to treatment with 5 per cent HCl for 10 min and it did not pass through a dialysis membrane. From the work of several other investigators including Linck and Blaydes (1960), Mascarenhas and Machlis (1962b), Miki (1954, 1955, 1959), and Rosen (1961), the chemotropic factor is known to be of small molecular size although it is associated with material of high molecular weight from which it can partly be dissociated by polar solvents. It is not soluble in lipid solvents and some workers report that it is heat stable and others that it is heat labile.

Although several early reports in the literature claimed chemotropic activity for specific compounds and crude preparations such as compressed yeast, sucrose, glucose, fructose, lactose, egg albumin, diastase and sodium malate (Brink, 1924; Lidforss, 1899; Miyoshi, 1894; Molisch, 1893) more recent work has failed to confirm these results (Brink 1924, Mascarenhas and Machlis, 1962a, b; Rosen, 1961; Tsao 1949). Two more recent papers (Schildknecht and Benoni 1963a, b) have reported that simple amino acid and amine mixtures coupled with sugars are responsible for the chemotropic attraction of pollen tubes in _Oenothera_ and _Narcissus_. The assay procedure used by Schildknecht and Benoni has, however, been criticized (Rosen, 1964) and neither Rosen (1961) with lily pollen nor Mascarenhas and Machlis (1962b) with snapdragon pollen were able to detect any chemotropic growth towards amino acid mixtures or sugars. In view of the recent interest in cyclic 3'5'-adenosine monophosphate this compound was tested in the author's laboratory in the depression assay over a wide concentration range (10^{-7} to 2×10^{-3} M) and was found to be chemotropically inactive.

In snapdragon (_Antirrhinum majus_) the calcium ion is the, or one of the, most important natural chemotropic factors for the pollen (Macarenhas and Machlis, 1962c, 1964). This effect is specific for the calcium ion and cannot be replaced by Mg^{2+}, Ba^{2+}, Sr^{2+}, Na^{+}, or K^{+}. Tropism of snapdragon pollen tubes to a source of Ca^{2+} was demonstrated in all the tests for chemotropism, such as the "surface" test, the "depression" test with both a large quantity of pollen and also with a single row of pollen, and the "slit" test (Mascarenhas and Machlis, 1962c, 1964). Rosen (1964) confirmed the chemotropic activity of calcium for snapdragon pollen with two different assays and also found that ashed snapdragon pistil was chemotropically active with snapdragon pollen in both the "surface" and "depression" tests. Analysis of the total calcium present in the pistil showed an overall gradient amounting to a four-fold increase in concentration between the upper third of the style and the ovules and placenta (Mascarenhas and Machlis, 1964). By labeling with ^{45}Ca it was shown that a large fraction of the calcium from the different parts of the pistil was readily diffusible into agar and hence must be soluble (Mascarenhas and Machlis, 1964). If the calcium ion were to be effective in vivo in directing the pollen tube to the micropyle of the ovule it would be necessary for the calcium to be present (1) in an ionic or soluble form and (2) in high enough concentrations in the tissues of the style and ovary through which the pollen tubes normally grow. Using the glyoxal-bis (2-hydroxy-anil) staining procedure (Kashiwa and Atkinson, 1963), the concentration of ionic calcium was found to be fairly low and almost constant throughout the length of the style, being slightly higher in the stigma and increasing in the region of the ovary, with the placenta and inside of the ovary wall containing an extremely high concentration of calcium (Mascarenhas, 1966). The stigmatoid tissue in the style and surrounding parenchyma cells contain a lower concentration of calcium than that found in the ovule and stigma. The cells of the ovule are comparatively low in calcium and there is no higher concentration of calcium in the region of the micropyle and embryo sac. Since this anatomical distribution of calcium would not be expected if a continuously increasing calcium gradient was important in directing pollen tubes all the way from the stigma to the ovule, it was suggested that some other factor(s) besides calcium might be involved, especially to direct the pollen tube to the micropyle (Mascarenhas, 1966). The question of gradients will be discussed again later. Other unpublished work from the author's laboratory indicates that some other factor, organic in nature, acts with calcium in causing tropism. This factor, however, seems to play a minor role in the process.

The calcium ion exerts a very pronounced stimulating effect on both pollen germination and tube growth of a large number of plant species (Brink, 1924; Brewbaker and Kwack, 1963). The chemotropic substance(s) from pistil tissues is known to have in addition to a tropic effect also a growth stimulating effect on pollen tubes (Knowlton, 1922; Beck and Joly, 1941).

Unfortunately, although Ca^{2+} might be the main chemotropic agent for snapdragon-pollen tubes, it is without any effect either on pollen tube growth in lily (Rosen, 1964) and corn (Cook and Walden, 1965) or on chemotropism in lily (Rosen, 1964). Thus, in these plants at least, some other factor plays the major role in chemotropism, and calcium may or may not be involved in the process. Since most pollens respond with enhanced growth to calcium (Brewbaker and Kwack, 1963) while pollen of corn and lily do not, this might indicate that these pollens contain an adequate store of calcium.

The chemotropic factor, as discussed earlier, is widely distributed in plant tissues and there might be several factors to which pollen tubes can react tropically. It has been suggested that there might be two or more factors that interact in causing chemotropism (Mascarenhas and Machlis, 1964; Rosen, 1964; Mascarenhas, 1966). For example, the optimum response of snapdragon pollen tubes to calcium is conditioned by the presence of boron (Mascarenhas and Machlis, 1964). Boron is a required growth factor for most pollens (Schmucker, 1932, 1933, 1935 and literature review in Vasil, 1964). Thus depending on the relative amounts present in the pollen of the different interacting factors, one or other factor that was limiting would be the one that would elicit a tropic response.

Any discussion of the mechanism of action of tropic factors has to take into consideration the special nature of growth of pollen tubes. Pollen tubes grow exclusively at their tips. The growth zone in Easter lily pollen, for example, is restricted to the tip-most 3 to 5 microns, (Dashek and Rosen, 1966). Growth of the tube at the tip region appears to take place by the fusion of polysaccharide-containing vesicles derived from either Golgi bodies or endoplasmic reticulum in the older parts of the tube (Dashek and Rosen, 1966).

For a tube growing straight, the growth zone at the tip is perpendicular to the long axis of the tube. For the tip to change its direction of growth all that is required is that there is a small shift in the angle made by the center of the growth zone with respect to the rest of the tube, in response to a directionally localized impinging of the chemotropic factor on the tip of the tube. At this point there may be a concentration gradient which need be, however, effective only over a very small distance. Once the direction of growth was changed and the tube tip was now in a uniformly distributed field of the tropic substance, the tube would continue to grow straight. No concentration gradient would be necessary to keep the tube growing in the direction it was already pointed towards. Any component contributing directly to the growth at the tip region could theoretically be the agent that could cause such a change in direction, i.e., be a tropic factor. One would accordingly expect that those factors required for normal metabolism of the pollen tube or for the synthesis of wall precursor material back of the tip, would contribute only to the growth of the tube, whereas those responsible for putting together the various components of the tube wall at the growth zone would in addition to being growth factors also be chemotropic factors.

The pollen tube is not a completely independent structure and depends for at least a part of its nutrition and growth requirements on the pistil tissue through which it grows. There is evidence for the movement of sugars, amino acids, etc. from the pistil tissue into the pollen tube (Linskens and Esser, 1959; Kroh, Miki-Hirosige, Rosen, and Loewus, 1970). Thus it is probable that for one or more of the requirements for tip growth the pollen tube is dependent on the pistil tissue and the missing component(s) would be the chemotropic factor(s).

If this hypothesis is correct there would be no necessity for having a continuously increasing concentration gradient of the tropic substance in the pistil along the pathway of the pollen tube from the stigma to the micropyle of the ovule. All that would be required would be the presence of the tropic factor in the tissues through which the pollen tubes grew in a concentration greater than a certain threshold value. Only in the region where a sharp change in direction occurred, such as, for example, from the placenta to the ovule and from the sides of the ovule into the micropyle, would a very restricted gradient of the chemotropic substance be of some use.

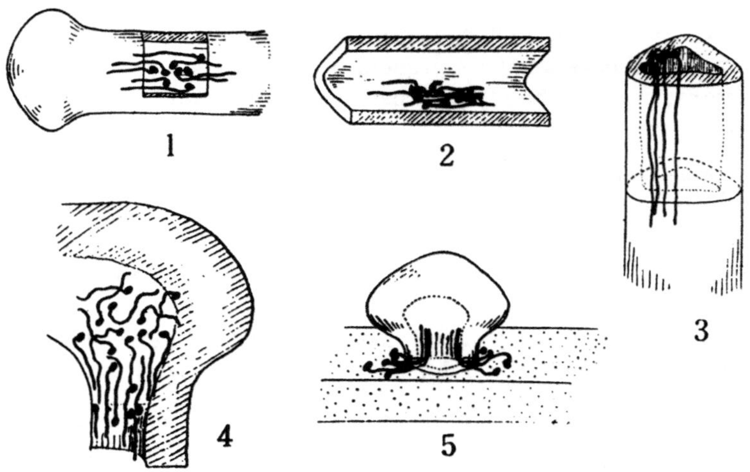

Figure 3. Diagrammatic representation of the direction of growth of pollen tubes in cut segments of the style of Lilium longiflorum. From Iwanami (1959) with permission. See text for details.

This hypothesis obtains some support from the following facts. In lily pistils, chemotropic activity is present in the stigma, style, and ovules and, seems to be localized in the stigmatoid tissue (Welk, Millington and Rosen, 1965). Iwanami (1959) has carried out some very elegant experiments with lily styles which are hollow with the insides being lined with stigmatoid cells. These experiments are described diagrammatically in Figure 3 taken from his paper. A hole was cut (Figure 3(1)) or an incision made (Figure 3(2)) in the middle of a style section and pollen spread on the inner wall. The grains germinated and very interestingly, about equal numbers grew towards the stigma and the ovary. When a style segment was cut and inverted with its stigma end down and pollen grains then spread at the top (Figure 3(3)), the tubes grew downwards over the stigmatoid tissue. If a portion of the style with the stigma was cut and placed with the cut surface on a gelatin layer and then pollen spread around the cut end (Figure 3(5)), the pollen tubes entered the style and grew upwards towards the stigma. All these experiments seem to indicate that there is no continuous increasing gradient of the chemotropic factor from the stigma to the ovary. If there was a gradient and it was important, then the pollen tubes would not have grown towards the stigma or stigma end of the style.

If this reasoning is correct then the fact that no continuous increasing gradient of calcium is found from the stigma to the ovary in snapdragon would not necessarily mean that calcium was not the chemotropic factor in vivo. One would also expect that in different pollen species there would be differences in the nature of the chemotropic factors.

The identification of chemotropic compounds in several additional species of plants and an understanding of pollen tube tip growth in molecular terms, would indicate whether the proposed hypothesis is correct or not.

ACKNOWLEDGEMENTS

I am grateful to Dr. W. G. Rosen for providing me with manuscripts of papers prior to publication and to Dr. Y. Iwanami for permission to reproduce Figure. 3.

REFERENCES

Beck, W. A. and Joly, R. A. (1941). Trans. Amer. Micros. Soc. 60, 149.

Brewbaker, J. O. and Kwack, B. H. (1963). Amer. J. Bot. 50, 859.

Brink, R. A. (1924). Amer. J. Bot. 11, 417.

Cook, E. S. and Walden, D. B. (1965). Can. J. Bot. 42, 779.

Dashek, W. V. and Rosen, W. G. (1966). Protoplasma 61, 192.

Esau, K. (1953). Plant Anatomy. John Wiley and Sons Inc., New York.

Iwanami, Y. (1959). J. Yokohama Municipal Univ. 116 (C-34, Biol. -13), 1.

Kashiwa, H. A. and Atkinson, W. B. (1963). J. Histochem. Cytochem. 11, 258.

Knowlton, H. E. (1922). Cornell Univ. Agri. Expt. Sta. Mem. 52, 746.

Kroh, M., Miki-Hirosige, H., Rosen, W., and Loewus, F. (1970). Plant Physiol. 45, 92.

Lidforss, B. (1899). Ber. d. deutsch. bot. Ges. 17, 236.

Linck, A. J. and Blaydes, G. W. (1960). Ohio J. Sci. 60, 274.

Linskens, H. F. and Esser, K. (1959). Proc. Kon. Ned. Akad. Wetensch; Amsterdam c62, 150.

Maheshwari, P. (1950). An Introduction to the Embryology of Angiosperms. McGraw-Hill Book Co., Inc., New York.

Mascarenhas, J. P. (1966). Protoplasma 62, 53.

Mascarenhas, J. P. and Machlis, L. (1962a). Vitamins and Hormones 20, 347.

Mascarenhas, J. P. and Machlis, L. (1962b). Amer. J. Bot. 49, 482.

Mascarenhas, J. P. and Machlis, L. (1962c). Nature 196, 292.

Mascarenhas, J. P. and Machlis, L. (1964). Plant Physiol. 39, 70.

Miki, H. (1954). Bot. Mag. (Tokyo) 67, 143.

Miki, H. (1955). Bot. Mag. (Tokyo) 68, 293.

Miki, H. (1959). Mem. Coll. Sci. Univ. Kyoto, Ser. B. 26, 61.

Miyoshi, M. (1894). Flora 78, 76.

Molisch, H. (1889). Sitz. Math. Naturw. Kl. Akad. Wiss. Wien (Anz. Akad. Wissensch). Wien 26, 11.

Molisch, H. (1893). Sitz. Math. Naturw. Kl. Akad. Wiss. Wien 102, 423.

Rosen, W. G. (1961). Amer. J. Bot. 48, 889.

Rosen, W. G. (1962). Quart. Rev. Biol. 37, 242.

Rosen, W. G. (1964). In Pollen Physiology and Fertilization Linskens, H. F., Ed., North-Holland Amsterdam, 159.

Rosen, W. G. (1968). Ann. Rev. Pl. Physiol. 19, 435.

Rosen, W. G. (1971). In Pollen : Development and Physiology, (Heslop-Harrison. J., ed.,) 177.

Rosen, W. G. (1971). In Pollen : Development and Physiology, (Heslop-Harrison. J., ed.,) 239.

Schildknecht, H. and Benoni, H. (1963a). Z. Naturforsch. 18b, 45.

Schildknecht, H. and Benoni, H. (1963b). Z. Naturforsch. 18b, 656.

Schmucker, T. (1932). Planta 16, 376.

Schmucker, T. (1933). Planta 18, 641.

Schmucker, T. (1935). Planta 23, 264.

Tsao, T.-H. (1949). Plant Physiol. 24, 494.

Vasil, I. K. (1964). In Pollen Physiology and Fertilization, Linskens, H. F., Ed., North-Holland, Amsterdam. 107.

Welk, M., Sr., Millington, W. F., and Rosen, W. G. (1965). Amer. J. Bot. 52, 774.

PHOTOTAXIS AND PHOTOKINESIS IN BACTERIA AND BLUE-GREEN ALGAE

W. Nultsch
University of Marburg,
Department of Botany,
Marburg,
Germany.

Bacteria and blue-green algae have some features in common: they lack a nucleus and all the cytoplasmic structures and organelles which are typical for eukaryontic cells, such as endoplasmic reticulum, golgi apparatus, and mitochondria. Although they also lack true plastids, in the phototrophic forms, i.e. the families athiorhodaceae, thiorhodaceae, and chlorobacteriaceae and in all blue-green algae the photosynthetic pigments are located in thylakoids, which are not surrounded by a plastid envelope.

In these microorganisms, in so far as they are motile, light can cause several different reactions in movement, which are summarized in the term "photomotion" (Wolken and Shin, 1958). Because there is a considerable confusion in the terminology of reaction types in photomotion of microorganisms, it seems to be necessary to give a clear definition of these reactions. The terms "phototaxis" and "photokinesis" were created at the end of the nineteenth century. The term "phototaxis", in its original sense, covers all photic reactions which lead to a distinct arrangement of microorganisms in space, while the term "photokinesis" denotes a change in the speed of movement, which depends directly on light intensity.

According to the observations of Rothert (1901) and Pfeffer (1904), we have to distinguish between two phototactic reaction types, which are called photo-topotaxis and photo-phobotaxis. The topotacic or topic reactions are defined as to be directed by light, while the phobotactic responses are due to sudden changes in light intensity $\frac{dJ}{dt}$. This conception has been confirmed by Buder (1917). Later the photo-phobotactic reaction was called "phobic response", "shock reaction", "stop response", or "motor response".

Photo-phobotactic reactions in purple bacteria were described for the first time by Engelmann (1882). He observed that in the so-called Bacterium photometricum, which is probably identical with the sulfur purple Bacterium

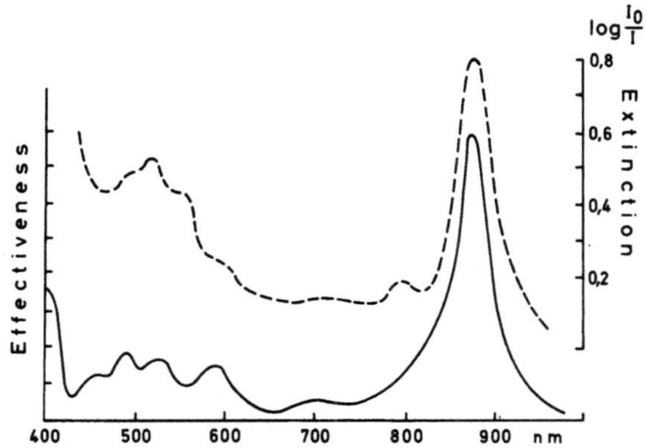

Figure 1. Photo-phobotactic action spectrum (——) and in vivo absorption spectrum (- - -) of Rhodospirillum rubrum. Abscissa: wavelength in nm; ordinate: quantum efficiency and extinction respectively (after Clayton, 1953a, from Haupt, 1966).

chromatium, a reversal of the swimming direction is caused by either a decrease in light intensity or exposure to a steep light gradient, e.g. by passing a boundary from light to dark. The reaction is positive, if the reversal is caused by a decrease, and negative, if it is caused by an increase in light intensity. Positive photo-phobotaxis results in an accumulation of the organisms in a bright light field projected onto a darkened preparation of microorganisms, the so-called Engelmann's light trap.

Since the classical work of Engelmann (1882, 1883, 1888) and Buder (1917, 1919) it is known that in purple bacteria radiation is photo-phobotactically active according to its absorption by the photosynthetic pigments. Later investigations, carried out by Manten (1948), Thomas (1950), Duysens (1952) and Clayton (1953 a, b), revealed that in Chromatium and Rhodospirillum the action spectra of positive photo-phobotaxis and photosynthesis are essentially identical and coincide with the absorption spectra of both species (Figure 1). These findings led to the conclusion that phobic responses may be due to sudden changes in the rate of photosynthesis.

This hypothesis was confirmed by investigations of Thomas and Nijenhuis (1950), who found that the saturation levels of photo-phobotaxis and photosynthesis are reached at the same light intensity. Clayton (1953) concluded from his experiments, that a sudden change in light intensity causes a transient change in the steady state of photosynthesis and this way initiates a phobic response. However, the question arose how this change could be transmitted to the locomtor apparatus. Links (1955) suggested a general hypothesis according to which phobic responses are due to sudden changes in ATP supply to the locomotor apparatus. This would mean that in case of photo-phobotaxis the reactions are caused by sudden changes in the ATP production of the photophosphorylation apparatus.

In blue-green algae, Dangeard (1910, 1911) found that red and far-red light was photo-phobotactically more active than blue light. Drews (1959).

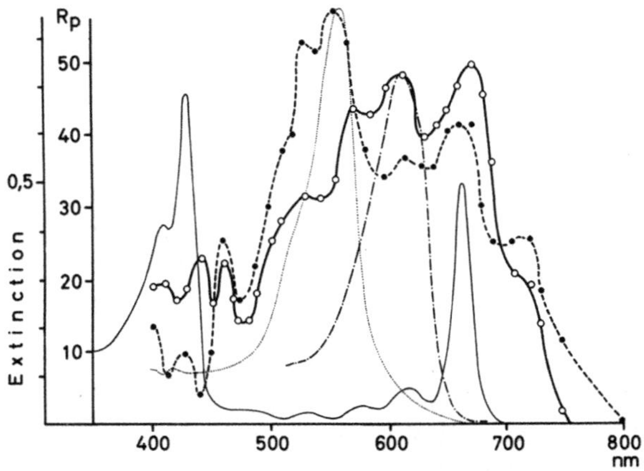

Figure 2. Photo-phobotactic action spectra of the blue-green algae Phormidium uncinatum (–●–●–) and Phormidium spec. (–○–○–). Absorption spectra of chlorophyll a (——), phycoerythrin (······), and phycocyanin (–·–·–). Abscissa: wavelength in nm; ordinate: phobotactic reaction (R_p) in relative units and extinction respectively (Nultsch, 1962 c).

using cut-off and interference filters, obtained similar results. However, the question remained undecided, whether or not there are correlations between photo-phototaxis and photosynthesis in blue-green algae, too.

This was the situation at the beginning of our investigations on phototaxis of purple bacteria and blue-green algae. Since photo-phobotactic action spectra of purple bacteria have been published repeatedly, the first step was to measure phobotactic action spectra of blue-green algae. For this purpose, we used some species of the genus Phormidium, which differ in their biliprotein content. As is shown in Figure 2, species which predominantly contain phycoerythrin display maximum phobotactic activity at about 560 nm, which only contain phycocyanin, a main maximum in the action spectrum lies at about 615 nm (Nultsch, 1962 b, c). Thus, the role of biliproteins as photoreceptors in photo-phobotaxis seemed to be proved. Moreover, in all species of blue-green algae investigated a second maximum exists at about 680 nm, which coincides with the red absorption maximum of chlorophyll a in vivo, while the effect of blue light is far out of proportion to its absorption by chlorophyll a.

Because of the striking similarity between these photo-phobotactic action spectra and some photosynthetic action spectra, which were measured by Duysens (1952) and Haxo and Norris (1953) in other species, the action spectra of photo-phobotaxis and photosynthetic $^{14}CO_2$ incorporation have been compared in Phormidium uncinatum (Nultsch and Richter, 1963), which turned out to be essentially identical. These results gave evidence that even in blue-green algae photo-phobotactic reactions are caused by changes in the rate of photosynthesis.

In order to obtain more information of the coupling between photo-phobotaxis and photosynthesis investigations on the effect of photosynthetic

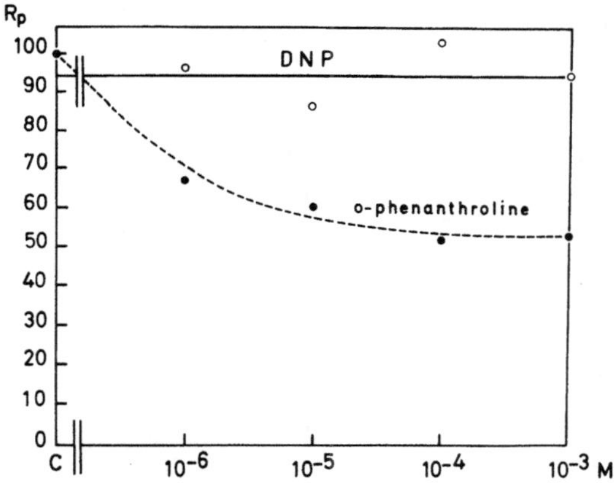

Figure 3. Effect of DNP and o-phenanthroline on photo-phobotaxis in Rhodospirillum rubrum. Abscissa: molarity of inhibitors; ordinate: photo-phobotactic reaction (R_p) as percent of the controls (C) (after Throm, 1968).

inhibitors and uncouplers upon photo-phobotactic responses have been carried out by Throm (1968) in purple bacteria. While photo-phobotaxis is not at all impaired by uncouplers, inhibitors of photosynthetic electron transport decrease the photo-phobotactic sensitivity with increasing concentrations (Figure 3), with the sole exception of DCMU. This is understandable in so far as purple bacteria lack the second light reaction which is sensitive to DCMU. The ineffectiveness of uncouplers, however, is a convincing argument against the hypothesis of Links, because it is rather unlikely that any reaction coupled with a phosphorylation process is insensitive to uncouplers. On the other hand, the strong effect of photosynthetic inhibitors favors the conception of correlations between photosynthesis and phobotaxis.

In blue-green algae, the effect of uncouplers such as dinitrophenol, sodium azide, imidazole, and arsenate has been investigated by Nultsch and Jeeji-Bai (1966). However, the results are not so clear as in purple bacteria. Since in these organisms uncouplers inhibit oxidative phosphorylation and, hence, the movement in the dark at very low concentrations, no phobic responses can occur, because the trichoms become immotile in the dark and are prevented from entering the light field as a result of immotility. Thus, the interpretation of these results meets considerable difficulties. More information may be obtained from investigations on the effect of uncouplers on the discrimination threshold, because in this case two fields of different light intensities are used, avoiding a dark surrounding field. This is important in so far as photosynthetic phosphorylation is less sensitive to uncouplers than the oxidative one and, as a result, movement in the light is maintained for a longer time than in the dark, if uncouplers are present. Such experiments are in progress.

Photosynthetic inhibitors such as phenylurethane, hydroxylamine, o-phenanthroline, 3-(3,4-dichlorophenyl)-1,1-dimethylurea (DCMU), salicylaldoxime, n-heptylhydroxyquinoline- N-oxide (HQNO), and antimycin A impair

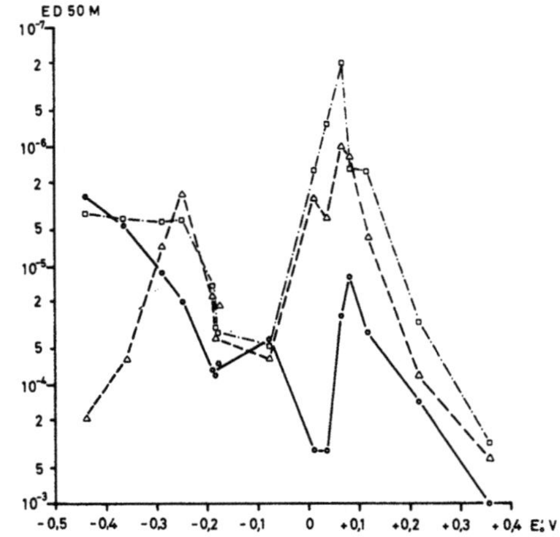

Figure 4. Effect of redox systems on photokinesis (–○–○–), dark movement (–△–△–) und phobotaxis (– □ –·– □ –) in Phormidium uncinatum. Abscissa: redox potential (E_0') in V; ordinate: ED_{50} in Mol (Nultsch, 1968).

the phobic response, as would be expected. However, phobotaxis is more sensitive to inhibitors of non-cyclic than to those of cyclic electron transport. Especially the sensitivity to DCMU is low compared with other inhibitors. Therefore, it was concluded that the coupling point between photosynthesis and phobotaxis is located in the second light reaction, but before the DCMU block (Nultsch, 1966).

However, more recent investigations on the inhibitory effect of externally added redox-systems on the phobic response have led to another interpretation of the aforementioned results. As shown in Figure 4, there are two maxima of inhibition, the first one below –0.25 V and a second one between ±0 and +0.1 V. These regions in the redox scale correspond with the regions of electron transfer from the two light reactions to the next electron acceptors. Although the main maximum is located at E_0' values of the electron acceptors of the second light reaction, the linkage, according to the aforementioned results, cannot be restricted to a distinct point of the electron transport chain.

Based on these results, Nultsch (1968, 1970) has concluded that, contrary to the hypothesis of Links (1955), in purple bacteria and blue-green algae photo-phobotaxis is coupled with the photosynthetic electron transport chain. He suggested that sudden changes in the steady state of electron transport, provided that they exceed a distinct threshold value, are transformed into bioelectric potential changes, e.g. action potentials, which are quickly conducted by the cytoplasmic membrane to the locomotor apparatus. This conception is consistent with the hypothesis of Clayton (1959), who postulated that phobic responses in purple bacteria are "mediated through the development of an excitatory state which is transmitted to the locomotor areas, causing a coordinated motor response."

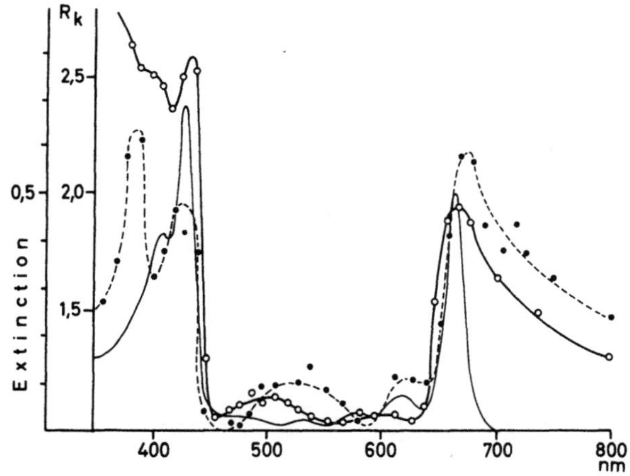

Figure 5. Photokinetic action spectra of the blue-green algae Phormidium uncinatum (-●-●-) and Phormidium spec. (-O-O-). Absorption spectrum of chlorophyll a (——). Abscissa: wavelength in nm; ordinate: photokinetic effect (R_k) in relative units and extinction respectively (Nultsch, 1962c).

In other microorganisms, as in flagellates (Haupt, 1959) and in diatoms (Nultsch, 1969), no correlations between photo-phobotaxis and photosynthesis seem to exist. This could be due to the existence of a chloroplast envelope, which seperates the thylakoids from the surrounding cytoplasm and this way prevents the immediate transmission of changes in the redox or electric potentials to the locomotor apparatus.

In course of his investigations Engelmann (1882, 1883, 1888) observed that purple bacteria, which had become immotile in the dark, resumed their movement after a short irradiation of some seconds to a few minutes, and that the speed of movement depended on light intensity. After a repeated darkening the bacteria continued to move for a while, but soon they became immotile again. From these observations Engelmann concluded that "a pool of any substance may be produced by irradiation which is necessary for movement and is consumed in the dark." He called this effect of light on motility "photokinesis". In the following decades photokinesis in purple bacteria has been observed occasionally, but no work has been done to elucidate this phenomenon.

According to the definition of Nultsch (1970) positive photokinesis is an acceleration of movement by light or, in organisms which are immotile in the dark, even an excitation of movement by light. Consequently, negative photokinesis is a light-induced decrease of the speed, in relation to the movement in the dark, eventually resulting in immotility.

In blue-green algae photokinesis was investigated for the first time by Nultsch (1962 a). In Phormidium autumnale he found light to be active in the

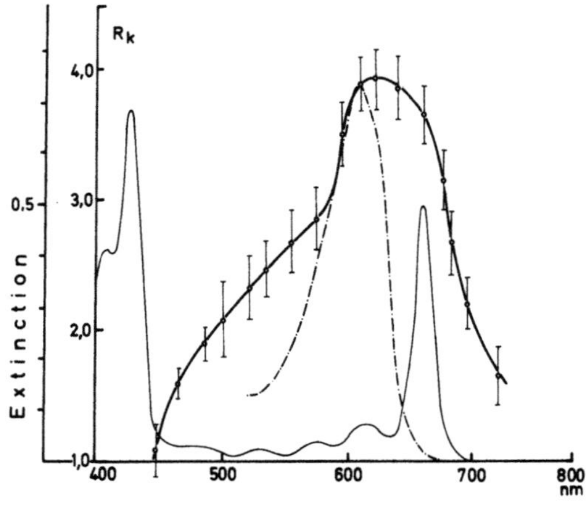

Figure 6. Photokinetic action spectrum of the blue-green alga Anabaena variabilis. Absorption spectra of chlorophyll a (——) and phycocyanin (–·–·–). Abscissa: wavelength in nm; ordinate: photokinetic effect (R_k) in relative units and extinction respectively.

sense of positive photokinesis in a wide range of intensities. However, beyond 20,000 lux, the speed was reduced with a further increase in light intensity, and movement was completely stopped at 40,000 lux.

In a series of investigations Nultsch and co-workers have studied photokinetic phenomena in several species of blue-green algae. As shown in Figure 5, in all species investigated the action spectra are very similar, independent of their biliprotein content. Two maxima of photokinetic activity have been found, one in the blue between 430 and 440 nm, and a second one in the red between 670 and 680 nm, which both coincide with the absorption maxima of chlorophyll a, while the activity of light between 450 and 650 nm is far out of proportion to its absorption by carotenoids and biliproteins.

From these results Nultsch (1962 a) has concluded that in the visible region chlorophyll a is the photoreceptor of photokinesis while carotenoids and biliproteins are scarcely effective if at all. He suggested that photokinesis is coupled predominantly with the first light reaction, and that the link between these two processes is ATP (Nultsch, 1965, 1966).

In order to confirm this conception and to locate the position of the coupling point between the two photoprocesses the effect of photosynthetic inhibitors such as phenylurethane, hydroxylamine, o-phenathroline, DCMU salicylaldoxime, HQNO, and antimycin A on photokinetic activity has been studied (Nultsch, 1965; Nultsch and Jeeji-Bai, 1966). As inhibitors of both non-cyclic and cyclic electron transport decelerate the movement, in principle both non-cyclic and cyclic phosphorylation can supply ATP for movement. However, under normal conditions, i.e. in air, cyclic phosphorylation may be the main energy source of photokinesis as the ATP produced by non-cyclic

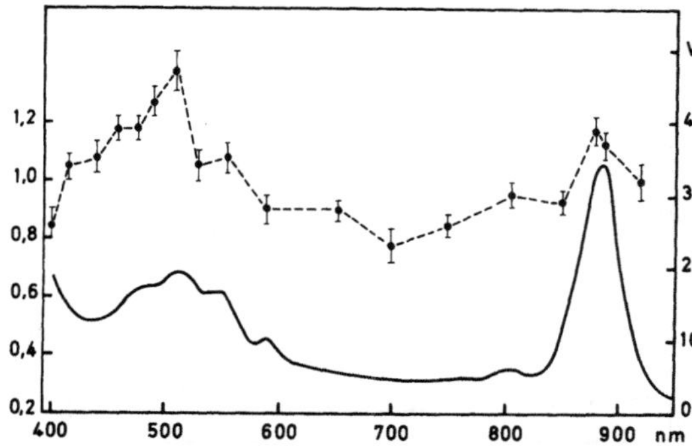

Figure 7. Photokinetic action spectrum (– ● – ● –) and in vivo absorption spectrum (———) of Rhodospirillum rubrum. Abscissa: wavelenth in nm; ordinate: absorbance (left) and velocity V in relative units (right) (Throm, 1968).

phosphorylation is consumed by CO_2-fixation to a large extent. For this reason, the photokinetic action spectrum of Phormidium resembles the absorption spectrum of chlorophyll a rather than the photosynthetic one.

This hypothesis was supported by investigations on the effect of uncouplers such as dinitrophenol, sodium azide, imidazole, arsenate, and ammonia on motility both in light and darkness (Nultsch, 1967). All uncouplers investigated more or less inhibit photokinesis, with the exception of ammonia, which has no effect at all. Moreover, the experiments have shown that movement in the dark is the result of an ATP supply from oxidative phosphorylation and, to a very small extent, from anaerobic phosphorylation in glycolysis.

Finally, the effect of redox substances, the E_0' values of which covered the range between −0.44 and +0.36 V, has been studied (Nultsch, 1968). As shown in Figure 4 all redox-systems which are able to trap electrons from the photosynthetic electron transport chain, more or less inhibit photokinesis. Maximum inhibition has been found at redox-potentials below −0.4 V, i.e. the range of viologens. A second smaller maximum lies between +0.06 and +0.08V (phenazine methosulphate, thionin). Thus, such redox-systems which, according to their redox-potentials, can trap electrons from the cyclic electron transport chain are most effective in inhibiting photokinesis. This is consistent with the conception that under normal conditions cyclic photophosphorylation is the main energy source of photokinesis and explains the lower activity of light absorbed by biliproteins.

However, the photokinetic action spectrum of the blue-green alga Anabaena variabilis, which has been measured most recently (Nultsch and Hellmann, unpublished), is quite different from the action spectra of the aforementioned Phormidium species. The maximum of photokinetic activity coincides with the absorption maximum of phycocyanin (Figure 6). While blue light absorbed by chlorophyll a is quite ineffective, the red region is slightly effective, although no distinct peak can be observed. Since this action spectrum was also measured in air, where the ATP produced by non-cyclic phosphorylation

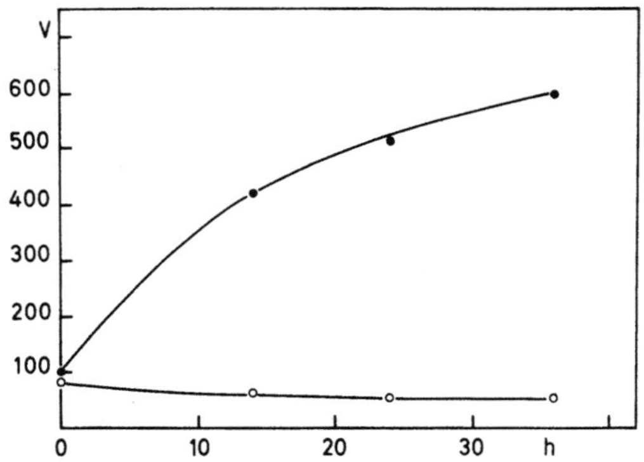

Figure 8. Effect of ATP on the speed of movement in Rodospirillum rubrum (-●-●-). Control (-○-○-). Abscissa: time (hours); ordinate: speed of movement in relative units (after Throm, 1968).

should be consumed by CO_2-fixation, it is suggested that the photokinetic effect may be due to ATP supplied from pseudocyclic phosphorylation. Consequently, the action spectrum resembles that of photosynthesis rather than the absorption spectrum of chlorophyll a. More detailed investigations on photokinesis of Anabaena are in progress.

In purple bacteria, photokinesis has been investigated by Throm (1968) and Nultsch and Throm (1968). Although the action spectrum of Rhodospirillum rubrum was measured under anaerobic conditions, the bacteria were motile also in the dark. Consequently, the photokinetic effect consists only in an increase of the speed. The action spectrum of photokinesis resembles that of photosynthesis, with the exception that the relative height of the two peaks in the blue-green and in the far red is inverse (Figure 7). This points to a stronger participation of carotenoids, especially of spirilloxanthin, in absorption of photokinetically active light. Thus, even in purple bacteria we find correlations between photokinesis and photosynthesis. However, contrary to the blue-green algae of the genus Phormidium there are no striking differences between the two action spectra, because there is only one light reaction system in purple bacteria. Because of its coupling to photophosphorylation, photokinesis of Rhodospirillum is sensitive to uncouplers and photosynthetic inhibitors as well.

If photokinesis is due to an additional ATP supply from photophosphorylation, it should be possible to simulate this effect by ATP. All attempts to increase the speed of blue-green algae and purple bacteria by externally added ATP have not been successful (Clayton, 1958; Nultsch, 1970). Throm (1968), repeating Clayton's experiments, also failed to demonstrate any effect of ATP on the speed of movement in short time experiments. However, in long time experiments he observed that the movement of Rhodospirillum rubrum in the dark was increasingly accelerated by 10^{-3} M ATP with increasing time (Figure 8). In these samples light had no more effect on the speed of movement, because the locomotor apparatus was energetically saturated. ATP cannot be

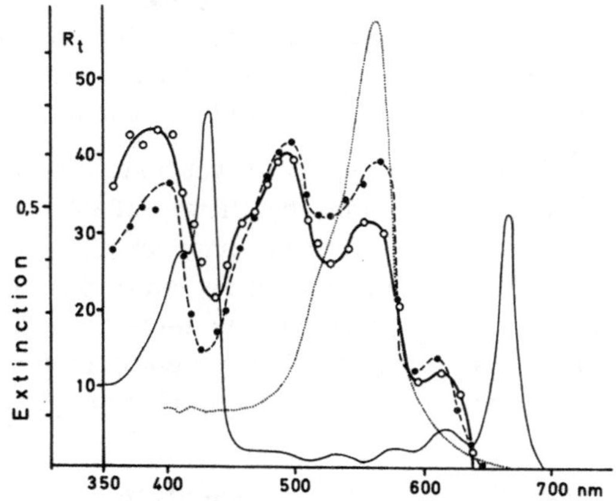

Figure 9. Photo-topotactic action spectra of the blue-green algae Phormidium autumnale (–○–○–) and Phormidium uncinatum (–●–●–). Absorption spectra of chlorophyll a (——) and phycoerythrin (......). Abscissa: wavelength in nm; ordinate: photo-topotactic reaction (R_t) in relative units and extinction respectively (Nultsch, 1961, 1962c).

replaced by GTP, CTP, ITP or other energy-rich phosphates, which decelerate the movement rather than accelerate it. Moreover, ADP and Adenosin are quite ineffective (Nultsch and Throm, unpublished). Obviously, in Rhodospirillum externally supplied ATP acts in the ATPase system of flagella after an adaptation time. Thus, we may conclude that light and ATP are equivalent in their ability to accelerate the movement.

Photo-topotactic reactions are positive, if the organisms move towards the light source, and negative, if they move away from it. Blue-green algae usually display positive reactions on unilateral illumination. However, the mode of topotactic reaction is different in both the families investigated, Nostocaceae and Oscillatoriaceae. While Nostocaceae show photo-topotactic reactions sensu strictu, i.e. an active orientation towards the light source by means of a steering mechanism, in Oscillatoriaceae the topotactic response is the result of trial and error motion rather than of a steering act. According to recent investigations of Throm (1968), purple bacteria, as Rhodospirillum rubrum, which were formerly reported to lack topotaxis at all, can also react topotactically, probably by means of trial and error motion.

In order to get some information about the photoreceptor, action spectra of photo-topotaxis were measured in blue-green algae in two species of the genus Phormidium (Nultsch, 1961, 1962 c), both containing phycoerythrin and phycocyanin. As shown in Figure 9 the action spectra of these two positively reacting species are very similar. The strong effectiveness of blue light with maximum activity at about 490 nm points to a participation of carotenoids in absorption of topotactically active light, while a second maximum between 560 and 570 nm is obviously due to phycoerythrin. Phycocyanin, only small amounts of which are present in both the species, is indicated by a small subsidiary maximum at 615 nm. Thus, in the species investigated both biliproteins and carotenoids seem to be active in mediation of the light stimulus, while the strong effectiveness of UV between 350 and 400 nm cannot be explained.

Action spectra of Nostocaceae have not yet been measured. According to preliminary experiments, carried out by Drews (1959), Anabaena variabilis and Cylinspermum spec., which only contain phycocyanin, seem to be sensitive mainly in orange light, i.e. in the absorption region of phycocyanin. Although more exact studies are necessary, biliproteins seem to be active in these organisms, too. In purple bacteria, the photoreceptor is unknown, because the photo-topotactic action spectrum of Rhodospirillum rubrum has not yet been measured.

Although the tracks of moving blue-green algae have been studied extensively (Drews, 1959; Nultsch, 1961), we do not understand the mechanism by which the photo-topotactic reaction is brought about. The same is valid for purple bacteria.

Summarizing the results we can say that in both purple bacteria and blue-green algae three types of photomotion are realized, which differ in their mechanism and, at least in some blue-greens, in the photoreceptor systems. However, many problems are still unresolved and offer a wide field for further research.

REFERENCES

Buder, J. (1917). Jb. wiss. Bot. 56, 529.
Buder, J. (1919). Jb. wiss. Bot. 58, 525.
Clayton, R. K. (1953a). Arch. Mikrobiol. 19, 107.
Clayton, R. K. (1953b). Arch. Mikrobiol. 19, 125.
Clayton, R. K. (1958). Arch. Mikrobiol. 29, 189.
Clayton, R. K. (1959). In W. Ruhland (Ed.), Handbuch der Pflanzenphysiologie, Vol. 17/1, Springer, Berlin, Göttingen, Heidelberg. pp. 371-387.
Dangeard, P. A. (1910). Bull. Soc. bot., France 57, 315.
Dangeard, P. A. (1911). C. R. A. Sc., Paris 152.
Drews, G. (1959). Arch. Protistenk. 104, 27.
Duysens, L. N. M. (1952). Diss. Utrecht.
Engelmann, Th. W. (1882). Pflügers Arch. ges. Physiol. 29, 387.
Engelmann, Th. W. (1883). Pflügers Arch. ges. Physiol. 30, 95.
Engelmann, Th. W. (1888). Bot. Ztg. 46, 661.
Haupt, W. (1959). In W. Ruhland (Ed.), Handbuch der Pflanzenphysiologie, Vol. 17/1, Springer, Heidelberg, pp. 318-370.
Haxo, F. T. and Norris, P. S. (1953). Biol. Bull. 105, 374.
Links, J. (1955). Diss. Leiden.
Manten, A. (1948). Antonie van Leeuwenhoek 14, 65.
Nultsch, W. (1961). Planta 56, 632.
Nultsch, W. (1962a). Planta 57, 613.
Nultsch, W. (1962b). Planta 58, 647.
Nultsch, W. (1962c). Ber. dt. bot. Ges. 75, 443.
Nultsch, W. (1965). Photochem. Photobiol. 4, 613.
Nultsch, W. (1966). In J. B. Thomas and J. C. Goedheer (Eds.), Currents in Photosynthesis, A. D. Donker, Rotterdam, The Netherlands, pp. 421-429.

Nultsch, W. (1967). Z. Pflanzenphysiol. 56, 1.
Nultsch, W. (1968). Arch. Mikrobiol. 63, 295.
Nultsch, E. (1969). Lecture at the XI. Internat. Bot. Congress. 24. Aug.-2. Sept. 1970, Seattle, Washington, USA.
Nultsch, W. (1970). In P. Halldal (Ed.), Photobiology Microoranisms. Wiley, in press.
Nultsch, W. and Jeeji-Bai (1966). Z. Pflanzenphysiol 54, 84.
Nultsch, W. and Richter, G. (1963). Arch. Mikrobiol. 47, 207.
Nultsch, W. and Throm, G. (1968). Nature, 218, 697.
Pfeffer, W. (1904). Pflanzenphysiologie, II. 2nd ed. Leipzig.
Rothert, W. (1901). Flora (Jena) 88, 371.
Thomas, J. B. (1950). Biochim. Biophys. Acta 5, 186.
Thomas, J. B. and Nijenhuis, L. E. (1950). Biochim. Biophys. Acta 6, 317.
Throm, G. (1968). Arch. Protistenk. 110, 313.
Wolken, J. J. and Shin, E. (1958). J. Protozool. 5, 39.

PHOTOTAXIS IN EUGLENA 1: PHYSIOLOGICAL BASIS OF PHOTORECEPTION AND TACTIC ORIENTATION

B. Diehn
The University of Toledo,
Department of Chemistry,
Toledo,
Ohio 43606, U.S.A.

As an introduction, perhaps a few words concerning the definition of the term "phototaxis" would be in order. At present, the most generally acceptable description of phototaxis defines it as orientation and subsequent oriented movement of freely motile organisms in response to light – towards the light in the case of positive, and away from it in the case of negative phototaxis. While in the past, some authors have distinguished between "topo-phototaxis" and "phobo-phototaxis", the former term actually means phototaxis proper while the latter refers to a light-induced nondirectional shock response (positive or negative, respectively, if occurring upon a decrease or an increase of light intensity). Since a nondirectional response is not a true taxis, I have proposed that the term "photophobic response" be used instead of "phobo-phototaxis" (Diehn, 1969 a, 1970 a), and will adhere to that terminology throughout this presentation.

The macroscopic results of these reactions of individual organisms have also been called "phototaxis", but should, of course, be termed phototactic or photophobic accumulation or expulsion from an illuminated region. If the mediating mechanism is now known, "photoinduced" would replace "phototactic" or "photophobic". The above terminology could be used to great advantage in the discussion of other taxes. The "avoidance response" of Dr. Adler's E. coli can, for instance, be described unequivocally by the term "positive chemophobic response".

The physiological basis of phototaxis is probably best understood in the unicellular green alga Euglena. This organism has roughly the shape of a prolate ellipsoid, with axes of about 70 and 15 μ (Figure 1, Leedale, 1967). Euglena propels itself by means of a flagellum that emerges at the anterior end, and usually assumes a trailing configuration during straight-line motion (Jahn and Bovee, 1968). Because of the torque resulting from the helical beat of the flagellum, Euglena rotates around its longitudinal axis as it moves in

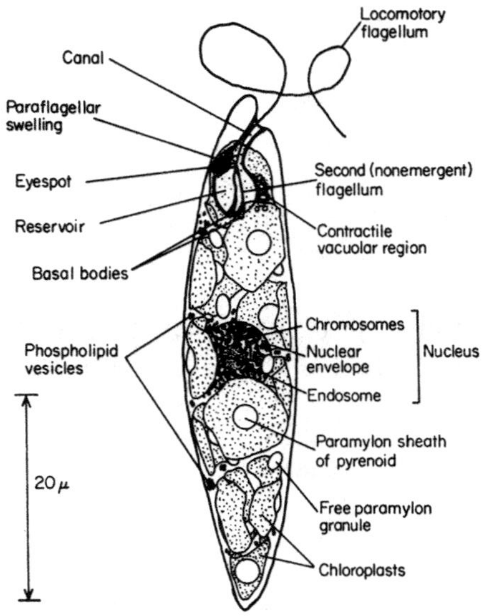

Figure 1. Schematic drawing of morphology of Euglena gracilis. After Leedale (1967).

the forward direction. Besides the flagellum, two other organelles are of special interest to us: the "paraflagellar swelling" at the base of the flagellum, and the "stigma", an orange-red pigment spot of about 4 μ^2 area at the anterior end of the organism on what has been defined as the "dorsal" side. On the assumption that the stigma is the photoreceptor of Euglena, it has been, and occasionally still is, called the "eyespot".

The first indication that the photoreceptor function actually resides in the paraflagellar swelling, was provided by the experiments of Engelmann (1882). He observed that Euglene exhibited a photophobic response upon shading of the anterior end of the cell while the stigma was still illuminated. Another line of evidence in support of this hypothesis was presented by Gossel (1957), who showed that a stigma-less mutant of Euglena still exhibited phototaxis, while Astasia, a colorless relative of Euglena possessing neither stigma nor paraflagellar swelling, showed none. A major obstacle to rigorous experimental proof that the paraflagellar swelling is indeed the photoreceptor lies in the fact that this organelle is very small (about 0.3 μ^2), and does not contain enough pigment for isolation or in vivo spectrophotometric identification.

The question now arises "If the stigma does not act as photoreceptor, what is its function, if any, in phototaxis?" Mast (1911) proposed more than 60 years ago that positive phototaxis, i.e. orientation and toward the light, is mediated by a shading action of the stigma with respect to the photoreceptor. This hypothesis has been considered off and on since then, but was generally thought to be very difficult to test experimentally (Jahn and Bovee, 1968). When we re-examined the problem in our laboratory last year, it became quite evident that the key to the solution lay in the photophobic responses which occur in Euglena upon changes in illumination intensity. Such changes are, after

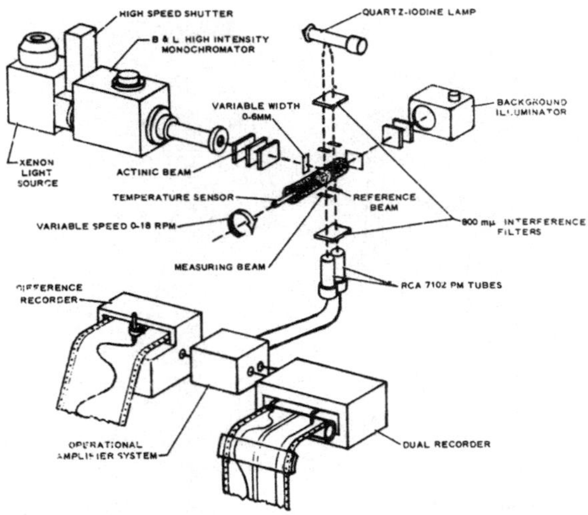

Figure 2. Schematic respresentation of the phototaxigraph Mk. III.

all, what occurs if a shading device is removed or interposed between photoreceptor and light source. The following is a summary of our microscopic observations of the photophobic responses in Euglena (Diehn, 1969 b, 1970 b):

The shock response appears as a rotation around the lateral axis which is normal to the dorsal/ventral plane. A "positive" photophobic response occurs in response to a sudden change toward a lower value of any light intensity which was initially below approximately 2×10^5 erg/cm^{2}sec (white light). The direction of rotation is toward the dorsal side, i.e. toward the stigma. In a "negative" photophobic response, the organism rotates in the opposite direction as the consequence of a sudden increase in light intensity from any initial value to beyond 2×10^5 erg/cm^{2}sec. Nothing happens if the light intensity is suddenly increased (or decreased, as the case may be) to 2×10^5 erg/cm^{2}sec. It appears as though Euglena were naturally adapted to this light intensity, which, incidentally, corresponds to the saturating intensity for photosynthesis (as well as to the normal intensity of the visible part of the solar radiation incident upon the surface of the earth in the Toledo area).

Depending on light intensity, the photophobic responses persist for up to 60 sec. Thereafter, adaptation has taken place, and the organisms resume their straight-line motion. If the illumination is from one side and exceeds 2×10^5 erg/cm^{2}sec, the direction of this movement will be away from the light (negative phototaxis). There is, besides adaptation, another way of terminating the photophobic responses, and that is by simple restoration of the previous lighting conditions. It is this observation which led us to a plausible hypothesis for a "periodic shading" mechanism of phototactic orientation. For this, one merely has to consider the following: In an organism that moves in a straight line path at right angles to the direction of the light (i.e. that has to perform a 90° turn for phototactic orientation), the stigma will shade the photoreceptor once every rotation. At the instant of shading, a positive photophobic response will commence. It will persist until the shadow of the stigma

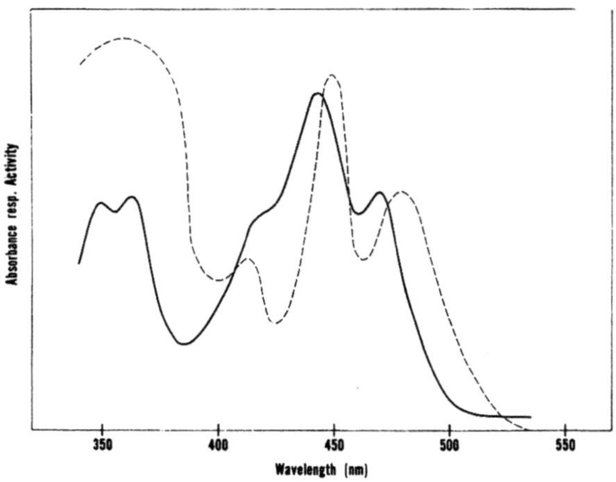

Figure 3. Composite action spectrum of the negative photophobic response in Euglena gracilis (broken curve), and absorption spectrum of riboflavin in 65 percent ethanol at 170 K (solid curve).

no longer falls upon the photoreceptor. A study of the geometry of the anterior end of Euglena indicates that shading would occur for one-third of each turn. Since a positive photophobic response results in a turn toward the stigma, which at the instant of shading was facing the light source, the net result is a fractional turn toward the light. This process is repeated until further shading is geometrically impossible, i.e. until the organism is oriented directly toward the light.

An entirely analogous mechanism would explain negative phototaxis. Upon high intensity illumination, Euglena experiences a negatively photophobic response which continues until the photoreceptor is permanently shaded. If permanent shading were indeed required, the shading function could not be performed by the stigma, though the posterior end of the cell could serve this purpose.

While the microscopically observed phototactic behavior of Euglena is entirely consistent with these hypotheses, independent experimental verification appeared to be very desirable. Such evidence has been obtained through the use of our "Phototaxigraph". This recording instrument for the measurement of phototaxis (Figure 2) is in essence a double beam infrared turbidimeter which measures the population density in an illuminated portion vs. the unstimulated part of an Euglena suspension. The actinic light enters the horizontally rotating sample cuvette at right angles to the measuring and reference beams. The processes occurring in the cuvette during a phototaxis experiment are complex and have been analyzed in detail (Diehn, 1970 a), and it must suffice here to point out that accumulation of cells in the actinic zone occurs in response to light scattered from cells already in that region, and that the "phototaxigram" produced by our apparatus allows the direct determination of the rate of phototactic in- or efflux. This rate may be expressed in, for instance, cells/cm^{2}sec. Feinleib and Curry (1967) have described a similar instrument in which the actinic light enters at the end of the cuvette. This arrangement has the advantage of having all organisms respond directly to the actinic light, but problems of screening and attachment of organisms to the window arise.

The "phototaxigraph" allows the study of the influence on photoinduced accumulation or expulsion of many parameters, such as temperature, chemical agents, circadian rhythms, and wavelength as well as intensity of the stimulating light. We have investigated all of these factors, and I think that Dr. Tollin will report on this in more detail. Because of time limitations, I will discuss only those experiments that have a direct bearing on the problems of orientation mechanism and photoreception in Euglena.

How would one test the "periodic shading" hypothesis of positive phototaxis with the phototaxigraph? Our approach has been to simulate periodic shading by using pulsed actinic light of varying frequency for stimulation. A resonance effect would then be expected as the repetition rate of the light pulses approaches the time it takes Euglena for one rotation. This is indeed what we did observe: if one plots the rate of positive phototaxis vs. pulse rate, a clear maximum appears at 1.05 sec. (Diehn, 1969 b).

The suggestion that the stigma is not involved in negative phototaxis is of great importance for the identification of the pigment molecule responsible for photoreception. As I have mentioned, the small size of the paraflagellar swelling would make it quite difficult to isolate this pigment, or to identify it by in vivo microspectrophotometry. This leaves the alternative route of identifying it through determination of the action spectrum of negative phototaxis. Bünning and Schneiderhöhn (1956), who determined the threshold action spectra of both positive and negative phototaxis for normally pigmented Euglenae, realized that no clear-cut interpretation of the action spectrum of positive phototaxis is possible, since here the absorption spectrum of the screening pigments in the stigma will be superimposed upon that of the photoreceptor pigment(s) proper. Since they determined the action spectrum of negative phototaxis at the threshold intensities at which inversion from positive to negative phototaxis occurred, the possibility of screening by the posterior end of the cell cannot be ruled out. Moreover, at the exposure time of 10 min. to the high light intensities which had to be used, modification of the photoreceptor pigment by bleaching could well have occurred.

Gössel (1957) determined the threshold action spectrum of negative phototaxis in a mutant of Euglena that lacked the stigma as well as chlorophyll. As you will hear from Dr. Tollin, the absence of a functioning photosynthetic apparatus has far-reaching consequences for the phototactic behavior of Euglena. Moreover, in a pigment mutant there is always the possibility that the invisible photoreceptor pigment has also been affected by the mutagenic agent.

The problem, then, was to determine the action spectrum for the negative photophobic response in a normally pigmented Euglena without resorting to the high light intensities that cause negative phototaxis. When we found ourselves confronted with these seemingly contradictory requirements, we were put on the right track for an experimental attack on this problem by an observation by Bound and Tollin (1967). They found that illumination with polarized white light whose plane of polarization was aligned such that the electric vector was perpendicular to the long axis of oriented Euglenae, would result in an efflux from the actinic zone of the phototaxigraph. They concluded that the stigma does not absorb polarized light of this orientation, and that for this to occur the pigment molecules in the stigma, which Batra and Tollin (1964) had shown to consist mainly of the carotenoids lutein and cryptoxanthin, would have to be aligned with their long axes parallel to the long axis of the cell. Having shown that the organisms leave the actinic zone of the phototaxigraph as the result of a series of negatively photophobic responses, we determined the rate of this phenomenon as a function of the wavelength of polarized light with the electric vector of its plane of polarization perpendicular to the long axes of oriented Euglenae (Diehn, 1969 c). The resulting action spectrum of the negative photophobic response, which according to our hypothesis should correspond to the absorption spectrum of the photoreceptor pigment(s), exhibited major peaks at 450 and 480 nm, and a minor peak around 412 nm. No activity was observed above 550 nm or below 350 nm.

The latter was a most puzzling result, since the cells exhibit strong positive phototaxis in this region, thus indicating that the photoreceptor is sensitive here. One possible explanation for the absence of the negative photophobic response is that, at the shorter wavelengths, the shading pigments are no longer transparent to the polarized light used. If this were true, then there had to exist another pigment system which fulfilled a shading function in the near ultraviolet. This system could not be located in the stigma, since according to Batra and Tollin (1964) a hexane extract of the stigma pigments does not show significant absorption below 400 nm. As it turned out, the negative response reappeared below 400 nm upon rotation of the plane of the polarized light by 90°. At present, the best explanation for this is that a separate short wavelength shading system does exist, and that its pigment molecules are aligned with their molecular transition moments perpendicular to the long axes of the cells. There is the alternative possibility that there are two oriented pigment systems operative in the photoreceptor rather than in the shading systems, but in that case one would have to abolish the by now quite firmly established "shaded photoreceptor" hypothesis which demands that the induction of the negative photophobic response by polarized light is due to loss of the shading function of the stigma pigments.

If one combines the long- and short-wavelength action spectra, the resulting curve very closely resembles the absorption spectra one obtains from flavins in nonpolar solvents (Kotaki et al., 1967). It is a reasonable conclusion that the photoreceptor pigment might well be a flavin derivative which is rigidly held in place in a hydrophobic environment. As shown in Figure 3, the composite action spectrum is indeed very similar to the absorption spectrum of riboflavin in 95 percent ethanol at 170 K, with a slight red shift in the long wavelength region.

Further indication that the photoreceptor pigment might be a flavin is provided by the work of Tollin and Robinson (1969) on photosuppression of phototaxis. Their action spectra, which can be interpreted as indicating photobleaching, resembled the absorption spectrum of the flavoprotein L-amino acid oxidase. As Song (1968) has pointed out, a comparison of the photochemical properties of the flavins with those of the carotenoids reveals that the former are more likely photoreceptor molecules than the latter, particularly if one considers that photoreception may be mediated by excited electronic states of the pigment molecule.

Iodide ion is known to quench the triplet excited state of flavins (Weber, 1950), while not affecting carotenoids. When we added KI at concentrations from 10^{-3} to 10^{-1}M to Euglena cultures before testing their phototactic response in the phototaxigraph, we found strong specific inhibition of positive phototaxis at concentrations to below 10^{-2}M (Diehn 1970 b). It appears that we can now state with some confidence that the photoreceptor pigment might be a flavin derivative.

I should now like to say a few words about the quantum efficiency of the phototactic receptor/effector system in Euglena. In recent experiments, we found the threshold for positive phototaxis at 475 nm to occur at an actinic beam intensity of 3.3 erg/cm^2sec. Having determined that the intensity of light scattered into the cuvette from the actinic zone was 0.9 percent of the incident intensity, and taking the photoreceptor area (from electron micrographs, Leedale, 1967) as $3 \times 10^{-9} cm^2$, one can calculate that without the stigma, 7 photons would impinge upon the photoreceptor in 0.3 sec. The stigma, which normally screens for 0.3 sec during each rotation, transmits about 40 percent at 475 nm (Strother and Wolken, 1960). Three photons would therefore impinge upon the photoreceptor during screening by the stigma. Hence, a difference in absorption of 4 photons results in a perceptible reaction. We are dealing with a very efficient system indeed!

Let me finally indicate what is apparently the next problem which demands an experimental solution. This is the question of how the phototactic stimulus is translated into flagellar motion. It has been suggested by Jahn and Bovee (1968) that the flagellum may have piezoelectric properties. If this were so, then an electrical impulse applied to the end of the flagellum will cause bending at that point, and the bend will be self-propagating because of the voltage generated when the elastic flagellum straightens. How can the initial potential be generated? Jahn (1963) has suggested that a photopigment, as the result of the absorption of light energy, might conduct electrons across a poised oxidation/reduction system. On the other hand, the primary photoact might simply cause abolition or reversal of a membrane potential that is ordinarily maintained by an ion gradient. If a product of the intramolecular or intermolecular photochemistry of riboflavin interferes with the K^+ or Na^+ pumps, then a depolarization or hyperpolarization wave might travel along the membrane that encloses both the flagellum and the paraflagellar swelling, in a fashion entirely analogous to the situation in the avoidance response of Paramecium (Naitoh and Eckert, 1969). At present, I am told, inserting a microelectrode into the base of the flagellum of Euglena is just beyond the state of the art. Nevertheless, this is exactly the challenge to our electrophysiologists with which I wish to conclude this presentation.

ACKNOWLEDGEMENT

Some of the work described herein was supported by Grants No. GB-7450 and GB-18701 from the National Science Foundation.

REFERENCES

Batra, P. P., and Tollin, G. (1967). Biochim. Biophys. Acta 79, 371.

Bound, K. E., and Tollin, G. (1967). Nature 216, 1042.

Bünning, E., and Schneiderhöhn, G. (1956). Arch. Mikrobiol. 24, 80.

Diehn, B. (1969 a). "Conference on Phototaxis and Photokinesis in Flagellated Cells", University of California, Santa Barbara, August 21-22, 1969.

Diehn, B. (1969 b). Exp. Cell Res. 56, 375.

Diehn, B. (1969 c). Biochim. Biophys. Acta 177, 136.

Diehn, B. (1970 a). Photochem. Photobiol. 11, 407.

Diehn, B. (1970 b). Unpublished observations.

Engelmann, T. W. (1882). Pflugers Arch. Ges. Physiol. 29, 387.

Feinleib, M. E. H., and Curry, G. M. (1967). Physiol. Plantarum 20, 1083.

Gössel, I. (1957). Arch. Mikrobiol. 27, 288.

Jahn, T. L. (1963). Vision Res. 3, 25.

Jahn, T. L., and Bovee, E. C. (1968). In D. Buetow (Ed.). The Biology of Euglena, Vol. I, Academic Press, N. Y., Chapt. 3.

Kotaki, A., Naoi M., Okuda, J., and Yagi, K. (1967). J. Biochem. 61, 136.

Leedale, G. F. (1967). Euglenoid Flagellates. Prentice-Hall, Englewood Cliffs, New Jersey.

Mast, S. O. (1911). Light and the Behavior of Organisms. Wiley, New York.

Naitoh, Y., and Eckert, R. (1969). Science 164, 963.

Song, P. S. (1968). Abstract Gf-2, 5th International Congress on Photobiology, Hanover, N. H., August, 1968.

Strother, G. K., and Wolken, J. J. (1960). Nature 188, 601.

Tollin, G., and Robinson, M. I. (1969). Photochem. Photobiol. 9, 411.

Weber, G. (1950). Biochem. J. 47, 114.

PHOTOTAXIS IN EUGLENA 11: BIOCHEMICAL ASPECTS

G. Tollin

The University of Arizona,
Department of Chemistry,
Tucson,
Arizona 85721, U.S.A.

1. INTRODUCTION

Phototaxis can be defined as a translational response of a freely moving organism to a light stimulus. In the alga Euglena, a sensory perception system is involved which is an easily recognized structure consisting of an eyespot (or stigma) and the paraflagellar swelling located at the base of the flagellum (Tollin, 1969). These organelles, functioning as a photosensitive device, allow the cell to become oriented with respect to the direction of a light source and to maintain its swimming motion in that direction. The physical mechanism by which this is accomplished is the subject of another paper to be presented at this symposium (Diehn, 1970 a) and thus will not be considered further here.

At the present stage of the investigation of phototaxis, there are two well-defined biochemical questions which can be asked and to which at least partial answers can be given. These are:

(1) What is the energy source which permits the organism to become oriented in the light beam?

(2) What is the identity of the pigment(s) responsible for photosensory perception? (The paper by Diehn also describes experiments dealing with this question.)

The remainder of this paper will be devoted to reviewing the present state of knowledge concerning these aspects of the phototactic process in Euglena.

*Supported in part by the U.S.Atomic Energy Commission, Contract No. AT(11-1)908.

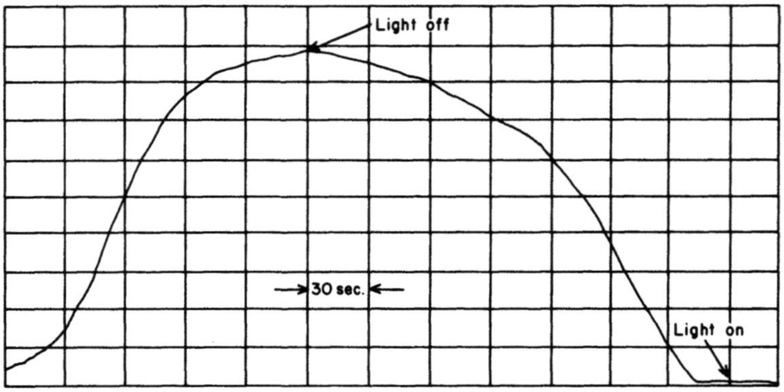

Figure 1. Typical phototactic accumulation curve for Euglena. Ordinate is proportional to number of cells.

2. Energy Source for Phototactic Orientation

There are three obvious sources from which Euglena could derive the energy required for achieving and maintaining an orientation which results in directed motion. These are: the light stimulus itself (this would imply an energy conversion system, perhaps analogous to photosynthesis), oxidative metabolism (locomotion, i.e., flagellar beating, derives its energy from this process), and photosynthesis (this must be the ultimate supply under autotrophic growth, of course, but what is meant here is a direct coupling of the phototactic and photosynthetic systems).

The first of these possibilities, i.e., energy conversion involving the light stimulus, is the easiest to test. This has been done (Diehn and Tollin, 1966 a) by determining the light intensity dependence of the phototactic response. Phototaxis was measured with a device, which we have called a phototaxigraph, which uses photoelectric recording to determine the rate of accumulation of cells in a small region of a cuvette in response to a stimulating light beam (Lindes et al., 1965). A typical response curve is shown in Figure 1. Phototactic rates are calculated from the maximum slope of the curve. The distance from the baseline to the top of the curve is a measure of the extent of accumulation. Figure 2 shows the results of a determination of the light intensity dependence of the rate and extent of phototaxis in Euglena. If the energy for the response is derived from the stimulating light, one would expect to obtain linear relationships at low intensities which saturate at some higher intensity, similar to what is observed for the photosynthetic process. However, in the case of phototaxis, a logarithmic dependency is found. We have also done experiments using white light as the stimulus and have observed that the logarithmic relationship holds over a considerable range of intensities (up to 140 ergs/cm^{2}sec., which was the highest intensity obtainable with our apparatus). Thus, the phototactic response in Euglena obeys the Weber–Fechner law, indicating that the stimulating light functions as a trigger which releases previously stored metabolic energy.

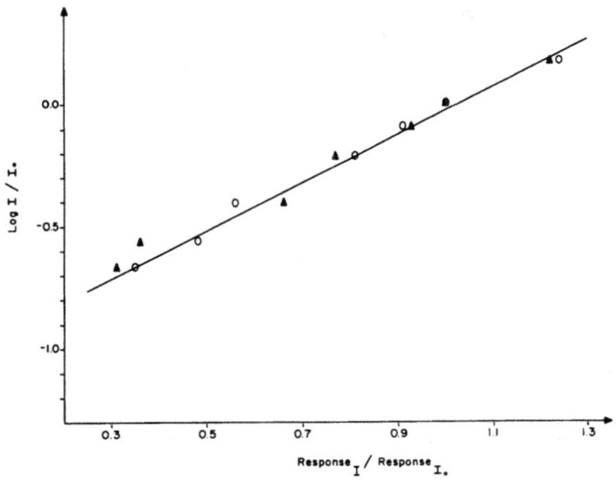

Figure 2. Light intensity dependence of rate and extent of phototaxis in Euglena. λ = 500 nm. I_0 = 0.5 erg/cm^{2}sec.

▲ extent of accumulation.
O rate.

The first indication that the photosynthetic apparatus might be involved in generating the energy required for phototaxis was obtained from experiments in which Euglena cultures were incubated in the dark and their phototactic ability measured (Diehn and Tollin, 1966 a). Normally, the cultures were exposed to a light–dark cycle and under these conditions phototaxis was maintained over long periods of time (several weeks). However, in the dark, the phototactic response of the culture persisted for about 24 hours and then decayed, being almost completely gone in 72 hours. This approximates the time course for chloroplast destruction found by Schiff et al. (1965) in Euglena. Also of significance is the fact that the dark incubation did not affect the motility of the culture (in these experiments, as well as in all of the following studies, the cultures were grown heterotrophically).

An additional experiment provided still further evidence for an interaction between phototaxis and photosynthesis (Diehn and Tollin, 1966 a). A Euglena culture was grown completely in the dark following the initial inoculation (from a normally grown culture). As expected, no chlorophyll formation or chloroplast development occurred (Wolken, 1961). Microscopic examination indicated normal eyespot pigmentation, however. The culture displayed no phototactic response, although again motility was apparently normal. When the organisms were subsequently placed in the light, it was found that chlorophyll formation and return of phototactic ability occurred simultaneously (Figure 3).

A similar effect was observed using a furadantin-bleached Euglena culture which had neither chloroplast nor eyespot pigmentation (Diehn and Tollin,

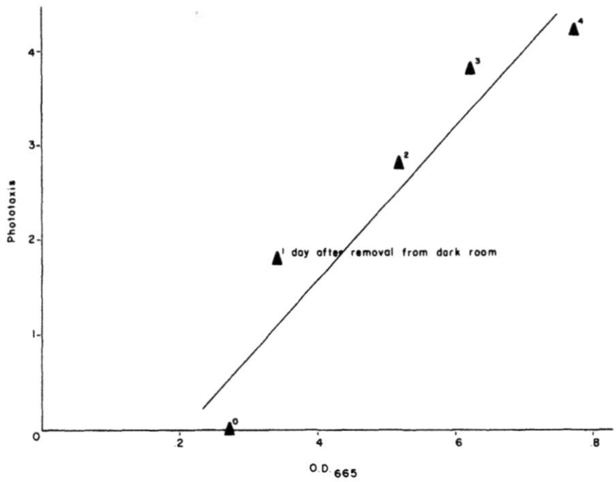

Figure 3. Relation between phototaxis and chlorophyll development in dark-grown Euglena after light incubation.

1966 b). These organisms, which were fully motile, did not respond phototactically to light stimulation.*

A more direct approach to this problem was pursued through the use of metabolic inhibitors (Diehn and Tollin, 1967). When substances such as cyanide (5×10^{-4}M), azide (10^{-8}M), and rotenone (5×10^{-7}M), which are known inhibitors of respiratory electron transport, were added to Euglena cultures, both motility and phototaxis were reduced to 50 percent of the control in about 30 minutes. Similar results were obtained with uncouplers of oxidative phosphorylation such as 2,4-dinitrophenol (5×10^{-5}M) and dichlorophenol indophenol (DCPIP, 10^{-5}M). This latter substance was metabolized by the organisms within 24 hours, as evidenced by the disappearance of the blue color, and both motility and phototaxis were fully restored. These results indicate that motility is required for phototactic orientation, although it is not a sufficient property as shown by the experiments with achlorophyllous cultures cited above.

3-(3,4-Dichlorophenyl)-1,1-dimethylurea (DCMU) is well known as a specific inhibitor of photosynthetic electron transport (Vernon and Avron, 1965). At concentration levels as low as 10^{-7}M, it strongly inhibits phototaxis without any apparent effect on cell motility. The time course of the effect of DCMU is quite interesting (Figure 4). Initially, a slight stimulation of the phototactic response is observed.† This is followed by inhibition and recovery. The rate at which the inhibitory effect is manifested depends on the DCMU concentration. The recovery effect is not due to depletion of DCMU by metabolic processes, because it occurs even when DCMU-saturated culture is left in contact

*More precisely, the culture did not respond positively (i.e., accumulate in the light-stimulated region). The organisms did, however, show negative phototaxis (a light-induced depletion of cells within the stimulated zone).
†This is somewhat variable. The reasons for this are not clear.

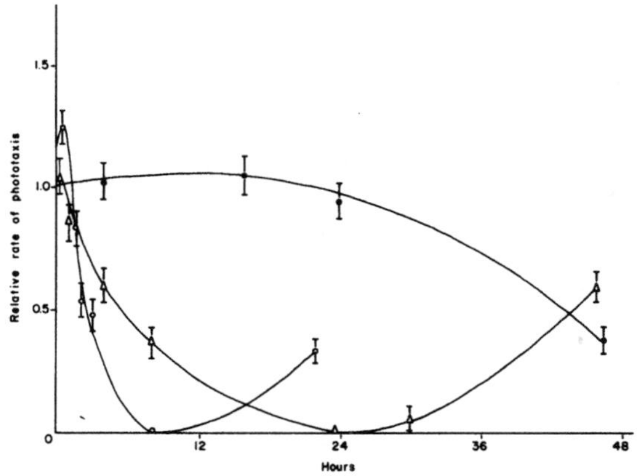

Figure 4. Effect of DCMU and darkness on phototactic rates in Euglena.

● darkness.
△ 10^{-7}M DCMU.
○ 5 × 10^{-7}M DCMU.

with crystalline material. It is also not due to the emergence of a DCMU-resistant strain, inasmuch as recovery can occur in much less than one generation time and, more importantly, DCMU prevents further growth of the culture. The most likely explanation of the recovery effect is that the organisms are somehow able to by-pass the DCMU-blocked step. Another of the selective inhibitors of photosynthesis, methyl octanoate (10^{-4} M) (Pedersen et al., 1960), gave results which were quite similar to those obtained with DCMU (Figure 5).

The fact that phototactic inhibition by DCMU occurs in the absence of any appreciable effect on motility provides suggestive evidence for the functioning of the photosynthetic system* in supplying energy for phototaxis. As a further test of this concept, we utilized the fact that the addition of external electron donors, such as reduced DCPIP, can restore photophosphorylation activity to DCMU-inhibited photosynthetic systems (Jagendorf and Margulies, 1966). When ascorbate (10^{-4} M) and DCPIP (10^{-5} M) or ferrocyanide (10^{-3} M) were added to Euglena cultures which were also treated with DCMU or methyl octanoate, no inhibition of phototaxis resulted (Figure 5).

It is significant that phototactic ability is also senstive to uncoupling of photophosphorylation. The substance carbonyl cyanide p-trifluoromethoxyphenylhydrazone (CCP) (Bamberger et al., 1963), at a concentration of 10^{-6} M, strongly suppresses Euglena phototaxis (Figure 6). This points directly to the involvement of photosynthetically generated high-energy compounds in providing energy for phototactic orientation.

*It is also possible, of course, that the phototactic energy source is actually not the photosynthetic apparatus but a separate system having the same inhibition spectrum as photosynthesis. However, Diehn (1970 b) has observed that a Euglena mutant impaired in photosystem II is only weakly phototactic.

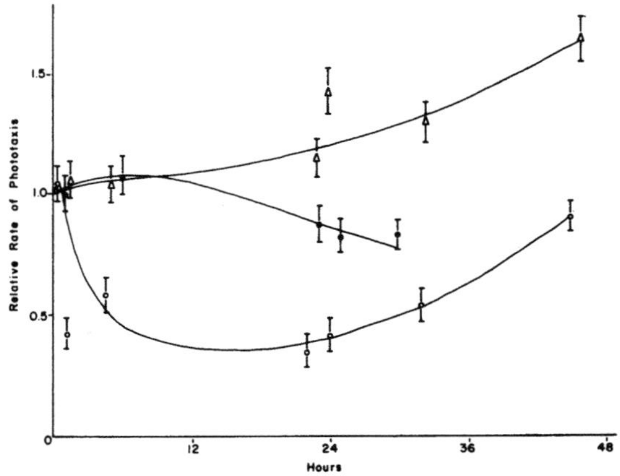

Figure 5. Effect of methyl octanoate on phototactic rates in Euglena.

○ 10^{-4}M methyl octanoate.
△ 10^{-4}M methyl octanoate plus 10^{-5}M DCPIP and 10^{-4}M sodium ascorbate.
● 10^{-4}M methyl octanoate plus 10^{-3}M ferrocyanide.

The next stage in our investigation of this aspect of the problem was an attempt to directly evaluate the suggested correlation between photosynthetic ATP production and phototaxis by simultaneously measuring both responses in a single culture (Tollin and Robinson, 1970). In order to do this, we developed a procedure for determining the ATP content of whole Euglena cells using the firefly bioluminescence assay (Strehler, 1953). The experimental protocol was as follows. A 1 ml. aliquot of Euglena suspension was removed from the culture into a 2.5 ml. hypodermic syringe. This was illuminated with red light for a given length of time and then quickly injected into a small volume (0.5 ml.) of boiling distilled water (it is important to do this quickly because of the apparent high ATPase activity present in Euglena), boiled for 1 min., and stored in an ice bath until the ATP assay was performed. An unilluminated sample was used as a control.

The effect of increasing illumination time on the ATP content of a normal Euglena culture is shown in Figure 7. Transients, similar to those observed with O_2 evolution and chlorophyll fluorescence (French, 1963; Kautsky and Hirsch, 1931), are found to occur during the first minute of illumination. After 5 min., the ATP level in the illuminated sample is invariably greater than in the dark control.

The effect of DCMU addition on phototaxis and photophosphorylation, measured on aliquots of the same culture, is shown in Figure 8. The kinetics of inhibition of the two responses are quite similar.

We thought it might be of interest to ascertain whether the delay in the response to DCMU (~2 hours) is due to the time required for the inhibitor to

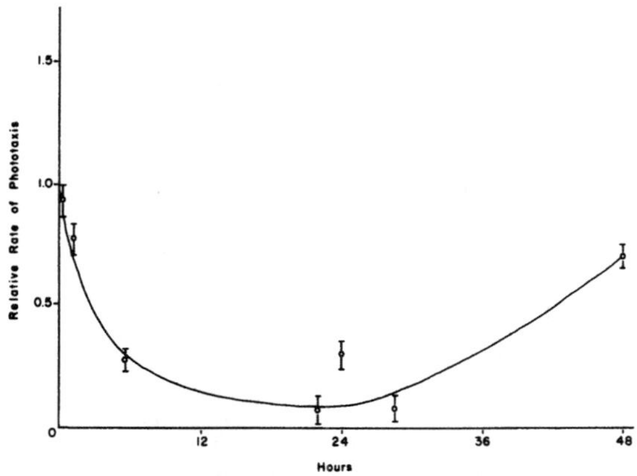

Figure 6. Effect of CCP on phototactic rates in Euglena.

enter the cell (or chloroplasts). Thus, we measured O_2 evolution rates and their response to DCMU addition. Figure 9 shows the results of an experiment in which DCMU was quickly injected into a Euglena culture whose O_2 evolution was being monitored with an oxygen electrode. The initial downward slope of the curve respresents dark respiratory O_2 uptake. As soon as the light is turned on, O_2 is evolved. Upon DCMU addition (arrow), inhibition of O_2 production occurs within 30 seconds. These results, considered in terms of the data shown in Figure 8, seem to indicate the presence of an endogenous pool of electron donors in Euglena, which allows photophosphorylation to proceed in the presence of a photosystem II inhibitor such as DCMU until the pool is depleted.

A similar experiment to that of Figure 8, using CCP as the inhibiting substance, is shown in Figure 10. Again, the kinetics of inhibition of ATP formation and phototaxis are similar, although the time course is different from that observed with DCMU. Particularly interesting is the fact that the CCP inhibition is manifested significantly more quickly than is the case with DCMU. This would be consistent with the suggestion of an electron donor pool, inasmuch as an uncoupling of phosphorylation caused by CCP would not be expected to allow such a pool to manifest itself as light-produced ATP.

Another way to test the existence of a relationship between ATP levels in Euglena and phototaxis would be to turn off the photosynthetic process, not with inhibitors, but with darkness. As was mentioned above, phototactic ability is maintained for about 24 hours under these conditions (Figure 4). In Table 1, the results of ATP determinations during the dark incubation are shown. Two points of interest emerge from these data. First, placing the organisms in darkness during the middle of a normal light period inhibits growth (as measured by turbidity). Second, ATP levels per cell in the dark culture actually increase over a 24 hour period (after 2-3 days, ATP levels decrease to quite low values). These results, along with the data shown in Figure 4, suggest the presence of a control system which acts to maintain phototactic energy reserves (and ATP levels) during an extended period of little or no photosynthetic activity, perhaps at the expense of cell growth and division.

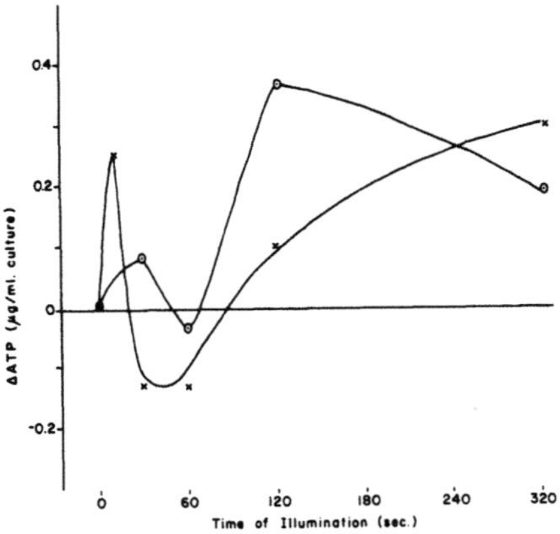

Figure 7. Effect of time of illumination with red light on ATP levels in Euglena. Ordinate represents difference in ATP between illuminated and un-illuminated aliquots. Two separate experiments are shown.

3. Identity of Pigments Involved in Photosensory Perception

As was pointed out above, one of the organelles implicated in phototactic light perception in Euglena is the eyespot or stigma. This structure consists of a cup-shaped cluster of bright orange-red globules located near the paraflagellar swelling, although physically separate from it. Most workers have assumed (Wolken, 1961) that the pigmentation was due to carotenoids, based partly on the appearance of the eyespot and partly on the action spectrum for the phototactic response.

We have taken a more direct approach to this question (Batra and Tollin, 1964) by isolating sufficient quantities of eyespot granules, using centrifugation techniques, to permit pigment extraction and identification. The absorption spectrum of a suspension of isolated eyespots is shown in Figure 11, along the spectrum of a hexane extract. The two spectra are in reasonable agreement (the eyespot spectrum is broadened and red-shifted, probably due to pigment –pigment and/or pigment–protein interactions) and strongly suggests the presence of carotenoids. This was confirmed by chromatographic analysis of the hexane extract. The pigment composition found is given in Table 2. This distribution of carotenoids is quite different from that present in whole cell extracts (Krinsky and Goldsmith, 1960). No evidence was obtained for significant quantities of any other pigment in the eyespot preparation. It is of interest to note that studies of phototaxis using polarized light (Bound and Tollin, 1967) have provided evidence for orientation of the carotenoid molecules within the eyespot. This has proven useful in investigating certain aspects of pigment involvement in phototaxis, as will be discussed by Diehn (1970 a) in this symposium.

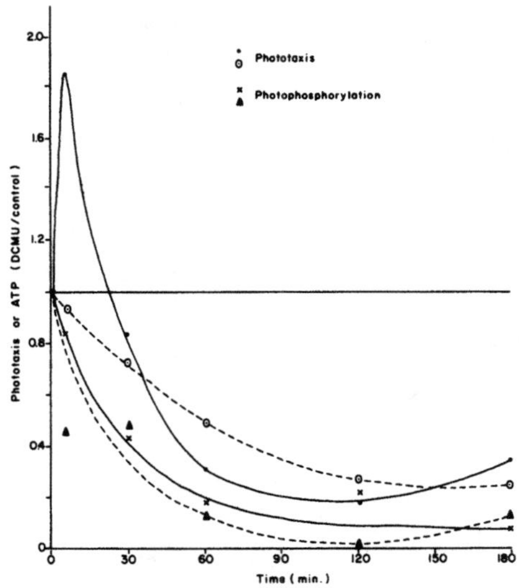

Figure 8. Effect of DCMU (2×10^{-6}M) on phototaxis and photophosphorylation in Euglena. Ordinate represents ratio of responses of DCMU-treated culture to control culture. The results of two separate experiments are shown; comparisons should be made between solid curves and between dashed curves.

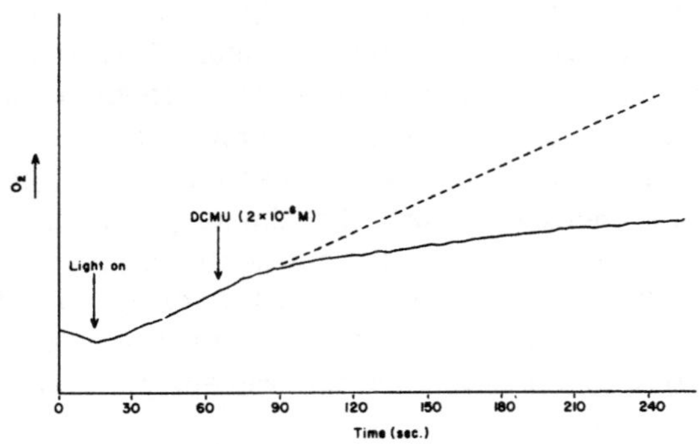

Figure 9. Effect of DCMU addition on photosynthetic oxygen evolution in Euglena.

The eyespot is believed to function merely as a light filter or shading device for the true photoreceptor, which is located within the paraflagellar swelling (Tollin, 1969). Thus, the primary phototactic light process does not occur within the eyespot and is not mediated by the eyespot carotenoids. This leaves open the question of the actual identity of the photoreceptor pigment. A phenomenon which we discovered while looking for photocontrol effects has given some insight into this problem (Tollin and Robinson, 1969). Pohl (1948), Bruce and Pittendrigh (1956), and ourselves (Diehn and Tollin, (1966 a) have shown that omission of a single dark cycle causes a markedly reduced level

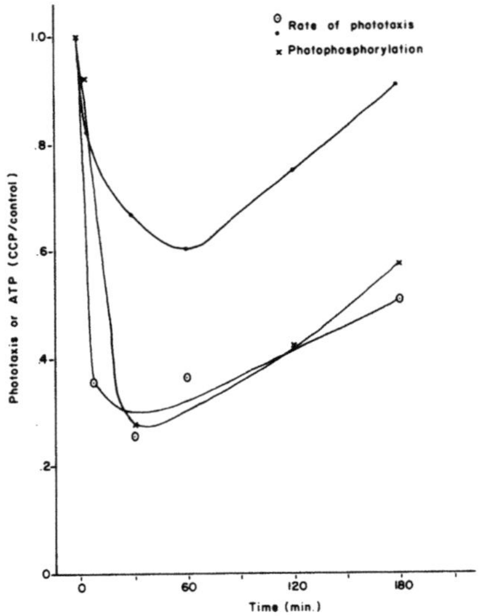

Figure 10. Effect of CCP (5×10^{-6}M) on phototaxis and photophosphorylation in Euglena. Ordinate represents ratio of responses of CCP-treated culture to control culture. The results of two separate phototaxis measurements are shown.

of phototactic activity in Euglena grown on a light–dark cycle. Subsequent exposure to darkness restores the response (Figure 12). If one takes a normally grown culture at any time during the light cycle and irradiates it with high intensity light of wavelength less than 650 nm, a marked suppression of phototaxis occurs (Figure 13). Microscopic examination of the culture immediately after such a treatment shows that the suppression is not due to a loss of motility. As in the continuous light experiment, placing an irradiated culture in the dark causes a return of phototactic ability. The time course of this effect is shown in Figure 14. The dark return of activity is not susceptible to acceleration by irradiation at any wavelength in the visible or near infra-red region.

A measurement of the light intensity dependence of the suppression phenomenon (Figure 15) shows that it is saturable, but that quite high intensities are required.

The action spectrum for photosuppression is shown in Figure 16, along with the absorption spectrum of a typical flavoprotein, L-amino acid oxidase. The similarities are striking, suggesting that perhaps a flavin chromophore is involved.

Experiments in which respiratory O_2 uptake was monitored during blue light irradiation, or in which irradiation was carried out under N_2, suggest that the respiratory system is probably not involved in photosuppression or in dark recovery. Furthermore, the fact that inhibition or cessation of photosynthesis requires periods of 30 minutes to several hours to become manifested

TABLE 1. Effect of Darkness on ATP Levels in Euglena

	Normal		Dark	
Time (hr.)	A_{800} nm	ATP (μg/ml)	A_{800} nm	ATP (μg/ml)
0	0.26	0.35	0.26	0.30
2	0.27	0.27	0.27	0.36
4	0.33	0.30	0.28	0.40
6	0.37	0.30	0.28	0.38
24	0.43	0.53	0.30	0.54
26	0.45	0.75	0.30	0.55
28	0.50	0.81	0.30	0.61
30	0.53	0.82	0.30	0.64

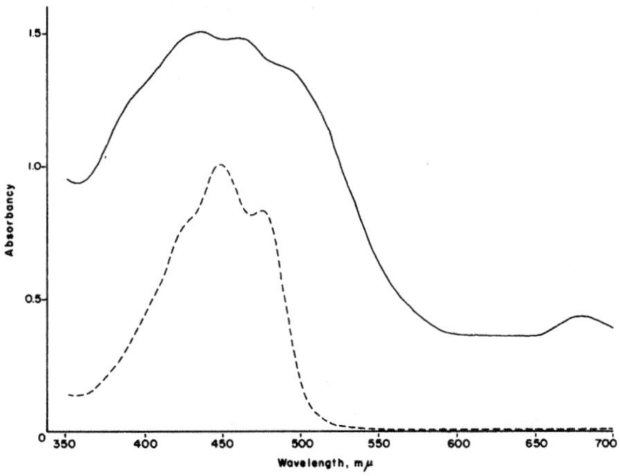

Figure 11. Spectral properties of Euglena eyespots.

—— suspension of isolated eyespot granules (the small peak at 675 nm is due to a slight chloroplast contamination).
- - - hexane extract.

in a suppression of phototaxis (see above), whereas blue light irradiation is effective in less than one minute after as little as 10 seconds of light, suggests that the photosynthetic system is also not mediating the photosuppression effect.

These phenomena caused by bright light irradiation are reminiscent of the bleaching and dark regeneration of visual pigment in higher organisms (Rushton, 1964). Thus, it is possible that we are observing the effect of photobleaching of the phototactic receptor pigment. If this is so, the implication is that this pigment is a riboflavin derivative. It is of interest that flavins can be reversibly photobleached in solution (Green and Tollin, 1968). The paper by Diehn in this symposium discusses other types of evidence supporting the role of flavin in phototactic light detection.

It is interesting to speculate about a possible physiological function for photosuppression as a control mechanism which reduces phototactic activity

TABLE 2. Absorption Maxima and Relative Amounts of the Carotenoids Isolated from Eyespot Granules

The pigments are listed in the order in which they were eluted from the column.

Fraction	% (V/V) acetone in petroleum ether required to elute from column	Relative amount %	λ_{max} (mμ) Petroleum ether	Ethanol	Chloroform
1. β-carotene	0	8	475, 447, 423	-	490-1, 462, 437
2. Cryptoxanthin	1.5	32	476, 448, 424	482, 452, 426	491-2, 461, 436
3. Unknown	4-5	9*(?)	475(?), 453, 430	482-4(?), 458, 432, 406(?)	490, 465, 439
4. Lutein	14-15	51	473, 446, 424	475, 447, 425	485-6, 457, 433

*This figure is based on the assumption that the extinction coefficient of this pigment is 1.4×10^5, which represents a median value for carotenoid pigments.

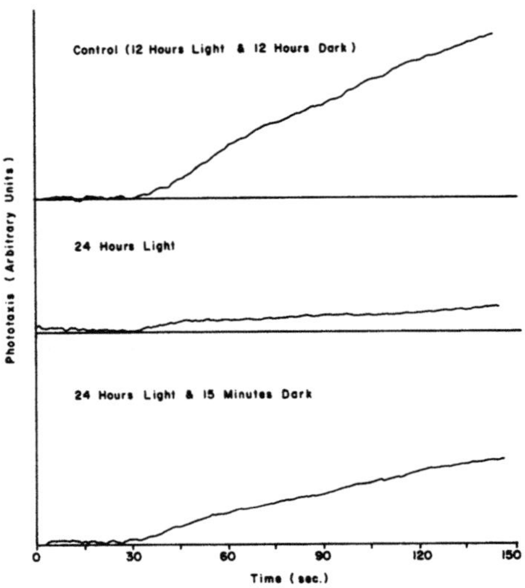

Figure 12. Phototactic responses of Euglena under various conditions of preillumination.

when the organisms have accumulated in a region of high light intensity. This would serve to decrease the likelihood that they would respond to stray light signals coming from other directions.

4. Conclusions

The experiments outlined in Section 2 of this paper strongly suggest that the photosynthetic phosphorylation system supplies the energy required by Euglena for phototactic orientation. This raises an interesting problem, however, inasmuch as the organelles which mediate these two phenomena (chloroplast and eyespot/paraflagellar swelling) are physically separate in this organism. Thus, it is necessary to postulate a transport system which carries

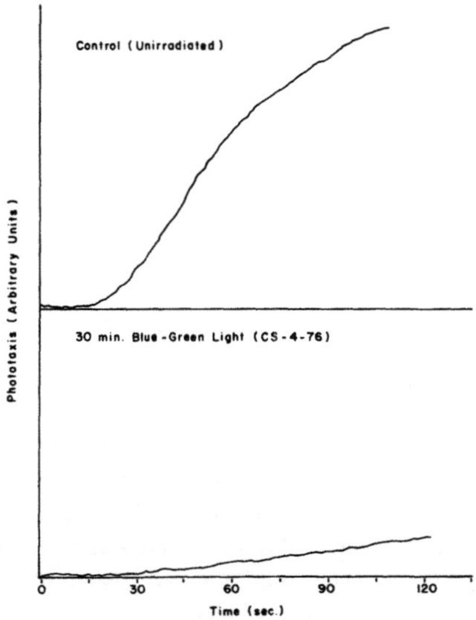

Figure 13. Photoactic response of Euglena before and after exposure to 30 min. of blue light (corning filter CS 4-76).

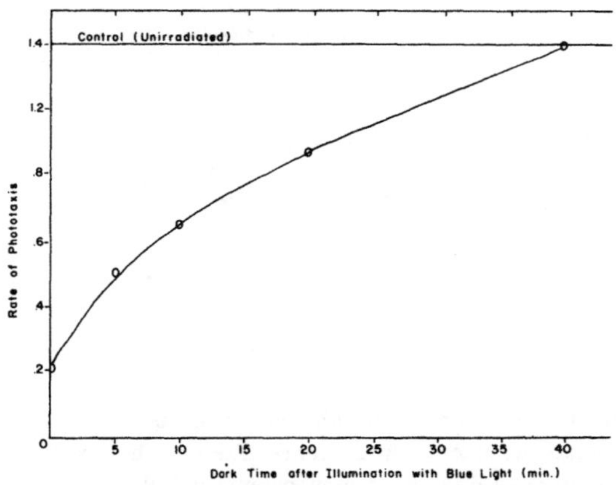

Figure 14. Dark recovery of phototaxis in Euglena after a 15 min. irradiation with blue light (corning filter CS 4-76).

ATP (or some other high-energy compound derived from the photophosphorylation system) from the chloroplast lamellae to some specific site in the flagellar apparatus. The release and/or utilization of this energy pool must then be controlled by the tactic photoreceptor. It is interesting to note that the euglenoid flagellates are the only algae in which the eyespot is external to the chloroplast. This would imply that, if the basic mechanisms of phototactic orientation are the same, a direct photocontrol of photosynthetic phosphorylation may be occurring in non-euglenoid species. However, it would still be necessary to have a transport system to carry high-energy materials from the chloroplast to the locomotive organelle.

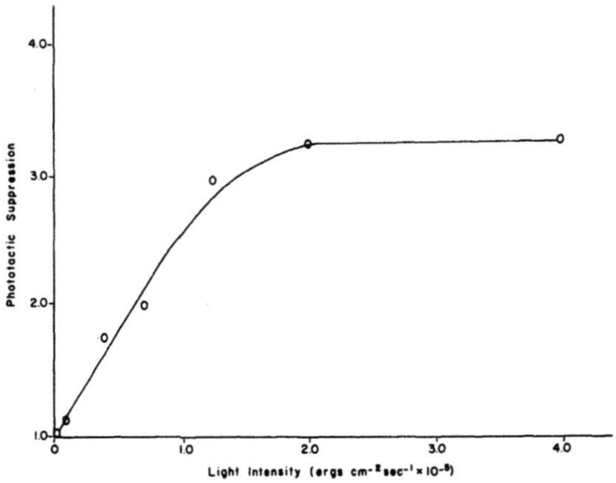

Figure 15. Light intensity dependence of photosuppression of phototaxis in *Euglena*. Ordinate represents ratio of maximum slope of accumulation curve prior to irradiation to that subsequent to irradiation.

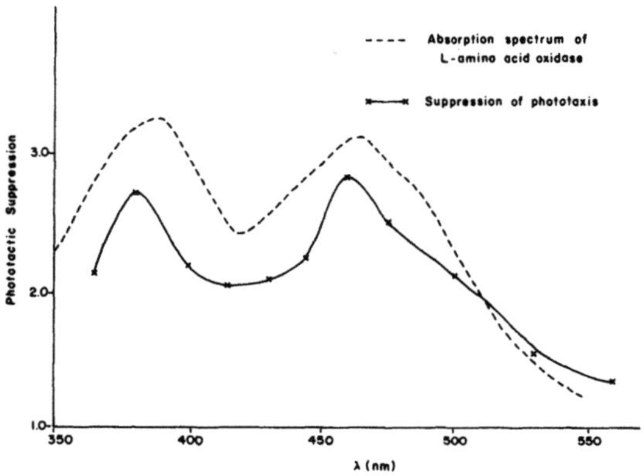

Figure 16. Action spectrum for photosuppression of phototaxis in *Euglena*. Interference filters (10 nm band-width) were used to obtain monochromatic light. Data are corrected for light intensity and are expressed on a quantum basis. Ordinate same as in Figure 15.

One of the fundamental questions still remaining to be answered about phototaxis is the nature of the linkage between light absorption and the change in flagellar motion which leads to a reorientation of the swimming pattern of the organism. The simplest hypothesis might be that a change in light intensity activates a "switch" which controls the flow of photosynthetically derived ATP to the flagellum. It seems reasonable to suppose that a cell which is moving in a straight line path as a result of the rhythmic beating of its flagellum can be made to change its direction by providing the flagellum with a "pulse" of ATP. This would cause an interruption of the normal motion of this organelle and hence a deviation in swimming direction.

An alternative to this type of mechanism could be one in which a membrane depolarization occurs in the paraflagellar swelling as a result of a change in photon flux. If this were propagated along the flagellum (perhaps as an alteration of conformation), a change in its beating pattern might be a consequence of the re-establishment of the initial state of polarization (and/or conformation).

Such ideas are, of course, highly speculative. They do, however, provide a physicochemical basis for the primary events in Euglena phototaxis which can perhaps be tested experimentally.

REFERENCES

Bamberger, E. S., Black, C.C., Fewson, C.A., and Gibbs, M. (1963). Plant Physiol. 38, 483.
Batra, P. P. and Tollin, G. (1964). Biochim. Biophys. Acta 79, 371.
Bound, K. E. and Tollin, G. (1967). Nature 216, 1042.
Bruce, V. G. and Pittendrigh, C. S. (1956). Proc. Nat. Acad. Sci., U.S. 42, 676.
Diehn, B. and Tollin, G. (1966 a). Photochem. Photobiol. 5, 523.
Diehn, B. and Tollin, G. (1966 b). Photochem. Photobiol. 5, 839.
Diehn, B. and Tollin, G. (1967). Arch. Biochem. Biophys. 121, 169.
Diehn, B. (1970 a). This Symposium.
Diehn, B. (1970 b). Personal communication.
French, C. S. (1963). In "Photosynthetic Mechanisms of Green Plants", p. 335, National Academy of Science, National Research Council, Washington, D.C.
Green, M. and Tollin, G. (1968). Photochem. Photobiol. 7, 129.
Jagendorf, A. T. and Margulies, M. (1966). Arch. Biochem. Biophys. 90, 184.
Kautsky, H. and Hirsch, A. (1931). Naturwiss. 19, 964.
Krinsky, N. I. and Goldsmith, T. H. (1960). Arch. Biochem. Biophys. 91, 271.
Lindes, D., Diehn, B., and Tollin, G. (1965). Rev. Sci. Instr. 36, 1721.
Pedersen, T. A., Kirk, M., and Bassham, J. A. (1966). Biochim. Biophys. Acta 112, 189.
Pohl, R. (1948). Z. Naturf. 3b, 376.
Rushton, W. A. H. (1964). In "Photophysiology", vol. II, p. 130, A. C. Giese, ed., Academic Press N. Y.
Schiff, J. A., Ben-Shaul, Y., and Epstein, H. T. (1965). In "Recent Progress in Photobiology", p. 147, E. J. Bowen, ed., Blackwell, Oxford.
Strehler, B. L. (1953). Arch. Biochem. Biophys. 43, 67.
Tollin, G. (1969). In "Current Topics in Bioenergetics", vol. 3, p. 417, D. R. Sanadi, ed., Academic Press, New York.
Tollin, G. and Robinson, M. I. (1969). Photochem. Photobiol. 9, 411.
Tollin, G. and Robinson, M. I. (1970). J. Bioenergetics, 1, 139.
Vernon, L. P. and Avron, M. (1965). Ann. Rev. Biochem. 34, 269.
Wolken, J. J. (1961). "Euglena", Rutgers Univ. Press, New Brunswick, N. J.

STUDIES IN MICROORGANISMAL BEHAVIOR BY COMPUTERIZED TELEVISION

D. Davenport
University of California,
Department of Zoology,
Santa Barbara,
California 93106, U.S.A.

Up to the present time behavior of motile microorganisms has been investigated in general by two methods. (1) "The mass movement" method and (2) the "individual cell" method. Quantitative "mass movement" techniques involve the principle of the measurement of optical density of cell suspensions (vide Pohl, 1948; Bruce and Pittendrigh, 1956; Feinleib and Curry,1967, etc.) As is well known, this method records changes in optical density resulting from the movement of cells into or out of the point being "watched". This is a good method to make measurements of the responses of populations of cells to changes in the environment (for example, studies of vertical or horizontal migration in gradients.) But the method is obviously not well suited to investigate the movement of the individual cell or to find out how such movements bring about the accumulation or dispersal that may be observed. A further weakness in the system results from the fact that mass movement takes time and this means that the observer may be monitoring movements of cells which are undergoing a change in physiological state when, indeed, he should be investigating them as nearly as possible in the steady state.

Direct observations of the movements of an individual cell have, of course, been made for more than a century by the use of the light microscope, with events recorded by standard photomicrographic techniques (Mast, 1911; Gebauer, 1930, etc.) Modifications of this method have involved the addition of electronic circuitry; among the most interesting has been the technique of Feinleib and Curry (1967) in their work on phototaxis in Chlamydomonas. For some years my own group conducted somewhat parallel studies with dinoflagellates, using what was essentially a flying-spot system with reduced optical elements (Hand, Collard, and Davenport, 1965). Although valuable advances were and are still being made with such systems on linear velocity, rate of change of direction, cell aggregation, etc. they do not allow discernment of the sequence of specific behavioral events which constitute the response of an individual cell to a particular stimulus. To date no investigator

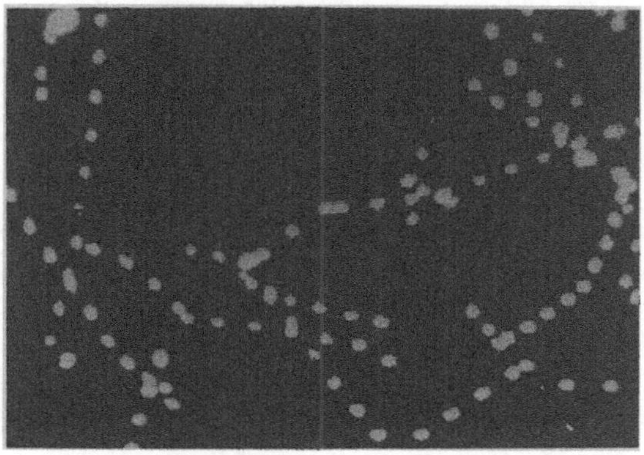

Figure 1. Bagwatcher-processed tracks of the dinoflagellate Gyrodinium. Each blip indicates the position of a cell at a given point in time. Optical magnification 40×. Scan rate 2/sec.

has succeeded in combining these in such a way as to allow him to observe and at the same time quantify mass movements, changes in linear velocity or rate of change of direction and at the same time with minor modifications of magnification etc. to record in detail what the individual cell does when it responds to a stimulus. Our system allows us to do all these things while allowing experimentation to conform to a basic criterion for any behavioral study, i.e. that controls be carried out under relatively unrestricted conditions as close to those encountered by the organism in nature as possible. In essence our system permits us to store and quantify data on all observable motion, either of the whole organism of its appendages, with speed and precision via a digital computer.

The System

The instrumentation, of which a film was shown, has been described in a popular article in the New Scientist (June 26, 1969, pages 692-693) while a more technical description has appeared in the Transactions on Biomedical Engineering of the Institute of Electrical and Electronics Engineers (Davenport, Culler, Greaves, Forward, and Hand, 1970).

In the course of the development of the instrumentation certain primary criteria were set up which are those demanded by all studies in behavior. First of all one wishes to be able to observe and record quantitatively the movement of a significant sample of individuals in an open unrestricted situation. The investigator demands freedom to change the conditions in the environment of the organisms during an experiment, altering illumination, salinity, temperature, or the concentration of chemical agents at will without restricting free movement. He wishes to be able to record resulting changes in velocity, both linear and angular, direction of movement, rate of change of direction and net displacement of the whole organism. The requirements for microorganisms are, then, precisely the same as those demanded by the behavioral physiologist who works with multicellular organisms.

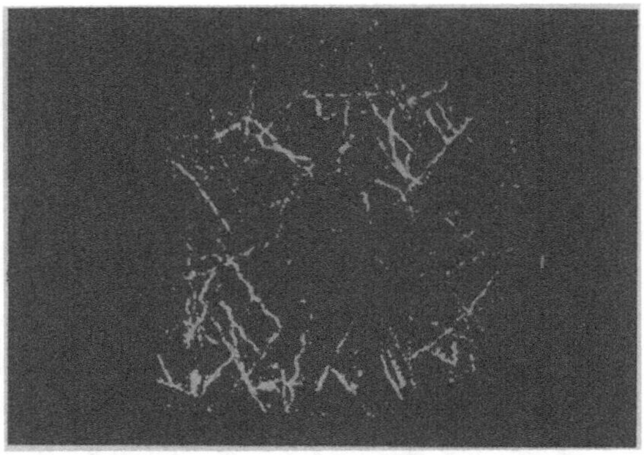

Figure 2. Cumulative pathways of dinoflagellates (Gyrodinium) returned by the computer to the Tektronics scope.

I quote from my New Scientist article:

"The basic optical element we use is the Nikon Model M inverted microscope with all magnifications from 20× to oil, with phase-contrast and dark field. This instrument has certain great advantages for the student of behavior. The illuminator is a long distance from the stage, reducing the possible effect of heat. The large open stage with objectives below it gives one maximum freedom to manipulate a free, open preparation. One can in effect put a small aquarium a few millimeters square on the stage and focus up into it either with low power or with a long-focus, high dry lens.

"The electronic elements of the 'pre-computerization' system consist of a Cohu Electronics Model 3000 TV camera with camera control (Model 3900) and monitors, and an Ampex Model 7500 video tape recorder. The TV camera views the optical image directly through the cine attachment of the microscope.

"There are numerous advantages in this combination of instruments. Because the TV camera is sensitive to a broad band of wavelengths (everything in the visible range) the experimentor can select for field illumination of his subjects any wavelength which he knows will not affect then, merely by placing a narrow-band filter on the microscope illuminator. This is extremely important for studies on such organisms as phytoplankters in which illumination at certain wavelengths, while not provoking any overt response, may have a very marked effect on the organism's response to other wavelengths." [As an example, in our studies of the dinoflagellate Gyrodinium we have been able to use a 620 mm filter in the field illuminator beam; this wavelength maintains the overt response to 470 mm (Forward and Davenport, 1968).] "The effect of directional light stimuli on organisms may be investigated in a controlled way by introducing one or more beams parallel to the microscope stage and at right angles to the field illuminator beam, without in any way affecting the TV image.

"The brilliance and contrast of images on the viewing screen (and hence on the tape) may be modified in a number of ways according to the aims of the

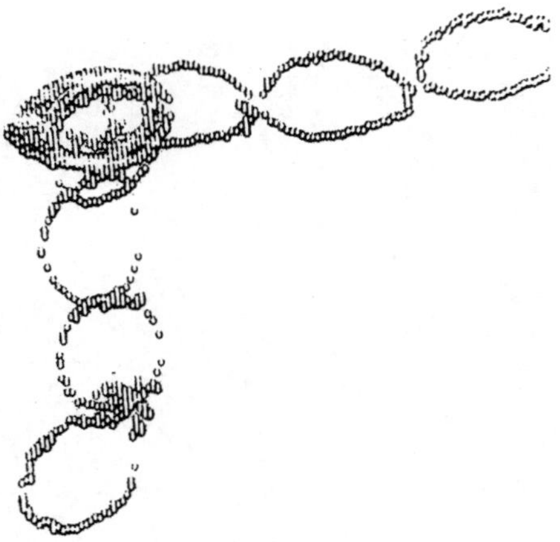

Figure 3. Bugwatcher-processed track of a Gyrodinium cell, showing the "stop-response" and reorientation. Each oval is made up of blips, each of which is the X–Y coordinate of a point on the periphery of the cell at a point in time. The cell enters from the right and exits below in the direction of the light stimulus. The area of overtrace indicates the occurence of the "stop-response". Optical magnification 200X. Photo by courtesy of William G. Hand.

experiment. Phase and dark field allow one to attain different visual ends at the final viewing screen. With the former, internal cellular structures may give one subjective clues to direction of movement in such a way that one can trace orientational changes very precisely. One may obtain image reversal on the video screen either by use of dark field optics or by electronic reversal of the phase of the image after the image has been stored on video tape. This image-reversal gives the worker without computer facilities the opportunity to store data easily if tediously merely by exposing film for a known interval to the brilliant track of the moving organism against the black background of the monitor screen (Figure 1). The film can then be processes and simple measurements made to determine the linear velocity of the organisms and other quantities.

"The next unit which has been of paramount importance to us is the tape recorder. We can record responses and replay them at our convenience without all the trouble involved in cinematography. We can select any part of the record for data analysis and we can slow down the tape so that particular elements of a behavioral act, such as the repetitive mid-course corrections of a Euglena cell when responding to a new light stimulus, become more apparent.

"We now face the problem of processing those data which have been stored on the television tape. A TV screen presents in one small area a mass of information that is almost beyond reckoning; pictures leap off the screen 30 times per second. Clearly if we feed information of the order of magnitude of that on a TV frame into a computer for some time it will soon produce a

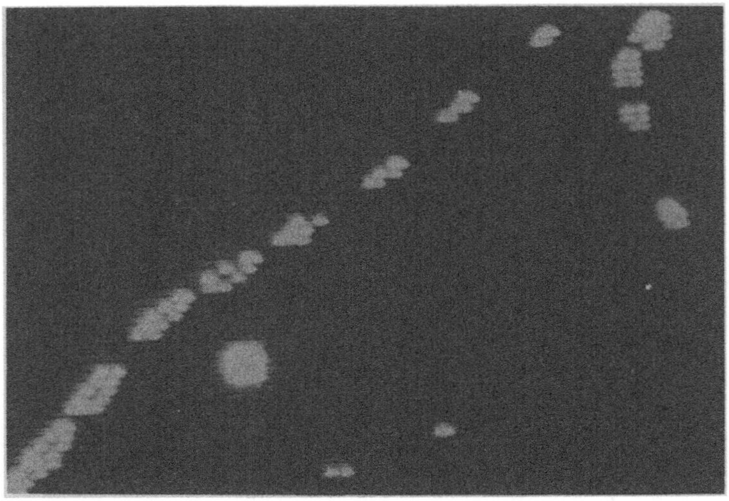

Figure 4. Tracks of echinostome miracidia, in "outline". Blips are the X - Y coordinates of points of the organisms' periphery. Opitical magnification 40x. Scene rate 15/sec.

state of information overload. The obvious answer is to design a video pre-processor that selectively strips off that portion of the picture in which we are interested and thus reduces the inflow of data of the computer. Dr. John O.B. Greaves, of the Department of Electrical Engineering at Santa Barbara has designed such a device for us. Christened the "bugwatcher", it is a pre-processing interface between the source of video information and a digital computer. The bugwatcher is connected to the digital input channel of an IBM 1800 computer. The 1800 is interfaced to a Ramo-Woolridge RW400 computer and its associated peripheral 'hardware'. The bugwatcher is designed to give a dynamic account of the position of moving organisms in the field of view of the video screen. The composite video signal has two information sources: the synchronization pulses rendering position and time data and the video information which describes the 'grayness' of a picture at a given position of the scan. We can realize a great amount of information reduction at the expense of a gray scale if we are content with only two levels of grayness, namely black and white, with freedom to choose the boundary which divides 'blackness' from 'whiteness' with appropriate controls.

"obviously we do not need to send a point to point description of each scan line of each frame to reproduce a picture. Instead we can send only the X and Y coordinates of those points on each scan line that transgress the boundary in black and white, and we can select either up-transitions or down-transitions by means of a single switch. If, for example, studies are being conducted on linear velocity, we need send to the computer only information about the position of each organism, in which case low optical magnification is used so that the organism appears merely as a point against a background (Figure 1).

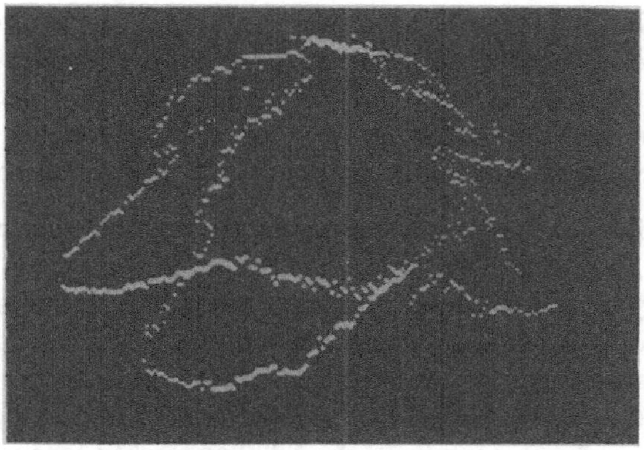

Figure 5. Curvilinear images indicating a positional change in the nauplius larva of the brine shrimp, Artemia, as returned by the computer to the Tektronics display scope. Each image is made up of the X–Y coordinates of points on the organism's periphery. Optical magnification was 40×.

"Experiments can be carried out with either dark field or bright field optics; in the former case transitions from black to white are sent to the computer and in the latter case, vice versa. In an experiment involving the detailed steps of a particular behavioral act by an individual cell, for example, orientation to a 'new' stimulus (Figure 3), we may, however, wish to quantify positional changes of the whole organism taped at high magnification levels. Under these conditions we send transitions from light to black and black to light, delivering an 'outline' drawing to the computer. For such studies it is obviously important to optimize by optical means the 'object versus background' contrast of the record on the tape and this we can vary by adjusting the optical elements and the TV camera controls.

"Finally the bugwatcher has two additional characteristics which are of value. The video source throws out a new picture every 1/16 of a second. It is obvious that slow moving organisms may not move an appreciable distance in this short time and that to read data points at the 60 frames per second rate would glut the computer with nearly redundant information. We can, however, select 13 different scan rates from 60/sec. down to 1/minute at convenient intervals. This process simply blanks out "in between" pictures, i.e. when scanning at 15 frames per second one out of every four pictures is sent". [Clearly this attribute of the instrumentation allows us to study motion in organisms with very different rates of movement, from the slowest moving protozoa to such forms as miracidia which move at a rate of over 1500 microns per second.] In addition we may, if we wish, transmit information which is not in motion by pressing a button which sends the next one (or two, depending on the switch position) frames to the computer, thus providing a simple graphical input 'snapshot' form.

"Doing playback through the bugwatcher an 8-bit descriptor word may be sent to the computer at the beginning of each frame, four of whose bits indicate the stimulus markers and four an encoding of the frame rate selector switch. Finally we may 'edit' a particular part of the experiment for computerization by recording on another audio channel of the tape recorder both audible information from the experimentor and a high frequency 'start–stop tone' which upon replay signals to the computer to begin and end its work."

Great flexibility is given to computerization by interfacing the RW 400 with the IBM 1800. From the RW 400 come the tools for experimentation in the mathematically oriented Culler on-line system. This system has the capability for building on-line programs in either or both computers and in particular for alphanumeric or curvilinear display on a Tektronics 600 storage scope (see Figures 2, 5). Programs for special display and analysis of data from the "bugwatcher" are written in the 1800 assembly language and can either be core-based or disc-based; they may be recalled manually via the keyboard input or by use of program control from the RW 400.

Prior to presenting a brief discussion of current investigations and those in press we would stress the point that the entire system, although dedicated to the recording and storage of mathematical information, nevertheless still permits that element without which no successful studies in behavior can be made, i.e. the personal, subjective evaluation of behavioral acts by the human observer. First of all it may be said that our ability to observe on a 25-inch viewing screen (in the pre-computerization chain) the much enlarged real images of microorganisms during the course of an experiment greatly enhances our perception of the chain of events involved in a response. We are not exactly sure thy this is so; the situation may perhaps be compared with the difference in information received by an observer who sees a tiger across a clearing through 10-power glasses and that of the observer who encounters the tiger at 10 feet face to face. This single element in our system, without exaggeration, puts us "directly into the medium" and brings us face to face with experimental subject. Frequently during our investigations a worker will observe something happen in the real image on the 25-inch screen, will have stored these events on tape and upon replay will say: "Now this phenomenon should be quantified." Comparison of the curvilinear image returned to the observer from the computer memory (Figure 5) with the real image on video tape indicates that the computer has a more than adequate "grasp" of events as they occur.

In order better to appreciate the versatility of the whole chain of instrumentation, we may, prior to a discussion of current investigations, present a series of photographs. Figure 1 shows the sort of data used in a standard linear velocity study. These are bugwatcher-processed images of positional changes in the dinoflagellate Gyrodinium taped at low magnification (40×). The tape was scanned by the bugwatcher, in this case at a rate of two scans per second. The discrete points making up an individual track are, of course, the X–Y coordinates of a single cell at a series of points in time. Figure 2 indicates a computer memory, as represented in curvilinear form on the Tektronics display scope, of accumulated pathways of moving Gyrodinium cells. As an example of the manner in which a specific behavioral response may be analyzed by the bugwatcher, we may observe Figure 3. Here we may see what happens when a single Gyrodinium cell moving in "from the right" is suddenly stimulated at 90° to its original course by a beam of 470 nm; as can be seen the cell briefly stops, makes a rapid 90° course correction and moves off at "standard" velocity in the direction of the light stimulus. In this case the behavioral event on the tape was processed by the bugwatcher at a rate of 5 scans per second, each oval consisting of the X–Y coordinates of points on the margin of the cell at a single point in time (events taped at 200×). Figure 4 shows the track of the miracidium larva of the trematode parasite Echinostoma revolutum. These organisms move approximately 8 times as fast as Gyrodinium (>1500 μ per second versus 200 μ per second) and consequently were scanned at the rate of 10/sec. Larger organisms can, of course, be quite as easily investigated as microorganisms. Figure 5 shows a computer memory (as seen on the Tektronics scope) of a single change in position over time in a nauplius larva of the crustacean Artemia, familiar to tropical fish fanciers.

Most recently Dr. Greaves has introduced a potentially extremely valuable element into the entire observer-instrumentation complex. It is now possible for the observer to trace with a "light-pen" any chosen part (or appendage) of an organism on the curvilinear display returned from the computer memory. The computer can then be asked to deal with that portion outlined alone and of course programmed to give information over a series of pages about the organ so identified. As can be seen, this introduction of a selective human element into the chain of instrumentation increases by orders of magnitude its versatility in the analysis of behavior.

In summary the instrumentation allows an observer to record and quantify any behavior of an organism or part of an organism which can be stored on a television tape.

Current Investigations

The vital chain in the pre-computerization link of the instrumentation, the "bugwatcher", was not brought to a state of operational efficiency until very recently; hence for all studies to be described below, data were obtained by photographing with a robot camera bugwatcher-processed images on a viewing screen. Currently Dr. Greaves is creating relatively simple programs to obtain such data as linear velocity, accumulation of cells, etc., and as time passes, will direct his attention to the more sophisticated programming necessary to analyze the machinery of cellular reorientation such as is exhibited in Figure 3.

Dr. Richard Forward, extended our information concerning the role of red light (Forward and Davenport, 1968) in mediating the response to blue in the dinoflagellate Gyrodinium. More specifically, he has conclusively demonstrated the existence of a circadian rhythm in the response of this phytoplankter to 470 nm. (Forward and Davenport, 1970). He showed that when cells which have been maintained under a 12-12 cycle are placed in constant darkness, sensitivity returns before dawn with maximum responsiveness one hour before dawn. Thereafter threshold rises sharply until at approximately five hours after dawn cells are no longer responsive. More interestingly, Forward was only able to demonstrate this rhythm in the response to blue when every sample subjected to the blue stimulus had been briefly irradiated by light of 620 nm.

The characteristic response of Gyrodinium which has been investigated for several years in the author's laboratory is the "stop-response", which is followed by orientation and movement toward the light source. My colleague and former student Dr. William G. Hand of Occidental College, who unfortunately could not be present at the symposium because of his absence on a summer postdoctoral in Germany with Dr. Haupt, has specifically investigated the orientation process, (Hand, 1970). He has used uni- and bi-directional stimulation to determine directional discrimination, which must, of course, effect orientation. Under unidirectional stimulation orientation is "complete" when the long axis of the cell is parallel to the axis of the light stimulus. If two beams 90° apart are introduced simultaneously, orientation is oblique to both stimuli; here orientation is complete when equilateral light stimulation is achieved. It is interesting to note that when two beams 180° apart are delivered simultaneously, no preferred orientation occurs. Hence there appears to be no position of the cell with respect to these beams that will produce an other than random orientational pattern. Hand presents an interesting the theoretical analysis of these events, which I believe worthy of quotation here.

"In Euglena, orientation is achieved by monitoring the stimulus beam at two points in time and space, through periodic shading of the photoreceptor by the stigma as the cell rotates during swimming (Jennings, 1906; Mast, 1911). Each shading event produces a small shift in orientation until the photoreceptor is no longer shaded (Diehn, 1969). At this time orientation is complete and the cell is swimming parallel to the axis of the stimulus. Such a process requires considerable time, as it is dependent upon swimming speed and cell rotation rate. In contrast, Gyrodinium requires a very short orientation time. Orientation can occur at the culmination of a stop-response where no cell movement including rotation occurs" [see Figure 3]. "Complete orientation requires only fractions of a second to occur. It must therefore be argued that orientation results from the comparison of the light stimulus at two or more points in space, but one point in time. . . . Such systems are classically considered to be those with bilateral photoreception (Fraenkel and Gunn, 1961)."

Hand analyzes the possiblilities in further detail and postulates that a shading body which shades two photoreceptors in association with the flagellae may "cue" the cell when to stop its axial rotation and thus initiate the process of reorientation.

The author has initiated long delayed studies to elucidate the interrelation of environmental factors in governing the behavior of the Gyrodinium cell. It has been possible to mount a microscope at right angles to the axis of a small optically clear glass pipette which is 3 mm square in cross section. We have created a steep but very transitory salinity interface between two media in this pipette by floating 75 percent culture medium on top of 100 percent culture medium. In both of these media Gyrodinium, an estuarine form, may be entirely successfully cultured and linear velocity is approximately the same, if Gyrodinium cells are in the 100 percent medium and are lured to the salinity interface by use of a light beam of 470 nm they "refuse" to pass through the interface until the interface has "broken down". Quantitative data on this phenomenon are not as yet at hand, but the indication is, of course, that the cells appear to have some sort of osmometer. The completion of this study should enable us to understand better the aggregation of such phytoplankters at specific depths in the sea.

Investigations have been initiated in the author's laboratory to create an "ethogramme" of the miracidia (Figure 4) of one or two digenetic trematodes (Echinostomatidae). Very little is known about the sum total of behavioral capabilities of these infectious agents. We have been so fortunate as to have the cooperation and support of Dr. Donald Heyneman, of the Hooper Foundation in San Francisco, who has made it possible for us to obtain material regularly from infected hamsters. The miracidia may be readily hatched out and they have proven themselves magnificent animals in terms of their suitability for investigation in our apparatus. Linear velocity studies have shown that two species of echinostomes, E. lindoense (BII) and E. revolutum, have linear velocities >1500 μ/sec. This is almost an order of magnitude faster than such a phytoplankter as Gyrodinium. In the ten hours of life of such a miracidium it would appear to be possible for the organism, if it were to travel continuously in a unidirectional manner (which it probably would not) to go as far as 72M. In any case this high rate of linear velocity enables the organism to move over relatively great distances in its "search" for the snail host. In this study we propose to investigate quantitatively the effects of varying wavelengths, the effects of temperature, and the effects of chemical agents including extracts from the host snail.

Finally, one student in the author's laboratory is investigating the behavior of the nauplius larvae of the interesting intertidal copepod Tigriopus. This copepod lives in the highest tide pools which are subject to very steep salinity changes during periods of evaporation or heavy rainfall; we are particularly interested in determining the extent to which the overt behavior of the organism is affected by the presence of salinity interfaces.

As can be seen, our instrumentation lends itself to the elucidation of the motile behavior of a wide variety of microorganisms from the size of nannoplankters of 2-3 μ upward. The construction of the instrumentation and investigations were supported by University Research Grant No. 12 (Santa Barbara) NSF Grant CB 7712 and ONR Contract No. N00014-69-A-0250-8003. Dr. Hand's investigations were supported by NSF Grant GB 8595, NSF-COSIP and a Hayes Grant in Biology from Occidental College.

REFERENCES

Bruce, V. G. and Pittendrigh, C. S. (1956). Proc. Nat. Acad. Sci. 42, 676.

Davenport, D., Culler, G. J., Greaves, J. O. B., Forward, R. B., and Hand, W. G. (1970). Trans. Biomed. Eng., I. E. E. E. BME-17, 230.

Diehn, B. (1969). Exp. Cell Res. 56, 375.

Feinleib, M. E. H. and Curry, G. M. (1967). Physiol. Plant. 20, 1083.

Forward, R. B. and Davenport, D. (1968). Science 161, 1028.

Forward, R. B. and Davenport, (1970). Planta. 92, 259.

Fracenkel, G. S. and Gunn, D. L. (1961). The Orientation of Animals: Kinese, Taxes and Compass Reactions. Dover, New York.

Gebauer, H. (1930). Beitr. Biol. Pflanz. 18, 463.

Hand, W. G., Collard, P., and Davenport, D. (1965). Biol. Bull. 128, 90.

Hand, W. G. J. (1970). J. Exper. Zool. 174, 33.

Jennings, H. S. (1906). The Behavior of Lower Organisma. (Reprinted 1964). The Univ. of Indiana, Bloomington.

Mast, S. O. (1911). Light and the Behavior of Organisms. Wiley, New York.

Pohl, R. (1948). Z. Naturforsch. 3b, 367.

ROLE OF THE CELL MEMBRANE IN BEHAVIOUR OF PARAMECIUM

ELECTRICAL MECHANISMS CONTROLLING LOCOMOTION IN THE CILIATED PROTOZOA

R. Eckert
University of California,
Department of Zoology,
Los Angeles,
California 90024, U.S.A.

ABSTRACT

The direction of swimming (forward or backward) in the ciliated protozoa depends on the orientation of the polarized cycle of ciliary movement. This orientation is coupled to membrane potential by membrane-limited movements of Ca^{2+} into the cell cortex and cilia. Stimuli which depolarize the cell cause the conductance of the membrane to Ca^{2+} to rise. As a consequence Ca^{2+}, driven by its electrochemical gradient, shows a net influx and accumulates in the cilia and cell cortex. The increasing Ca^{2+} concentration activates the mechanism for ciliary reversal. As depolarization subsides and Ca^{2+} diffuses away from the cortex and/or is actively transported out of the cell, the cilia resume their forward-swimming orientation.

1. Introduction

The amazing capabilities of metazoan nervous systems in generating and coordinating locomotor behavior depend on the anatomical organization and specific interconnection of large numbers of neurons, the functional properties of these units, and integrative processes between neurons at specialized junctions called synapses. Unicellular organisms do not possess nervous systems composed of interacting cellular units. Thus it is not surprizing that their behavioral capabilities are far more limited than those of the metazoa. Nevertheless, one must ask how, in the absence of a nervous system, the locomotor activity of the protozoa is controlled. I will consider some aspects of this problem in the ciliates.

Experiments over the past three decades at the University of Tokyo, and more recently in our laboratory, provide strong evidence that the electrophysiological organization of a ciliate is fundamentally no different from that of individual metazoan receptor, nerve, or muscle cells, and that the behavior

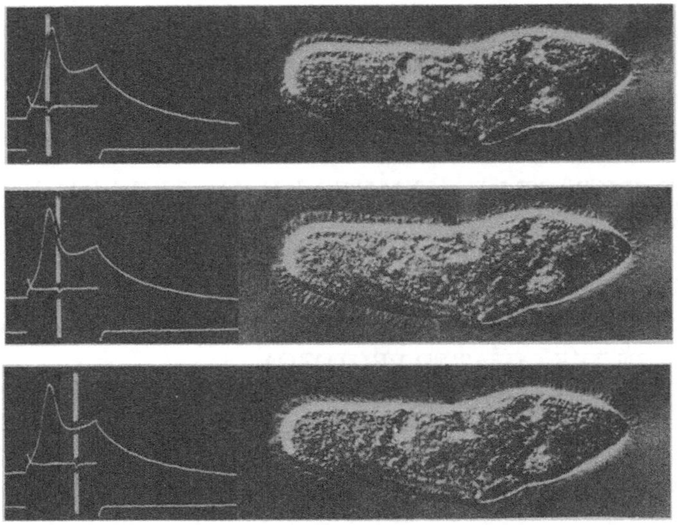

Figure 1. Orientation responses of cilia to changes in membrane potential. Treatment with 1 mM $NiCl_2$ eliminated ciliary beat in P. caudatum, permitting simple visualization of ciliary orientation. Duration of current pulses (lower traces) was 60 msec each. Potential change (upper traces) from resting level to peak of response was 39 mV. Corresponding flash photos were taken during recording at the times indicated by the vertical white bars. Anterior end is facing left. Forward shift of cilia in response to membrane excitation corresponds to reversal of power stroke in beating cilia. Hyperpolarization produced no response. From Eckert and Naitoh, 1970; permission of Rockefeller University Press.

of the ciliates is controlled by mechanisms far simpler in organization than those which would require subcellular analogues of neuronal nets and synapses. This paper presents the thesis that locomotor behavior in the ciliate is controlled primarily through familar electrical properties of cell membranes. A new hypothesis, consistant with old and new data, relates ciliary reversal to membrane potential. By regulating intracellular concentrations of Ca^{2+}, to which the locomotor apparatus is sensitive, the cell membrane controls locomotor activity.

Ciliary Reversal Regulated by Ca^{2+}

Paramecium responds to electric current (Ludloff, 1895) and application of cations such as K^+(Jennings, 1906; Kamada and Kinosita, 1940) with reversal of the ciliary beat. Both stimuli produce depolarization of the cell membrane correlated with ciliary reversal. More recent intracellular stimulation and recording techniques have been used to show that depolarization of the cell membrane produces a reversal in direction of the beat in addition to an increase in frequency (Kinosita, 1954; Eckert,and Naitoh, 1970). Further evidence implicates the calcium ion in activating the reversal of ciliary beating (Naitoh, 1969, 1972).

How is the reversal of ciliary beating regulated by depolarization of the cell membrane? I propose that the primary membrane-related event which activates reversal is not displacement of calcium from binding sites as proposed by Jahn (1962) and Naitoh (1968), but instead an influx of calcium ions

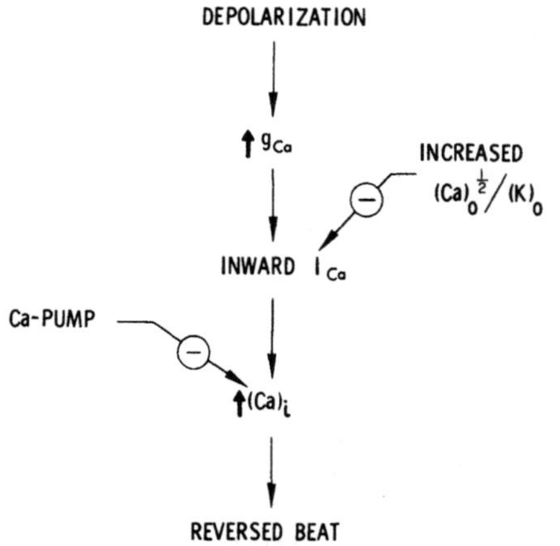

Figure 2. Schema of ciliary reversal controlled by membrane regulated calcium influx. The key points in the sequence are: i) calcium conductance, g_{Ca}, of the membrane increases with depolarization, ii) in the steady state ($dVm/dt = 0$) inward calcium current, I_{Ca}, cannot exceed the simultaneous efflux of positive charge. Thus I_{Ca} is limited by the potassium conductance, which decreases as the ratio $[Ca]_0^{\frac{1}{2}}/[K]_0$ increases. iii) The intensity of reversal depends on the maximum level of $[Ca]_{in}$, and the duration of reversal depends on the rate at which $[Ca]_{in}$ is subsequently lowered by active extrusion or sequestering.

across the cell membrane during stimulus-evoked excitation according to the equation

$$I_{Ca} = g_{Ca}(Vm - E_{Ca}) \qquad (1)$$

I_{Ca} is that part of the membrane current carried by the net flux of Ca^{2+} across the membrane, g_{Ca} is the conductance of the membrane to calcium current, Vm is the membrane potential, and E_{Ca} is the potential at which Ca^{2+} is in electrochemical equilibrium across the membrane as given by the Nernst relation (See Katz, 1966, for theory). The intracellular concentration of free Ca^{2+} is very low in most cells ($< 10^{-6}$ M), so in experimental concentrations (circa 10^{-3} M) of extracellular calcium E_{Ca} may be about +100 mV, while Vm is in the range of −30 mV. Since the resting membrane of Paramecium is known to be permeable to Ca^{2+} (Naitoh and Eckert, 1968a) there must be a steady state inward calcium flux at rest equal to the rate of calcium extrusion by active transport. Under those conditions net calcium current, I_{Ca}, equals zero even though $[Ca]_{out}$ is much higher than $[Ca]_{in}$ and the intracellular concentration remains stable.

The calcium conductance, g_{Ca}, increases as a result of depolarization (Eckert and Naitoh, 1969). According to Eq. 1 this will produce a rise in I_{Ca}. Calcium influx will then exceed metabolically driven efflux until g_{Ca} returns to normal or until the rate of pumping Ca^{2+} out of the cell increases to compensate. The result is a temporary increase in $[Ca]_{in}$.

Evidences that membrane-regulated inward flux of extra-cellular calcium couples ciliary reversal to membrane depolarization include the following:

i) Intracellular Ca^{2+} is required for ciliary reversal. This conclusion is based on Naitoh's demonstration that the cilia of glycerinated paramecia swing into an anterior-pointing orientation when Ca^{2+} is added to the activation medium consisting of ATP and Zn^{2+}. This has recently (Naitoh, 1972) been significantly extended by experiments in which specimens, previously extracted in a Triton X-100 solution and swimming forward in a solution of ATP, Mg^{2+} and EGTA, reverse ciliary beat and swim backwards when the concentration of

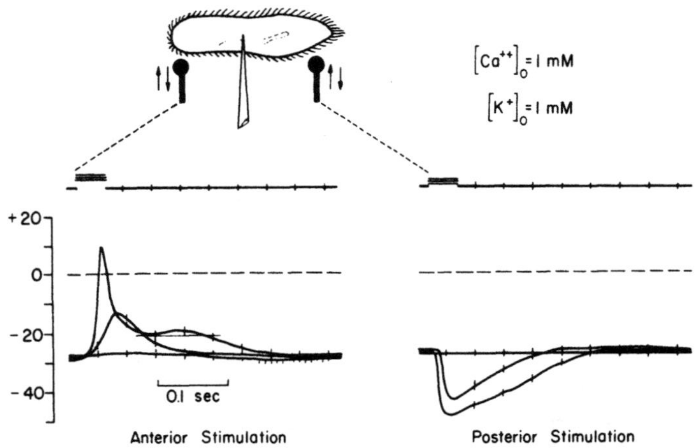

Figure 3. Responses to mechanical stimulation of anterior and posterior ends of P. caudatum. Both signals are recorded equally well from all parts of the cell because of cable spread. From Naitoh and Eckert, 1969a; copyright 1969, American Association Advancement of Science.

free Ca^{2+} in the solution is raised above 10^{-6} M/liter. Since the cell membrane is destroyed by the Triton extraction, the ambient concentrations of Ca^{2+}, Mg^{2+}, and ATP represent the concentration to which the ciliary apparatus is exposed, and is therefore equivalent to an intracellular concentration. The low level of $[Ca]_{in}$ effective in producing reversal is commensurate with concentration shifts which might be transiently attained at the cell cortex by a membrane-regulated calcium influx.

ii) Extracellular Ca^{2+} is essential for reversal in the living cell. Reversal is blocked by calcium precipitating agents in the bath (Ueda, 1961), and in solutions of low calcium concentration (Kinosita, 1954; Naitoh, 1968).

iii) Membrane depolarization causes an increase in calcium conductance and inward calcium current (Eckert and Naitoh, 1969). Stimuli which cause depolarization also produce ciliary reversal. Reversal occurs in response to outward (depolarizing) current injected into the cell with a microelectrode (Naitoh, 1958; Eckert and Naitoh, 1970; Figure 1 in this paper); depolarization of the cell with a variety of cations (Kamada, 1940; Kamada and Kinosita, 1940; Naitoh and Eckert, 1968a); depolarizing receptor current evoked by mechanical stimulation (Naitoh and Eckert, 1969a, b) and spontaneous depolarization (Kinosita, 1954; Kinosita et al., 1965; Naitoh, 1966; Naitoh and Eckert, 1969b; Machemer, 1970). However reversal does not occur with depolarization if $[Ca]_{out}$ is too low (point ii, above).

iv) It can be predicted from Eq. 1 that I_{Ca} will reverse sign (calcium will flow out across the membrane against its concentration gradient) if Vm is made more positive than E_{Ca}. This should be accompanied by absence of reversal. This, indeed is the case. Naitoh (1958) found in Opalina that low and moderate outward current produced reversal, but that at very high intensities of outward current (strong intracellular positivity) the normal stroke continues without reversal during the passage of current. Instead, reversal occurs at the "break" of the high intensity current pulse. Under these conditions Ca^{2+} must flow outward during the current pulse, and the transiently inward as the membrane potential drops exponentially past values more negative than E_{Ca} at the end of the pulse. The analagous behavior occurs in the Ca-dependent release of transmitter from the presynaptic terminal of the giant synapse of squid (Katz and Miledi, 1966). Naitoh also reported that sufficiently strong inward current (intracellular negativity increased) produces reversal. This is also predicted from Eq. 1 if it is assumed that g_{Ca} undergoes little or no reduction with hyperpolarization.

Once initiated, how is the activation of reversal terminated? It is reasonable to suppose that the accumulated Ca^{2+} is removed from the cytoplasm by an active process, a "calcium pump", which maintains $[Ca]_{in}$ below levels sufficient to activate reversal. If such an active process utilizing metabolic energy is involved, reversal in response to a given stimulus should be prolonged at low temperatures, since the rate of extrusion of calcium will be reduced. It is significant, therefore, that Oliphant 1930) found the duration of reversal to vary inversely with temperature with a Q_{10} of about 2.0.

This hypothesis, with Ca^{2+} acting as the agent coupling ciliary reversal to membrane potential is outlined in Figure 2. It is similar in concept to modern theories of excitation–contraction coupling in muscle. Experiments are now required to test quantitative relations between membrane stimulation, calcium fluxes and ciliary reversal.

Ion Antagonism and Ciliary Reversal

Ciliary reversal has traditionally been induced by transferring paramecia from an "equilibration medium" to a "stimulation medium" of different ionic strength (e.g., increased KCl). In this case the duration of reversal is complexly related to the relative concentrations of the monovalent cation (usually K^+) and calcium in the equilibration and stimulation media (Kamada and Kinosita, 1940; Jahn, 1962; Kuznicki, 1966; Naitoh, (1968). As first noted by Jahn (1962), the duration of reversal is related to the ratio $[X^+]/[Ca^{2+}]^{1/2}$ of the stimulation medium. Reversal lasts longest at an optimum value of this ratio characteristic for the stimulating cation. This is reminiscent of the antagonism exhibited by extracellular Na^+ and Ca^{2+} in amphibian cardiac muscle (Lüttgau and Niedergerke, 1958).

Data obtained by this approach are difficult to interpret because of the number of uncontrolled variables and complexities inherent in that approach. Interpretations must take into account that membrane-associated calcium affects membrane resistance and excitability (Frankenhaeuser and Hodgkin, 1957; Hagiwara and Nakajima, 1966; Naitoh and Eckert, 1968a), and that increased concentrations of cations depolarize the membrane (Kamada, 1934; Naitoh and Eckert, 1968a).

The observations on cation antagonism can be explained in terms of membrane-limited calcium current. Several reasonable assumptions enter

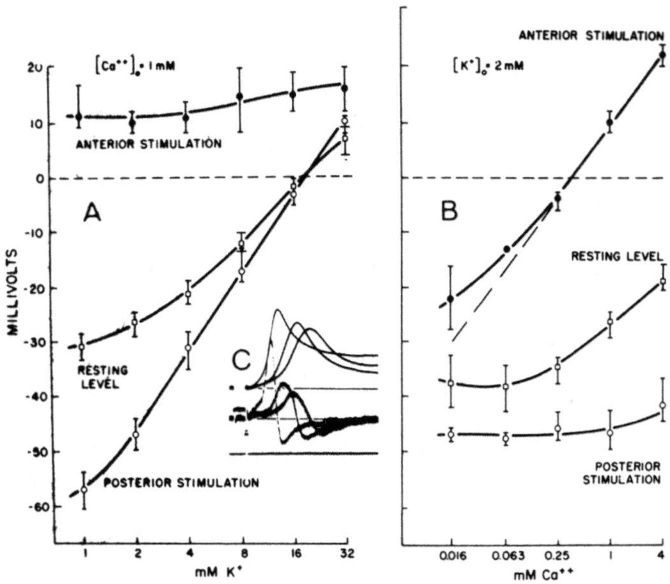

Figure 4. Ionic requirements of electrical responses to mechanical stimulation of anterior and posterior ends of Paramecium. Anterior response has a strong $[Ca]_{out}$ dependence and approaches the theoretical slope for a calcium electrode. The posterior response is insensitive to $[Ca]_0$, but has a slope of about 50 mV for a ten-fold increase $[K]_0$, which approaches the theoretical slope for a K^+ electrode. Two components of anterior response are evident in differentiated signals (middle trace) of membrane potentials (upper trace). The initial component is the receptor potential and the second component is the regenerative Ca^{2+} spike. Different intensities of mechanical stimulation (bottom trace) were applied in three separate sweeps.

into this interpretation. First, it is assumed that there is an increase in calcium conductance, g_{Ca}, when the membrane is depolarized by increased cation concentrations (Naitoh and Eckert, 1968a), just as there is when the membrane is depolarized by an outward current delivered with a microelectrode. Second, it will be assumed that differences in membrane conductance at different $[K]/[Ca]^{1/2}$ result entirely from differences in g_k (A simultaneous increase in g_{Ca} would serve only to reinforce the argument in favor of the hypothesis). Finally, the simplifying assumption will be made that charges are carried across the membrane primarily by cations, since the membrane shows a low permeability to anions such as Cl^- (Dunham, 1971).

If all else remains equal, an increase in extracellular calcium will increase the driving force on Ca^{2+} ($Vm - E_{Ca}$). A depolarization which produces a given increase in calcium conductance will then be accompanied by a stronger influx of Ca^{2+} (Eq. 1), and this will produce a more intense and/or more prolonged reversal of ciliary beating.

It is important to note that the trend for increased $[Ca]_{out}$ to raise Ca^{2+} influx due to an increased electrochemical gradient is modified by an effect of $[Ca]_{out}$ on the membrane conductance. The membrane conductance remains relatively constant with changes in ionic strength providing the ratio $[K]/[Ca]^{1/2}$ is held constant throughout. However, the conductance drops as the ratio increases (Naitoh and Eckert, 1968a). The total membrane conductance becomes important to calcium current when the membrane potential is constant following a depolarization. At that time net membrane current is zero, and therefore charge influx must equal charge efflux. Since K^+ has the proper electrochemical gradient to carry charge out of the cell (Naitoh and Eckert, 1969a) charge efflux is limited by K^+ conductance. Since Ca^{2+} influx must equal K^+ efflux during the post-stimulatory steady state, any factor (such as an increase in relative concentration of Ca^{2+}) which decreases the conductance of the membrane to K^+ can potentially reduce Ca^{2+} influx indirectly by slowing K^+ efflux. Thus, the effects of increasing $[Ca]_0$ at constant $[K]_0$ are at least two-fold: i) E_{Ca} undergoes a positive shift (Eq. 1) which exceeds the concomitant shift in Vm, and so that term $Vm - E_{Ca}$ in Eq. 1 becomes larger, ii) g_K drops. Thus, an increase in $[Ca]_0$ affects I_{Ca} positively according to Eq. 1 while a decrease in the ratio $[K]_0/[Ca]_0^{1/2}$ affects I_{Ca} negatively by reducing g_K. As a result, inward calcium current (and thus the intensity and/or duration of ciliary reversal) can either increase or decrease when $[Ca]_0$ and/or $[K]_0$ are changed, depending on which effects predominate at various combinations of calcium and potassium. The depressant effect on calcium influx of increasing the relative calcium concentration is indicated in Figure 2.

The dual effect of $[Ca]_0$ on the duration of reversal is apparent in Naitoh's (1968) Figure 9. At very low calcium concentrations the electrochemical gradient for calcium $(Vm - E_{Ca})$ is too low to drive calcium into the cell at a rate sufficient to initiate reversal (Eq. 1). Toward the right hand end of the abscissa the membrane conductance drops sufficiently to limit the rate at which K^+ can leave the cell in exchange for Ca^{2+} entering the cell. As a result, calcium influx is reduced and the duration of ciliary reversal is reduced. When the ratio $[K]_0/[Ca]_0^{1/2}$ is kept constant Naitoh, 1968, (Figure 10) membrane conductance remains constant, and the duration of reversal increases monotonically with increased depolarization and increased $[Ca]_0$.

Differences in [K] and [Ca] of the equilibration medium prior to potassium depolarization also affect the duration of reversal (Naitoh, 1968). This is not unexpected, since external cation concentrations affect internal ion concentrations during equilibration (Dunham and Child, 1961).

Membrane Excitability

Sensory excitability to mechanical stimuli is exhibited by the membranes of ciliates (Naitoh and Eckert, 1969a, b). The ciliate shows a transient hyperpolarization when mechanically stimulated at the posterior end, and a transient depolarization when stimulated at the anterior end (Figure 3). The potential change produced in direct response to transduction of stimulus energy is analagous to the receptor potentials recorded in metazoan receptor cells (Mellon, 1968). Receptor potentials are graded with stimulus intensity, are nonregenerative, and spread electrotonically.

Figures 4a and 4b show the relation between membrane potentials and the extracellular concentrations of K^+ and Ca^{2+}. The maximum potential produced by mechanical stimulation of the rear depends on $[K]_0$ and the maximum potential produced by mechanical stimulation of the anterior depends on $[Ca]_0$. This indicates that the mechanical stimulus applied to the rear renders that part of the membrane temporarily more permeable to K^+, and when applied to the anterior end produces an increase in permeability to Ca^{2+}. In the standard solution (1 mM KCl +1 mM $CaCl_2$ +1 mM Tris–HCl) the electrochemical gradient for K^+ is outward, and when the K^+ permeability increases potassium ions carry current out of the cell, with a resulting increase in intracellular negativity. As $[K]_0$ is raised the electrochemical gradient across the membrane drops accordingly and the maximum value of the posterior potential becomes more positive (Figure 4a).

The depolarization evoked by mechanical stimulation of the anterior is more complex than the pure receptor potential evoked at the posterior end. As shown in Figure 4c, it consists of two components: i) a depolarizing receptor potential which gives rise to ii) a regenerative depolarization due to the electrical excitability of the membrane. The second component is identical to the regenerative graded excitation evoked by artificially applied outward current (Eckert and Naitoh, 1969). Thus, a small mechanical stimulus to the anterior end of the ciliate evokes a small receptor potential, and this elicits an additional small regenerative depolarization over the entire cell membrane. Stronger mechanical stimulation produces a larger receptor current and this elicits a larger regenerative depolarization as it spreads electrotonically throughout the cell. In this way the amount of calcium entering the cell through the excited cell membrane is related to the intensity of the stimulus.

Mechanical deformation is only one form of stimulus encountered. Protozoa also show locomotor responses to radiant energy, temperature and various chemicals (Jennings, 1906; Rose, 1964). This is not necessarily the result of a specific receptor mechanism. When, for example, a specimen encounters a region of increased cation concentration the intracellular potential becomes more positive (Kamada, 1934; Kinostita, 1954; Naitoh and Eckert, 1968a).

Behavioural Correlates of Bioelectric Responses

The sensory capability of the membrane at the anterior end of the cell is instrumental in producing the classical "avoiding reaction" first described by Jennings (1906). The sequence of steps leading from a stimulus to the avoiding reaction is summarized in Figure 5. Deformation of the membrane at the anterior end by a mechanical stimulus causes that region of membrane to produce a depolarizing receptor current which spreads to depolarize the remaining surface membrane by electrotonic spread (Eckert and Naitoh, 1970). This causes a regenerative increase in calcium conductance of the cell membrane (Eckert and Naitoh, 1969). The regenerative inward calcium current produces an increase in the cortical concentrations of free Ca^{2+}, and the

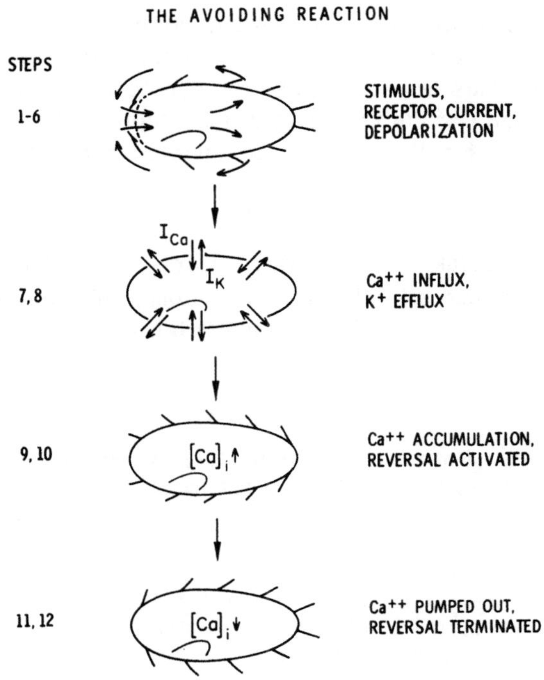

Figure 5. Sequence of events between mechanical stimulus and avoiding reaction. 1) Stretch of anterior membrane. 2) Local increase in calcium conductance of anterior membrane. 3) Local inward receptor current through membrane of anterior end. 4) Electrotonic spread of receptor current and 5) outward current return through rest of membrane. Arrows show current flow. 6) Depolarization of cell membrane by receptor current produces 7) distributed increase in calcium conductance. 8) Inward Ca^{2+} current, outward K^+ current. 9) Intracellar [Ca] increases. 10) Cilia reverse beat. 11) Ca^{2+} pumped out. 12) Original $[Ca]_{in}$ restored; cilia resume normal orientation. Copyright 1972, American Association Advancement of Science.

increase in intracellular Ca^{2+} produces a temporary reversal in the direction of the ciliary power stroke.

The avoiding reaction is highly stereotyped and can be understood in terms of three genetically programmed classes of organization. First, there are the metabolic and physical properties of the cell membrane which regulate the active and passive transport of ions. Second, there is the sensitivity of individual cilia to intracellular regulatory ions and molecules. Third, there is the anatomical organization of membrane properties over the cell surface. The genetic control of electric excitability was recently demonstrated in P aurelia (Kung and Eckert, 1972). The increased calcium conductance produced in the wild type by membrane depolarization was eliminated by genic mutation, leaving the mutant incapable of producing a regenerative inward calcium current. The absence of an inward calcium current is accompanied by the inability of the mutant to respond to a depolarizing stimulus with a reversal of ciliary beating. This is predicted by the hypothesis presented above that membrane-regulated Ca^{2+} is the agent which couples ciliary reversal to electrical responses of the cell membrane to environmental stimuli.

ACKNOWLEDGEMENTS

I thank Drs. Yutaka Naitoh, Akira Murakami and Miles Epstein for many instructive and stimulating discussions. Work in our laboratory was supported by grants from the National Science Foundation (GB-7999) and the U.S. Public Health Service (NB-08364).

REFERENCES

Dunham, P. (1971). In Biology of Tetrahymena, A. M. Elliott, Appleton-Century Crofts, Inc. New York.

Dunham, P. B. and Child, F. (1961). Biol. Bull. 121: 129-140.

Eckert, R. and Naitoh, Y. (1969). Abstr. 3rd Int. Biophys. Congr. Int. Union Applied Biophysics, Cambridge, Massachusetts, p. 257.

Eckert, R. and Naitoh, Y. (1970). J. Gen. Physiol. 55: 467-483.

Frankenhaeuser, B. and Hodgkin, A. L. (1957). J. Physiol. 137: 218-

Hagiwara, S. and Nakajima, S. (1966). J. Gen. Physiol. 49: 807.

Jahn, T. L. (1962). J. Cell. Comp. Physiol. 60: 217-228.

Jennings, H. S. (1906). Behavior of the Lower Organisms. Columbia University Press, New York.

Kamada, T. (1934). J. Exptl. Biol. 11: 94-102.

Kamada, T. (1940). Proc. Imp. Acad. (Tokyo). 16: 241-247.

Kamada, T. and Kinosita, H. (1940). Proc. Imp. Acad. (Tokyo). 16: 125-130.

Katz, B. (1966). Nerve, Muscle and Synapse. McGraw-Hill, New York.

Katz, B. and Miledi, R. (1966). Nature. 212: 1242-1245.

Kinosita, H. (1954). J. Fac. Sci. Univ. Tokyo, Sect. IV. 7: 1-4.

Kinosita, H., Murakami, A., and Yasuda, M. (1965). J. Fac. Sci. Univ. Tokyo, Sect. IV. 10: 421-425.

Kung, C. and Eckert, R. (1972). Proc. Nat. Acad. Sci. 69: 93-97.

Kuznicki, L. (1966). Acta Protozool. 4: 241-256.

Ludloff, K. (1895). Pfluger's Arch. ges. Physiol. 59: 525-554.

Lüttgau and Niedergerke, R. (1958). J. Physiol. 143: 486-505.

Machemer, H. (1970). Naturwissenschaften 8: 398-399.

Mellon, DeF. (1968). Physiology of Sense Organs. W. H. Freeman Co. San Francisco.

Naitoh, Y. (1958). Annot. Zool. Japon. 31: 59-73.

Naitoh, Y. (1966). Science. 154: 660-662.

Naitoh, Y. (1968). J. Gen. Physiol. 51: 85-103.

Naitoh, Y. (1969). J. Gen. Physiol. 53: 517-529.

Naitoh, Y. (1972). Science. (in press).

Naitoh, Y. and Eckert, R. (1968a). Z. vergl. Physiologie. 61: 427-452.

Naitoh, Y. and Eckert, R. (1968b). Z. vergl. Physiologie. 61: 453-472.

Naitoh, Y. and Eckert, R. (1969a). Science. 164: 963-965.

Naitoh, Y. and Eckert, R. (1969b). Science. 166: 1633-1635.

Oliphant, J. F. (1938). Physiol. Zool. 11: 19-30.

Rose, W. (1964). Z. Tierpsychol. 21: 257-

Ueda, K. (1961). Annot. Zool. Japon. 34: 99-110.

Also see Eckert, R. (1972). Bioelectric control of ciliary reversal. Science 176:473,481 and Naitoh, Y. and Kaneko, H. (1972). Reactivated Triton — extracted models of Paramecium: modification of ciliary movement by calcium ions. Science 176:523-527. — J. Adler.

ROLE OF BOUND CALCIUM IN THE CONTROL OF CILIA

Y. Naitoh
University of California,
Department of Zoology,
Los Angeles,
California 90024, U.S.A.

ABSTRACT

Ciliary reversal induced by application of cations was investigated in Paramecium caudatum. Ca^{2+}, Mg^{2+}, Ba^{2+}, K^+, Rb^+ are bound by anionic binding sites on the specimen in a manner consistent with the law of mass action, though their binding affinities vary. Ciliary reversal occurs when calcium ions bound by the sites are liberated in exchange for externally applied cations other than calcium. Thus, the effectiveness of cations in inducing reversal depends on their affinities to the binding sites. Factors which affect the duration of ciliary reversal are (a) initial amount of calcium bound by the anionic sites, (b) final amount of calcium bound by the sites after equilibration with the stimulation medium, and (c) concentration of Ca^{2+} in the stimulation medium. Cilia in glycerol-extracted Paramecium reorient to a reversed position in the presence of calcium, ATP, and zinc. The following hypothesis is proposed for ciliary reversal: Calcium ions liberated from the cation exchanger system activate a contractile mechanism energized by ATP. Contraction of this component results in the reversal of direction of effective beat by a mechanism not yet understood. The duration of reversal is related to the time course of release of bound calcium.

1. INTRODUCTION

Several decades ago, Jennings (1906) made exhaustive observations on various kinds of taxis in Paramecium. He found that all kinds of tactic behavior in ciliates were based on a series of ciliary responses to a stimulus or by repetition of responses in a "trial and error" manner. He named the response an "avoiding reaction". When a forward-swimming Paramecium encounters a stimulus of any kind with its anterior end, it transiently reverses beat direction of its cilia toward the anterior, causing it to swim backward a short distance. It then pivots aborally about its posterior end due to the anatomical

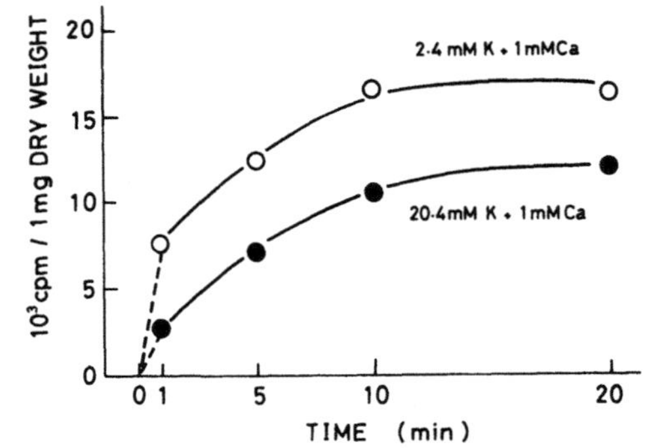

Figure 1. Time course of $^{45}Ca^{2+}$ binding by live Paramecium caudatum and the effect of coexisting K ions in the equilibrum medium on the binding (open circles, 2.4 mM K^+; solid circles, 20.4 mM K^+). Ca^{2+} concentration in the media was 1 mM ($^{45}Ca^{2+}$, 10 μc/ml).

sequence with which forward-swimming ciliary orientation is restored, and finally resumes forward locomotion in a new direction. If the specimen encounters the same stimulus again, it repeats the response until it continues forward without encountering the stimulus. Thus, the specimen avoids noxious stimuli.

Mast and Nadler (1926) transferred Paramecia into solutions of salts in various concentrations, and determined the duration of backward swimming due to ciliary reversal. They found that the effectiveness of monovalent cations to induce reversal depended on the identity and concentrations of the stimulating ions. On the other hand, divalent cations antagonized the effects of monovalent cations. This led them to conclude that the reversal induced by cation stimulation might be related to an adsorption of the cations on the membrane of Paramecium. They proposed that the cations produce a change in electrical potential of the membrane, which acts on an hypothetical neuromotor center to trigger impulses through a cortical fibrillar system which controls the direction of the power stroke.

Oliphant (1938, 1942) obtained similar results, and assumed that an increase in protoplasmic viscosity by a specific action of monovalent cations causes an activation of the fibrillar neuromotor system to evoke ciliary reversal (cf. Heilbrunn, 1952).

The implication of an hypothetical nerve-like function of the neuromotor system is based on Taylor's proposal of a conductile function of the "neuromotor" system in Euplotes for coordinating the orientation of widely separated ciliary organelles (Taylor, 1920; Rees, 1922). Recent experiments (Okajima and Kinosita, 1966; Naitoh and Eckert, 1969) have failed to support Taylor's conclusions, and it now appears that the fibrils have little if anything to do with ciliary coordination. Rather it is clear that the electrical activities of the plasma membrane play an essential role in coordinating ciliary orientation (Kinosita, 1954; Naitoh, 1958, 1961, 1966; Naitoh and Eckert, 1968a, b; Eckert and Naitoh, 1970).

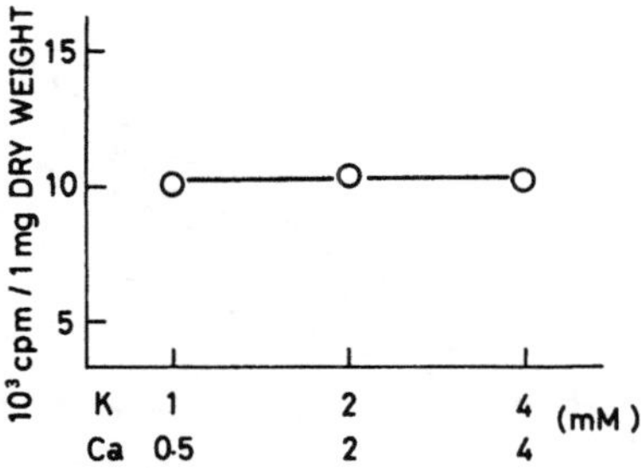

Figure 2. Amount of $^{45}Ca^{2+}$ bound by live P. caudatum during 1 min of equilibration in three kinds of solutions having the same ratio, $[K^+]/\sqrt{[Ca^{2+}]} = 1.41$.

Kamada (1929) found that the effectiveness of K ion for inducing ciliary reversal in Paramecium was dependent not only on extracellular Ca ions (antagonize against K) but also on the [Ca]/[K] ratio of the solution in which the specimens were equilibrated prior to stimulation. Thus, Kamada and Kinosita (1940) examined the quantitative relations of the duration of ciliary reversal to the [Ca]/[K] ratio and their concentrations in both equilibration and stimulation media, but they did not note any simple quantitative relations. However, the duration of reversal exhibited in a given test solution was generally longer in specimens equilibrated in the media with higher [Ca]/[K] ratio. They suggested that previous accumulation of Ca ions in the cell might promote ciliary reversal by subsequent K stimulation.

These results, together with the observation that an injection of oxalate into cytoplasm of Paramecium induces ciliary reversal (Kamada, 1938)* led Kamada (1940) to propose an hypothesis for the mechanism of ciliary reversal. He assumed a hypothetical anion in the cytoplasm, which acts to induce reversal when the anion is liberated from its calcium compound upon a decrease in cytoplasmic calcium concentration. Internal calcium dropped, according to Kamada, because of cation exchange with externally applied K ions through the membrane.

No attempts had been made to analyze the mechanism underlying ciliary reversal until Jahn (1962) noted an important relation between the duration of reversal in the experiments of Kamada and Kinosita and relative concentrations of K and Ca in their solutions. He assumed that reversal is correlated with the physiological state of the membrane, which depends on the amount of ions bound by the membrane in accordance with the Gibbs–Donnan rule (cf. Wilson and Wilson, 1918). According to the Gibbs–Donnan equation, the ratio of [K]/[Ca] on the membrane is proportional to $[K]/[Ca]^{\frac{1}{2}}$ in the surrounding solution, and is independent of ionic concentrations. Jahn analyzed the data of Kamada and Kinosita (1940) and found the duration of reversal related to $[K]/[Ca]^{\frac{1}{2}}$ instead of [K]/[Ca]. An increase in the $[K]/[Ca]^{\frac{1}{2}}$ ratio of the surrounding medium was responsible for inducing reversal. The maximum duration of reversal in specimens equilibrated in a given medium occurred in

*Ciliary reversal by an injection of oxalate was always followed by death of the specimen. According to Oliphant (1942), ciliary reversal was always associated with death of the specimens, irrespective of the cause of death. The reversal in this case appears to be different in its mechanism from that induced by cations.

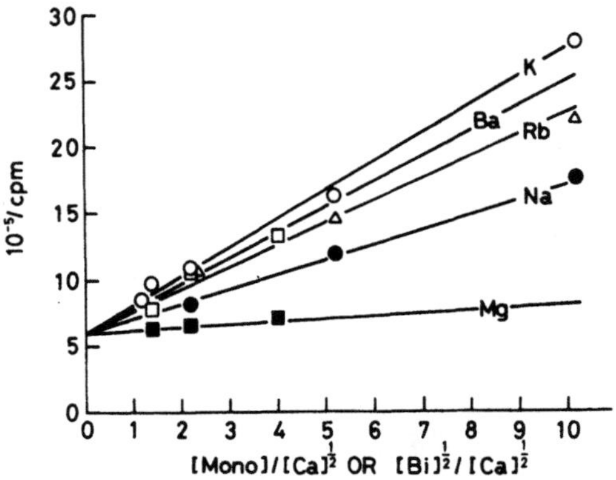

Figure 3. Effects of various coexisting ions in the equilibrium medium (○, K^+; △, Rb^+; ●, Na^+; □, Ba^{2+}; ■, Mg^{2+}) on the binding of $^{45}Ca^{2+}$ by live P. caudatum.

stimulation media having a given $[K]/[Ca]^{\frac{1}{2}}$ ratio, and was largely independent of the absolute concentrations of these ions. From these relations Jahn proposed that a Gibbs – Donnan equilibrium is established between Paramecium, K^+, and Ca^{2+}. Furthermore, he suggested that reversal is caused by the removal of calcium ions from the cell surface.

Grebecki (1964, 1965) confirmed the relations discovered by Jahn (1962), and, on the basis of his experiments with EDTA suggest that removal of calcium was responsible for ciliary reversal only when the amount of bound calcium was within a certain range.

Jahn's proposal stimulated us to study ciliary reversal in Paramecium in relation to bound cations. Our data led to a new hypothesis for the mechanism of ciliary reversal by chemical stimulation. The mechanism involved liberation of Ca from the membrane binding sites, and activation of a contractile system which governs the orientation of cilia by Ca ions and ATP. The control of reversal by Ca ions is reminiscent of its role in muscle, where Ca is thought to be released from intracellular membrane sites to activate the contractile mechanism.

In the first series of experiments the binding affinites to the anionic binding sites on Paramecium relative to that of Ca ions were determined for several common cations by making use of ^{45}Ca. This enabled us to calculate the amount of ions bound on Paramecium equilibrated in various mixtures of these ions (Naitoh and Yasumasu, 1967). In the next series of experiments the relations between duration of ciliary reversal and the amount of bound ions, and the change in relative amounts bound were examined (Naitoh, 1968). In the last series of experiments (Naitoh, 1969), I examined the requirements of ciliary reversal for Ca ions as well as ATP in glycerol-extracted paramecia.

2. Materials and Methods

Specimens of P. caudatum (Mating type 1 of Syngene 1) reared in hay infusion were thoroughly washed with an equilibration solution for more than 30

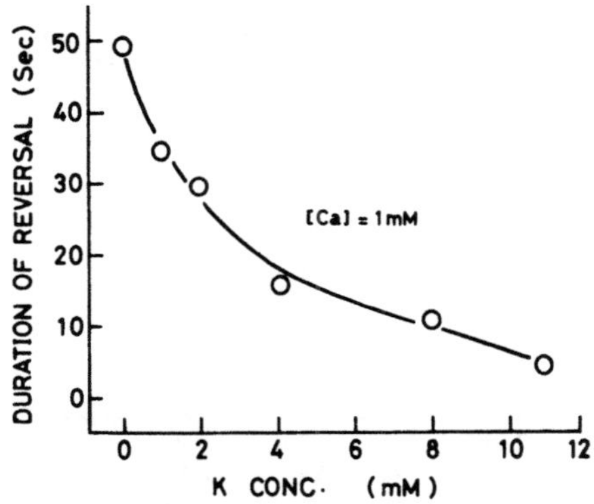

Figure 4. The influence of $[K^+]$ in the equilibration medium on the duration of ciliary reversal.

minutes prior to experimentation. Details of experimental methods will be described at the beginning of each following section. All the experiments were performed at 19-21°C.

3. Binding of Cations by Paramecium

Washed specimens were suspended in a solution, of 20 mM KCl plus 0.1 mM $CaCl_2$, buffered to pH 7.2 by 1 mM Tris-HCl in a density of 1.0 mg of specimens in dry weight/ml. A 1-ml aliquot of the suspension was pipetted into a glass filtrating vessel and 10 ml of solution containing ^{45}Ca and other ions was pipetted into the vessel and mixed. After a given time, the suspension medium was rapidly removed through a Millipore filter. The ^{45}Ca remaining in the filter was then washed out with an unlabeled mixture of an ionic composition identical to that of the labeled suspension medium. The filter was dried, and the radioactivity due to ^{45}Ca accumulated by Paramecium was counted.

The time course of ^{45}Ca binding was determined in two different concentrations of potassium. The results shown in Figure 1 indicate that much greater amounts of ^{45}Ca accumulated within a 1 min-equilibration period in the presence of low (2.4 mM) K than in high (20.4 mM) K concentration. This rapid uptake was followed by a slow phase which seemed to be independent of K concentration. It is reasonable to assume that the rapid initial compoent of ^{45}Ca uptake is due to binding of ^{45}Ca by anionic sites on Paramecium, and the K ions compete for the same binding sites.

If a cation exchanger type system is involved in the rapid binding of calcium, the equilibrium between the binding sites, Ca^{2+} and K^+ may be formulated according to the law of mass action as:

$$PCa_{\frac{1}{2}} + K^+ \rightleftharpoons PK + \tfrac{1}{2}Ca^{2+} \tag{1}$$

$$[PK]/[PCa_{\frac{1}{2}}] = k[K^+]/[Ca^{2+}]^{\frac{1}{2}} \tag{2}$$

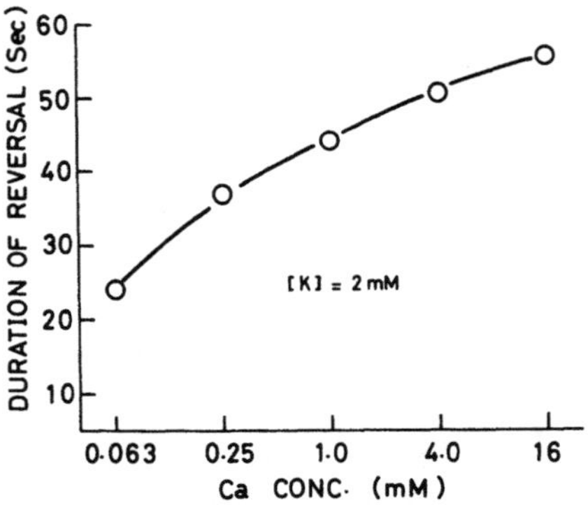

Figure 5. The influence of $[Ca^{2+}]$ in the equilibration medium on the duration of ciliary reversal.

in which P represents the binding site of Paramecium; $[PCa_{\frac{1}{2}}]$ represents the concentration of Ca bound by Paramecium; [PK] represents the concentration of K bound by Paramecium; $[K^+]$ and $[Ca^{2+}]$ represent the concentrations of K and Ca ions in the equilibrium medium; and k represents the equilibrium constant.

If it can be assumed that all the binding sites are filled with K and Ca, the total binding capacity of Paramecium, Pt, can be represented as:

$$Pt = [PK] + [PCa_{\frac{1}{2}}] \tag{3}$$

and the following expression for the amount of bound calcium can be derived from Eqs. (2) and (3):

$$[PCa_{\frac{1}{2}}] = Pt/kJa + 1 \tag{4}$$

in which Ja represents the ratio $[K^+]/[Ca^{2+}]^{\frac{1}{2}}$ in the equilibrium medium. By rearranging, Eq. (4) can be put in the form of a straight line:

$$1/[PCa_{\frac{1}{2}}] = kJa/Pt + 1/Pt \tag{5}$$

Equations (4) and (5) show that if Ja in the equilibrium medium is kept constant, the amount of bound Ca should remain constant, regardless of ionic concentrations in the medium. In order to test this prediction, the initial rapid binding of ^{45}Ca was determined in three equilibrium media having different concentrations but the same Ja value.

The results shown in Figure 2 indicate that the initial rapid phase uptake of ^{45}Ca by Paramecium was almost identical in each of these solutions. This is strong evidence for the applicability of the law of mass action to the equilibrium between Paramecium, Ca, and K ions, and saturation of the assumed binding sites with Ca and K ions.

Equation (5) implies that the reciprocal value of the amount of bound Ca must have a linear relationship with Ja in the equilibrium medium, the slope of which correlates with the value of k. In order to determine whether

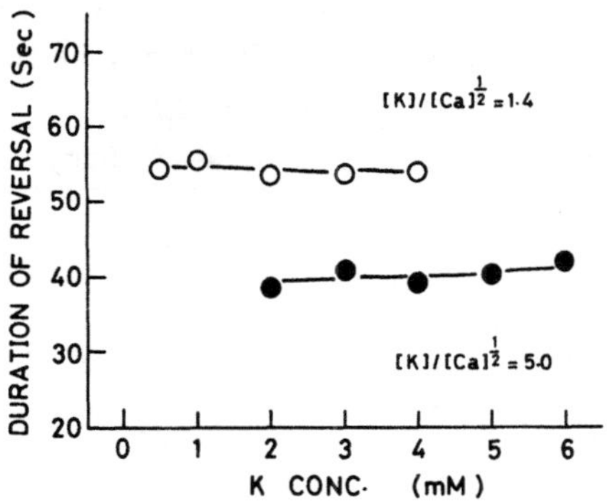

Figure 6. Antagonism between Ca^{2+} and K^{+} in the equilibration medium with regard to the duration of ciliary reversal.

cations other than K, such as Na, Rb, Mg, and Ba, compete for the same calcium–potassium binding sites, rapid ^{45}Ca uptake was measured in several media, each of which consisted of 1 mM $CaCl_2$ plus one of these ions in each of several concentrations. The reciprocal values of the radioactivities were plotted against the Ja value in each medium*. All the data showed linear relations with Ja, and each ion species gave a line with a different slope (Figure 3). All the lines crossed the ordinate at a point which corresponds to 1/Pt, as is expected from Eq. (5). These findings indicate that the law of mass action also applies to the equilibrium established between the binding sites, Ca ions and other ions used in the present experiments.

From the value of 1/Pt and the slope of each plot, k for each ion species was calculated, and listed in Table 1.

It is interesting to note here that these cations other than calcium having relatively high affinities, such as K, Rb, and Ba iduce prolonged ciliary reversal of Paramecium when applied externally, whereas the ciliary response to sodium is significantly shorter, and Mg, which has a very low affinity, does not induce ciliary reversal. These facts will be considered later in relation to the mechanism of reversal.

4. Ionic Control of Ciliary Reversal

In this series of experiments we examined several ionic factors which influence the duration of reversal. Our experimental results can be explained in terms of numbers of ions bound by Paramecium, and the change in that number.

A specimen was pipetted from an "equilibration medium" into a large volume of "stimulation medium". Duration of the reversed swimming in the stimulation medium was measured with a stop watch. Hereafter, this duration will be called "duration of reversal".

a) Ionic Factors in Equilibration Medium which Affect Duration of Reversal.

1. [K] changed at constant [Ca]. Specimens were equilibrated in a series of media containing 1 mM Ca plus K in several concentrations, then were

*The Ja values in the present case were calculated as [monovalent ion]/$[Ca^{2+}]^{1/2}$ or $[\text{divalent ion}]^{1/2}/[Ca^{2+}]^{1/2}$.

TABLE 1. Binding Affinities of Some Cations Relative to that of Calcium Ions to the Anionic Sites on Paramecium

Ionic species	Relative affinity
Sodium.	0.19
Potassium	0.35
Rubidium	0.28
Magnesium	0.033
Calcium.	1.0
Barium.	0.32

transferred into a stimulation medium which consisted of 20 mM K plus 1 mM Ca, and the duration of reversal determined. Duration of reversal was shorter when equilibration occurred in the media with the higher K concentration (Figure 4).

2. [Ca] changed at constant [K]. Specimens were equilibrated in 2 mM K plus Ca in several concentrations, then were transferred into a stimulation medium (20 mM K + 1 mM Ca). Reversal was shorter in the specimens equilibrated in the media with the lower Ca concentration (Figure 5). The effect of decreasing the Ca concentration in the equilibration medium was the same as that of increasing K.

3. Changes in [K] and [Ca] at constant $[K]/\sqrt{[Ca]}$. Specimens were equilibrated in a series of media of differing concentration but a constant ($[K]/\sqrt{[Ca]}$) and stimulated with 20 mM K + 1 mM Ca. As shown in Figure 6, the duration of ciliary reversal remained constant throughout. This indicates that the initial amount of bound ions on Paramecium is a major factor determining the duration of reversal induced by a subsequent stimulation. Specimens with more bound calcium (equilibrated in lower Ja) exhibit a reversal of longer duration.

b) Ionic Factors in Stimulation Medium Affecting Duration of Reversal.

Specimens were equilibrated in 1 mM K + 1 mM Ca, and were then transferred into stimulation media of different ionic compositions.

1. [K] changed at constant [Ca]. Equilibrated specimens were transferred into a series of 1 mM Ca plus K of several concentrations. Duration of reversal was longer in stimulation media of higher K concentration (Figure 7). A slight tendency to decrease in the duration with K concentrations higher than 40 mM is thought to result from deterioration of the specimen due to osmotic shrinkage.

2. [Ca] changed at constant [K]. Equilibrated specimens were transferred into a series of stimulation media which consisted to 20 mM K plus Ca of several concentrations. Duration of reversal increased with decreasing Ca concentration to about 0.33 mM (Figure 8). The effect of a decrease in [Ca] appears to be the same as that obtained with an increase in [K]. The duration of reversal, therefore, is dependent on the Ja value of the stimulation

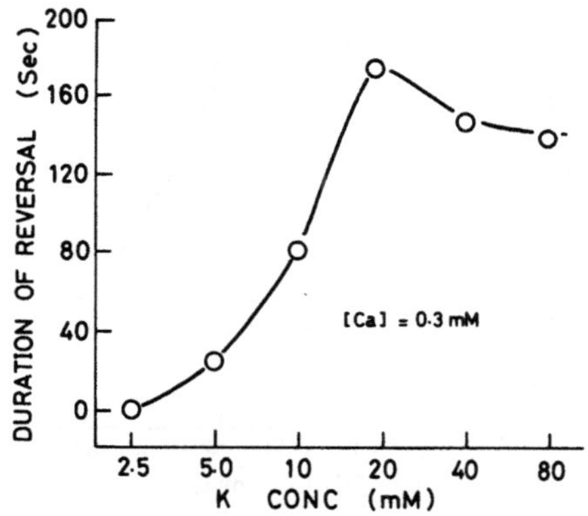

Figure 7. The influence of $[K^+]$ in the stimulation medium on the duration of ciliary reversal.

medium, being longer in media of larger Ja. In other words, the greater change in the amount of bound ions (decrease in bound Ca and increase in bound K) is responsible for the increased duration of reversal. The duration tended to decrease, however, with further (<0.33 mM) decrease in Ca concentration. In this range of Ca concentration the effect of Ca ions must be mediated by another mechanism than that which involves ionic binding.

3. [Ca] changes at constant $[K]/\sqrt{[Ca]}$ ratio. Determinations of reversal times were made in a series of stimulation media with a given $[K]/\sqrt{[Ca]}$ ratio (20) and different Ca concentrations ranging from 0.016 to 4 mM. The logarithm of the duration varies linearly with a logarithmic increase in Ca concentration (Figure 9). The duration, T, can be represented as:

$$T = T_1[Ca]_s^{a} \qquad (6)$$

Where $[Ca]_S$ is the Ca concentration (mM) in the stimulation medium; T_1 the duration of reversal at a $[Ca]_S$ of 1 mM; and a the slope of the logarthmic plot (=0.15 ± 0.01; mean of six measurements and its S.E.).

4. Various alkaline and alkaline earth metal salts. An increase in Ja value causes K ions to bind to anionic sites on Paramecium in exchange for equal mole equivalents of bound calcium to establish a new equilibrium dependent on the final Ja values. Is it liberation of Ca or the binding of K which is effective in initiating and sustaining ciliary reversal?

Solutions of 1 mM Ca plus 20 mM of various alkaline and alkaline earth metal salts ($NaCl$, KCl, $RbCl$, $MgCl_2$, and $BaCl_2$) were tested to determine to what extent they induce reversal.

The results shown in Table 2 indicate that reversal can be induced by monovalent cations (Na, Rb) other than K, and by Ba ions although the durations vary. Note that the duration of reversal such as K, Rb, and Ba (see Table 1) was significantly longer than that induced by the ions with low affinites, such as Na. Magnesium, which has a very low affinity, did not elicit

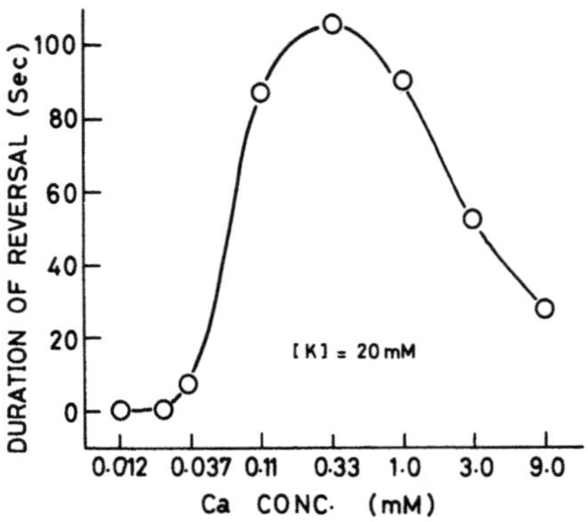

Figure 8. The influence of [Ca^{2+}] in the stimulation medium on the duration of ciliary reversal.

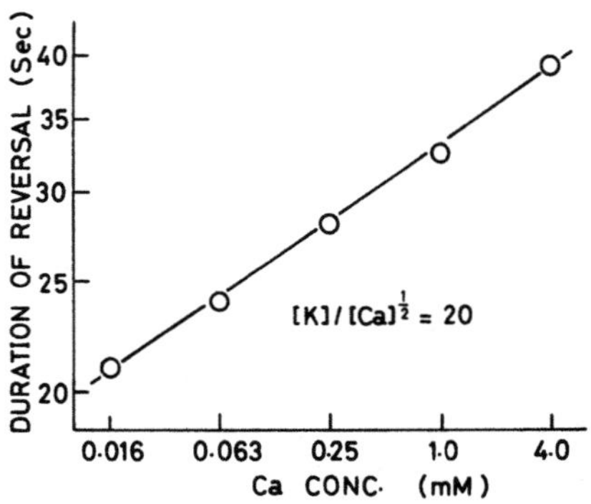

Figure 9. The influence of [Ca^{2+}] in the stimulation medium on the duration of ciliary reversal. The [K]/√[Ca] ratio of each stimulation medium was kept at 20.

reversal. The lack of ionic specificity in inducing ciliary reversal, and the common effect of these ions in displacing calcium from the anionic sites suggest that they evoke reversal by liberating calcium.

(c) Does Liberation of Divalent Cations Other than Ca^{2+} Cause Reversal?

Specimens were equilibrated in a series of media, which consisted of 1 mM Ca plus Ba in several concentrations, so that all the binding sites were filled by Ca or Ba. Specimens were then transferred to a stimulation solution rich in K (20 mM K + 1 mM Ca) to liberate Ba and Ca from the sites. If the liberated Ba ions induce reversal like Ca ions do, the duration of reversal might remain constant independent of the degree of the binding of Ba on the sites. However, the duration became shorter with an increase in bound Ba (Figure 10). Liberated Ba ions are apparently not as effective as calcium in inducing ciliary reversal. Magnesium cannot substitute for calcium either, for it has a very low affinity to the sites.

TABLE 2. Duration of Ciliary Reversal in Paramecium Elicited by Applications of 20 mM Alkaline and Alkaline Earth Metal Ions

Ion species	Na^+	K^+	Rb^+	Mg^{2+}	Ba^{2+}
Duration (sec)	2.0 ± 0.1	77.4 ± 1.9	72.4 ± 2.0	0	159.6 ± 1.7

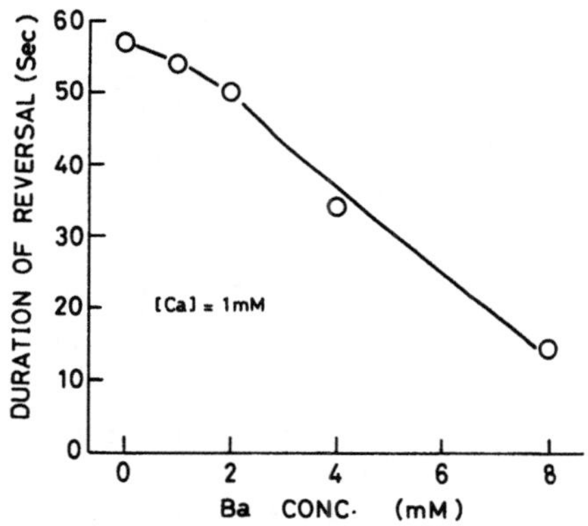

Figure 10. The influence of $[Ba^{2+}]$ in the equilibration medium on the duration of ciliary reversal.

(d) Quantitative Relations between the Duration of Reversal and $[K]/\sqrt{[Ca]}$ Ratios in Both Equilibration and Stimulation Media

The factors affecting the duration of ciliary reversal (T), as shown above, are the initial amount of calcium bound by the anionic sites ($[PCa_{\frac{1}{2}}]_i$) and final amount of calcium bound by the sites ($[PCa_{\frac{1}{2}}]_f$) after establishment of an equilibrium with the stimulation medium, providing the Ca concentration in the stimulation medium ($[Ca]_S$) is kept constant.

Five groups of specimens obtained from the same culture were equilibrated in five different media having different $[K]/\sqrt{[Ca]}$ ratios. Each was then stimulated by five different media of different $[K]/\sqrt{[Ca]}$ ratios but identical Ca concentration (1 mM)

The logarithm of the duration of ciliary reversal was plotted against the logarithm of the amount of change in the bound calcium associated with the transfer of the specimen from the equilibration medium to the stimulation medium. ($[PCa_{\frac{1}{2}}]$) were calculated from Eq. (2) by introducing the value of k(0.35) and Ja of both equilibration and stimulation media, and are given as percentage of the total binding capacity of Paramecium (Pt).

Figure 11 shows that log T is proportional to log ($[PCa_{\frac{1}{2}}]_i) - [PCa_{\frac{1}{2}}]_f$, and that the slope of this proportionality depends on $[PCa_{\frac{1}{2}}]_i$, being steeper at higher values of $[PCa_{\frac{1}{2}}]_i$. Each line was extrapolated to the abscissa and the values of the intercepts were plotted against $[PCa_{\frac{1}{2}}]_i$ in Figure 12. The logarithm of the intercept is related linearly to the logarithm of $[PCa_{\frac{1}{2}}]_i$, and the slope of this plot (b) is about 2.5. These findings, together with the relations in Eq. (6), can be related by the equation:

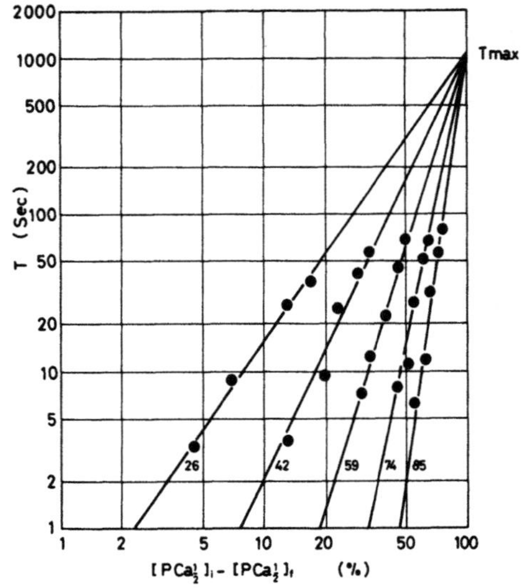

Figure 11. Relation between the duration of ciliary reversal (T in sec) and the difference between the initial ($[PCa\frac{1}{2}]_f$) amounts of bound calicum (as percentage of total binding capacity, P_t). Each straight line on the figure corresponds to a different initial amount of bound calcium, $[PCa\frac{1}{2}]_i$, as indicated in percentage of P_t by the numerals beside each line.

$$T = [Ca]_s^a \left(\frac{[PCa\frac{1}{2}]_i - [PCa\frac{1}{2}]_f}{c\,[PCa\frac{1}{2}]_i^b} \right)^{\frac{\log T_{max}}{\log \frac{P_t}{c.\,[PCa\frac{1}{2}]_i^b}}} \qquad (7)$$

in which the constant T_{max} is the maximum duration of cliary reversal (sec) for the maximum possible change in bound calcium (Pt); the constant C is a value of $(PCa\frac{1}{2}]_i - [PCa\frac{1}{2}]_f$ (percent of Pt) for a unit duration of reversal (1 sec) in specimens with a unit amount of bound calcium (1 percent of Pt); both constants are for a $[Ca]_s$ of 1 mM.

The values of both T_{max} and C were found to fluctuate, apparently according to the condition and age of the culture (T_{max}; 631-3160 sec, C; 5.1-30 $\times$ 10^{-4} percent). The duration of reversal under given conditions differed among groups of the specimens obtained from different cultures.

Although the physicochemical significance of this equation is presently unclear, it will be explored after the time course of bound calcium release in response to ionic stimulation has been investigated.

5. Orientation of Cilia in Response to ATP and Ca in Glycerol Extracted Specimens

The results of the preceding experiments suggest that calcium ions displaced from the anionic binding sites on paramecium may activate a contractile

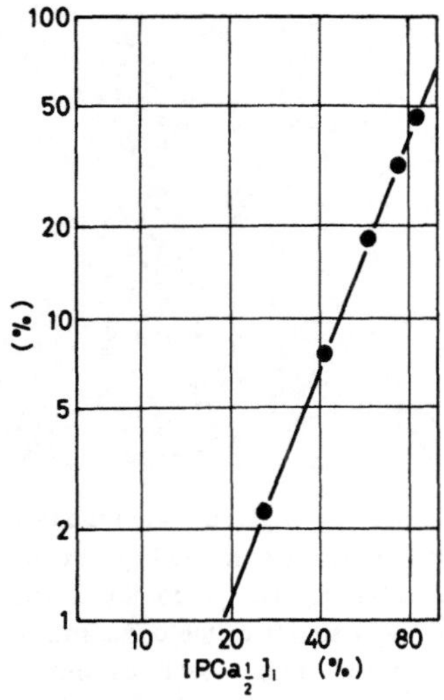

Figure 12. Relationship between value of $[PCa\frac{1}{2}]_i$ (abscissa) and the value of the intercept (ordinate) of each line with abscissa on Figure 11.

system which results in the reversal of the direction of ciliary beat. In order to test this hypothesis, the effects of Ca ions on the orientation of cilia were examined in glycerol-extracted Paramecia, in which the cell membrane is believed to be disrupted. The results show that reorientation of cilia, which is thought to be homologous with ciliary reversal in the live speciment, is caused by the addition of calcium, ATP, and a small amount of zinc.

Paramecia were extracted in a glycerol medium consisting of 50 percent (V/V) of glycerol, 50 mM KCl, 10 mM EDTA (4K-salt), and 10 mK Tris—HCl buffer (pH 7.4) for 10-15 days at −15°C. Serveral extracted specimens, washed with a solution containing 50 mM KCl buffered to pH 7.4 by 10 mM Tris—HCl buffer for at least 15 minutes, were pipetted into a large volume of test solution. This consisted of test substances plus the basic 50 mM KCl solution at 20° to 23°C. The specimens were then photographed, and the angle between the ciliary axis and the cell surface at the anterior aboral edge of the specimen was measured in the photographs.

(a) Reorientation Response

Figure 13 A is a photograph of a glycerinated Paramecium in 50 mM KCl solution (pH 9.0), showing the cilia pointing posteriorly, which approximates the orientation of beating cilia in the forward-swimming live specimens (Naitoh, 1966; Eckert and Naitoh, 1970). Preliminary experiments showed that with the addition of ATP (10 mM), calcium (10 mM), and zinc (0.1 mM) the cilia changed orientation to point more anteriorly. The position of cilia approximates the

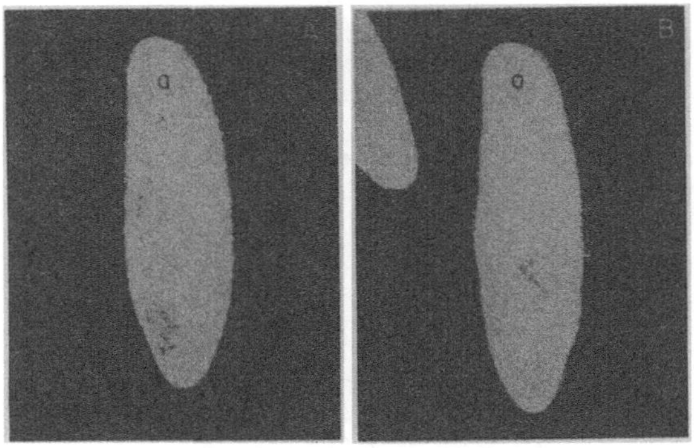

Figure 13. Photographs of glycerinated models of Paramecium caudatum. A, an extracted specimen suspended in 50 mM KCl solution. The predominant orientation of cilia is toward the posterior of the organism. B, a model after transfer into a mixture of ATP, calcium, and zinc. The cilia have become reoriented perpendicular to the cell surface or toward the anterior.

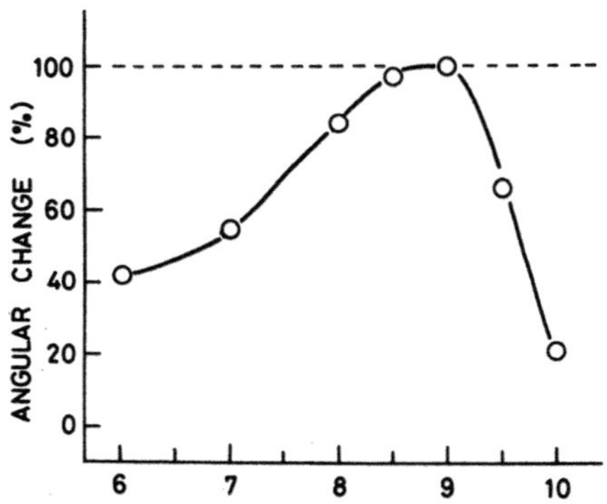

Figure 14. Effect of pH in a mixture of ATP, calcium, and zinc on the reorientation of cilia. Angular changes of ciliary axis in each test solution are plotted as percentage of the maximum change at pH 9.0.

orientation of cilia in a live backward-swimming specimen. This is shown in Figure 13 B.

(b) Influence of pH

The angular change of the ciliary axis in the presence of ATP, Ca, and Zn was determined in a series of media with pH varying from 6 to 10. The maximum angular change was obtained at pH 8.5-9.0.

The remaining experiments were all performed with the pH adjusted to 9.0 with 10 mM Tris–HCl buffer.

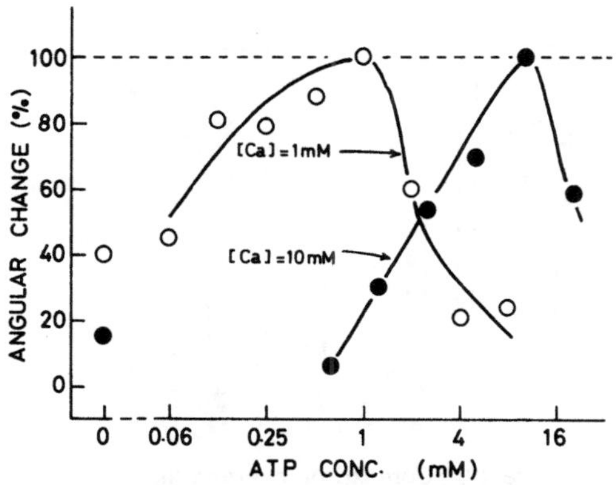

Figure 15. Effect of ATP concentration on the reorientation of cilia.

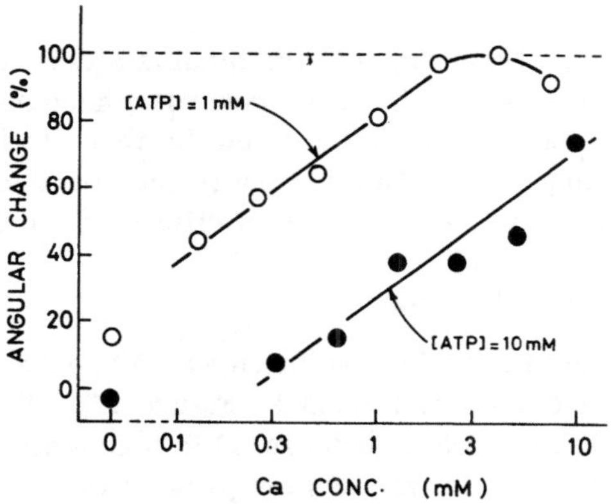

Figure 16. Effect of [Ca^{2+}] on the reorientation of cilia.

(c) Effect of ATP Concentration

Reorientation of the cilia was examined in two series of solutions with varying ATP concentration. The Ca concentration was 1 mM in one series and 10 mM in the other. The maximum response occurred at an ATP concentration which was dependent on the Ca concentration (Figure 15). The response increased with ATP concentration until the latter equalled the Ca concentration, and showed a decline with further increase in ATP.

(d) Effect of Ca Concentration

The degree of the angular change was examined in two series of test solutions with varying Ca concentration. ATP concentration was 1 mM in one series and 10 mM in the other series. The degree of the angular change increased with increased Ca concentration to a plateau in the 1 mM ATP series at approximately 4 mM Ca (Figure 16).

The degree of ciliary reversal in response to a cationic stimulus in live specimens is graded, being greater under conditions that cause a larger amount

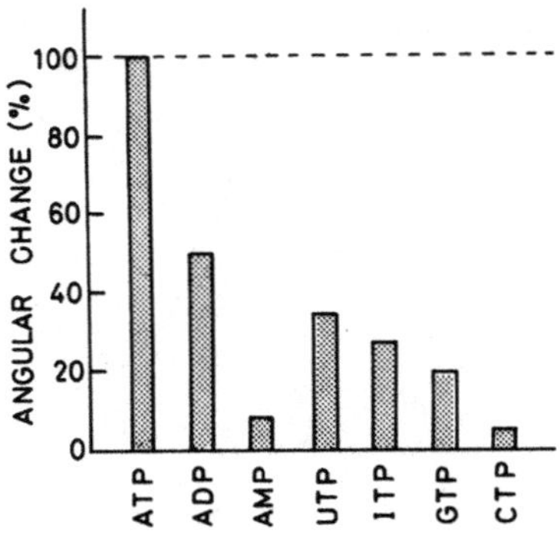

Figure 17. Comparison between the effects of various nucleotide phosphates on the ciliary reorientation response.

of calcium to be liberated from the cellular binding sites. Local concentration of liberated Ca ions near the inferred reversal mechanism of live specimen is assumed to depend, at least in part, on the rate at which calcium is released from the binding sites. This is consistent with the graded effect of calcium concentration on the reorientation of cilia in glycerinated specimens.

(e) Nucleotide Phosphates Other than ATP

The angular change in the ADP solution was 50 percent of that in ATP, while almost no response occurred in AMP (Figure 17). These results suggest that the energy-rich phosphate bond in ATP is essential for reversal, and that there is an adenylate kinase system present in the extracted Paramecium. UTP, ITP, GTP, and CTP showed only limited effectiveness.

(f) Effect of EDTA

The reorientation response was reduced in test solutions containing EDTA. This may be due to its chelation of calcium. Most interesting was the observation that cilia previously reoriented with an ATP–Ca–Zn mixture resumed their original posterior orientation when the extracted cells were washed with an EDTA solution. When the ATP-treated extracted cells were washed with 50 mM KCl solution, there was no effect on the orientation of their anteriorly pointing cilia. Furthermore, the extracted cells once treated with an EDTA solution, exhibited reorientation in response to the Ca–ATP –Zn test solution. Induction of the response and its subsequent reversal with EDTA could be repeated several times.

In live specimens ciliary reversal elicited by a cationic stimulus is always temporary. This suggests a relaxing system present in live specimens which acts to return the reversed cilia to the normal posteriorly pointing direction. This may be accomplished by chelation of calcium (and/or zinc) in a manner analogous to the effect of EDTA on the glycerinated specimen.

6. Proposal of "Calcium Hypothesis"

On the basis of these findings I propose the following hypothesis for the mechanism of ciliary reversal in response to cationic stimuli. Externally applied cations bind to the anionic sites in exchange for bound calcium according to the law of mass action. The Ca ions thus liberated are effective in activating, directly or indirectly, a mechanism energized by ATP, which results in the reversal of direction of effective beat of the cilia. The duration of reversal is thought to be correlated with the time between the onset of calcium release and the time when the rate of the calcium release (and hence the local concentration of free calcium near the contractile system) drops below a threshold level as the binding system approaches equilibrium with the medium. There may be a relaxing system which acts to return the reversed cilia to normal posteriorly pointing direction by chelating calcium from the ATP–Ca-activated contractile system.

The effect of Ca concentration on the duration other than that due to Ja factor may be due to an influence on the rate of diffusion of the liberated calcium into the external medium. The inhibition of ciliary reversal associated with low Ca concentration in the external medium, and the lack of the response in an EDTA solution can be explained as due to a decrease in the amount of liberated calcium available to activate the reversal mechanism because of increased leakage of the calcium into the Ca-poor external medium.

As is well known, the external application of calcium ions to live *Paramecium* never elicits ciliary reversal. It is not known why only those calcium ions liberated from the cellular binding sites activate the reversal system. One of the reasons may be a difference in the effective diameter of liberated and free Ca ions resulting from a difference in the degree of hydration.

7. Some Thoughts on the Coupling of the Electrical Behavior of the Membrane to Ciliary Reversal

Recent advances in electrophysiology of protozoans (cf. Eckert and Naitoh, 1970; Eckert, 1970) revealed that a depolarization or a hyperpolarization of the membrane occurred spontaneously or in response to certain stimuli in ciliates. The depolarization is always associated with reversal, while the hyperpolarization with an acentuation of ciliary orientation in normal direction, or inhibition of reversal. The mechanism by which the electrical events in the membrane are coupled to ciliary behavior is a matter of central interest. Does a depolarization of the membrane cause liberation of calcium from the anionic binding sites to induce ciliary reversal? It is noteworthy that effect of a depolarizing current in eliciting ciliary reversal is counteracted by a simultaneous increase in Ca concentration or decrease in K concentration of the medium. Conversely, the effect of an increase in K or a decrease in Ca concentration in eliciting reversal is diminshed by simultaneous application of a hyperpolarizing current (Nagahashi, 1964). It is probable that depolarization of the membrane, or an outward current through the membrane, may act to liberated calcium from the anionic binding sites, whereas a hyperpolarization, or an inward current, may act to accelerate the binding of calcium.

The question of whether a change in membrane potential associated with an increase in external Ja value has an effect on the degree of the resulting reversal is still unclear. In this regard it is interesting to note that transfer of the specimen into a medium with high Ja value always causes reversal even though the cationic strength of the medium is reduced so as to cause a hyperpolarization upon transfer. The duration of the ciliary reversal, however, is less than that elicited in a medium with the same Ja but more concentrated. This suggests that hyperpolarization antagonizes the effect of increased Ja. However, dilution of the medium brings about a decrease in Ca concentration which in itself acts to reduce the duration of reversal (Eq. (6)). Therefore, it remains unclear whether the effect of dilution to suppress the duration is due to hyperpolarization or to calcium deficiency.

REFERENCE

Eckert, R. (1972). This volume.

Eckert, R. and Naitoh, Y. (1970). J. Gen. Physiol. 55, 467.

Grebecki, A. (1964). Acta Protozool. 2, 69.

Grebecki, A. (1965). Acta Protozool. 3, 175.

Heilbrunn, L. V. (1952). An Outline of General Physiology. W. B. Saunders, Philadelphia.

Jahn, T. L. (1962). J. Cell. and Comp. Physiol. 60, 217.

Jennings, H. S. (1906). Behavior of the Lower Organisms. Columbia Univ. Press, New York.

Kamada, T. (1929). J. Fac. Sci. Univ. Tokyo. Sect. IV. Zool. 2, 123.

Kamada, T. (1938). Proc. Imp. Acad. Tokyo. 14, 260.

Kamada, T. (1940). Proc. Imp. Acad. Tokyo. 16, 241.

Kamada, T. and Kinosita, H. (1940). Proc. Imp. Acad. Tokyo. 16, 125.

Kinosita, H. (1954). J. Fac. Sci. Univ. Tokyo. Sect. IV. Zool. 7, 1.

Mast, S. O. and Nadler, J. E. (1926). J. Morphol. 43, 105.

Nagahashi, M. (1964). Zool. Mag. (Tokyo). 73, 355.

Naitoh, Y. (1958). Annot. Zool. Jap. 31, 59.

Naitoh, Y. (1961). Zool. Mag. (Tokyo). 70, 435.

Naitoh, Y. (1966). Science (Washington). 154, 660.

Naitoh, Y. (1968). J. Gen. Physiol. 51, 85.

Naitoh, Y. (1969). J. Gen. Physiol. 53, 517.

Naitoh, Y. and Eckert, R. (1968a). Z. vergl. Physiol. 61, 427.

Naitoh, Y. and Eckert, R. (1968b). Z. vergl. Physiol. 61, 453.

Naitoh, Y. and Eckert, R. (1969). Science (Washington). 166, 1633.

Naitoh, Y. and Yasumasu, I. (1967). J. Gen. Physiol. 50, 1303.

Okajima, A. and Kinosita, H. (1966). Comp. Biochem. Physiol. 19, 115.

Oliphant, J. F. (1938). Physiol. Zool. 11, 19.

Oliphant, J. F. (1942). Physiol. Zool. 15, 443.

Rees, C. W. (1922). Univ. Calif. Publ. Zool. 20, 333.

Taylor, C. V. (1920). Univ. Calif. Publ. Zool. 19, 403.

Wilson, J. A. and Wilson, W. H. (1918). J. Am. Chem. Soc. 40, 886.

Also see Naitoh, Y. and Kaneko, H. (1972). Reactivated Triton — extracted models of Paramecium: modification of ciliary movement by calcium ions. Science 176; 523-524 — J. Adler

BEHAVIORAL MUTANTS OF PARAMECIUM AURELIA

C. Kung
University of California,
Department of Biological Sciences,
Santa Barbara,
California 93106, U.S.A.

A Paramecium can be viewed as a eucaryotic organism capable of behavior, but it can also be regarded as a unicell comparable to excitable cells, such as hair cells, neurons, etc. in multicellular forms. The genetics of behavior in Paramecium aurelia makes use of both its organismic and cellular properties. The behavior of Paramecium directly reflects the state of the excitable membrane of the same cell with no compensation or other complication by other cells, as is possible in multicellular animals. As will appear, we succeeded in producing by mutation molecular lesions in this system of excitation. We have also begun to characterize the mutants electrophysiologically, thus raising the prospect of "dissecting" this system at a basic level and in a way which seems to be impossible or impracticable by other means.

Such study must rely on our knowledge of the behavior, the electrophysiology and the genetics of the subject organism. Fortunately, the wealth of information on protozoa in these three areas concentrates on the genus Paramecium.

Jennings chose Paramecium as the representative of infusoria in his monumental work Behavior of Lower Organisms (1906). It was on the basis of this study that his concept of an action system was formulated. The most important feature of the action system in Paramecium is the well-known avoiding reaction in which the animal swims backward, pivots on the posterior end and then resumes forward swimming, usually in a new direction. By a single avoiding reaction or a series of such reactions – trial and error, the animal may escape the stimulus which was the initial cause of the reaction. The avoiding reaction can be elicited by a large number of stimuli, e.g., obstacles, chemicals, temperature stress, etc. This reaction is stereotypic only in the sense that it occurs in various situations but not in the sense that the reaction is uniform. It is a misconception to think that Paramecium, and for that

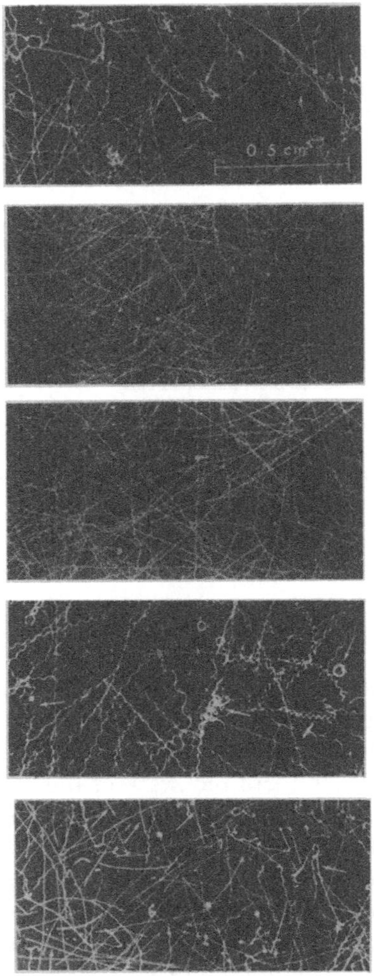

Figure 1. Swimming patterns of wild type and mutants of P. aurelia in a thin film of culture fluid.

Swimming patterns were recorded with the dark field macrophotographic method of Dryl (1958). Each white line is the trajetory by one animal in the 9 seconds of light exposure. The shutter of the camera was opened for 9 seconds immediately after the liquid film became steady. Since the animals had just been handled and were confined to the thin liquid film, these records actually show the behavior of different strains upon mild mechanical disturbances.

(A) Wild type animals of stock 51. Normal spiral course of forward movement. Arrows point to avoiding reactions.

(B) Fast of the first type. The fainter traces are partly due to their smaller bodies and partly to their higher speed. Notice also the lack of avoidance in this condition.

(C) Fast of the second type. Rapid movement is also recorded. Avoiding reactions, though present (arrow), are much less frequent than among normal animals.

(D) Pawn. Although many cells show wide spiralling or other more complicated trajectories (arrows), no avoidance is observed since no "kinks" are seen in the curves.

(E) Paranoiac. Besides the normal path and the transient reversals as in wild type, long distance backward swimming (continuous ciliary reversal, CCR (Grebecki, 1965) is recorded (arrows). CCR is registered as tight spirals due to the much more rapid rotation during the backward swimming.

matter, other ciliates and flagellates, behave identically when stimulated by different agents of any suprathreshold strength. Jennings has written:

> "The avoiding reaction varies greatly under different conditions, though its characteristic features are maintained throughout. But its different phases vary in intensity depending on circumstances. The backward movement may be long continued, or may last but a short time; or there may be merely a stoppage or slowing of the forward movement."

He also pointed out other variations of the avoiding reaction such as variations in the degree of swerving and rotation.

More recently, Grebecki (1965) has classified different modes of behavior of Paramecium. Besides the normal movement (NM) (= forward left spiralling (FLS)), three types of reactions, namely, periodic ciliary reversal (PCR), continuous ciliary reversal (CCR), and partial ciliary reversal (PaCR) have been recognized. His terminology and abbreviations are used throughout the rest of this article.

Our knowledge of the basic mechanism of normal ciliary beat is incomplete. In fact, the traditional doctrine of the form of the beat has recently been challenged by Kuznicki, Jahn, and Fonseca (1970). The works of Kamade and Kinosita (1940), Jahn (1962), Grebecki (1964), Naitoh and Yasumasu (1967), and Naitoh (1968) show that a system of ion exchange in the membrane controls the ciliary action and reaction. Ca^{2+} displaced from the anionic binding sites may activate the reorientation of cilia (Naitoh 1968) although the physical entity which directly controls the orientation is not yet identified. Information on the membrane properties and the correlation between the membrane state and behavior is accumulated by using intracellular microelectrodes. (Kamada 1934; Kinosita, Murakami, and Yasuda, 1965; Kinosita, Dryl, and Naitoh 1964a, b; Naitoh and Eckert 1968a, b). The reader is referred to the contributions of Drs. Dryl, Eckert, and Naitoh to this symposium for review and discussion of the behavior of Paramecium and its physiological bases.

The foundation of the genetics of Paramecium is our understanding of its life cycle and the discovery of mating types (Sonneborn 1937). Since the two gametic nuclei in conjugation are not direct products of meiosis but identical mitotic products of a haploid nucleus, the zygotic dipoloid nuclei in the two conjugants of a pair are necessarily identical. On the other hand, environments of the zygotic nuclei, such as the general cytoplasm, the cytoplasmic inclusions and cortical structures, of each exconjugant can be strictly controlled and identified. This, in combination with our ability to manipulate the nuclei (as in macronuclear regeneration), the cytoplasm (as in cytoplasmic transfer) and the cortex (as in cortical grafting), has proved most fruitful in our understanding of cytoplasmic inheritance (Beale, 1954; Sonneborn, 1959; Preer, 1970) and the more recent cortical genetics (Sonneborn, 1970). Autogamy (Diller, 1934; Sonneborn, 1939), an almost unique process of P. aurelia, also offers great advantages in genetic research. In this process the gametic nuclei (the mitotic products of a single haploid nucleus as in conjugation) fuse within one cell. Since the two gametic nuclei here are necessarily identical, autogamy is thus a one step jump to complete homozygosity. In other diploid organisms, a recessive trait can only result from crossing parents both carrying the corresponding genes. Bringing out recessive mutant traits in mutagenesis would usually require at least three generations. In P. aurelia, however, induced recessive mutations can be brought to expression by this easily controlled process of autogamy. This makes work on mutagenesis in P. aurelia almost as easy as in haploid organisms.

Previous work on the genetic control of motility and behavior in Paramecium has not been extensive. Cooper (1965) reported a case of a fast swimmer designated as "51-fast". Although this mutant occurred spontaneously in culture of stock 51 of P. aurelia and serotypic study also indicated its resemblance to stock 51, 51-fast would not mate with other stocks of the same syngen including 51. Cronkite (personal communication) using the technique of chemical induction of mating (Miyake, 1968) also could not induce

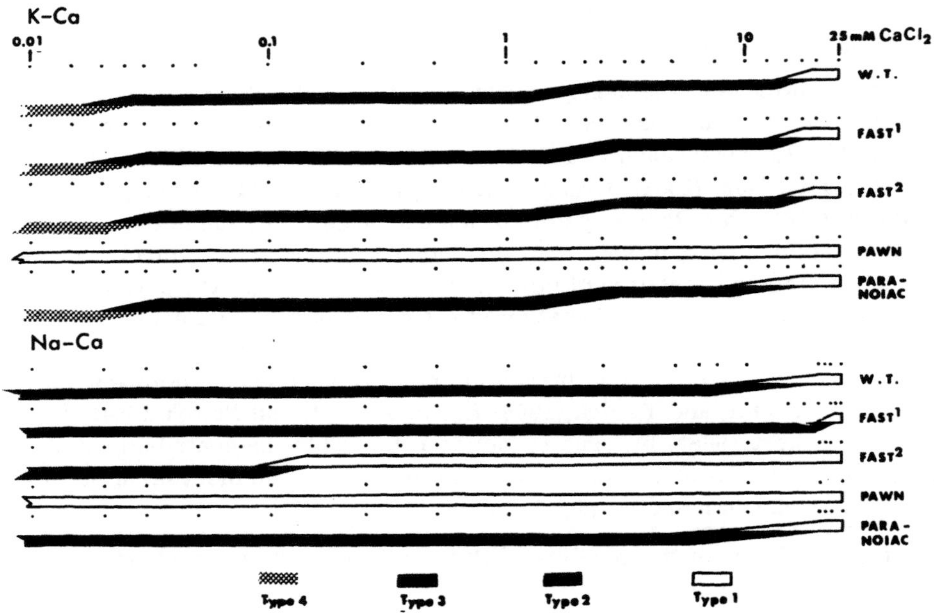

Figure 2. Broad Range Tests of K – Ca and Na – Ca Stimulation.

The increase of [Ca^{2+}] in the test solution is arranged from left to right on a logarithmic scale. [K^+] or [Na^+] decreases correspondingly to give a total concentration of 25 mM besides the 1 mM Tris (pH 7.2). The horizontal bars represent different types of reactions which occurred when cells were transferred from the equilibration medium into the test solution of the concentration covered by the bars. Each bar represents tests on a different strain, as labeled. W. T. stands for wild type. The points above the bars mark the concentrations actually tested. The upper group is the result of the K – Ca test and the lower that of the Na – Ca test.

The description of the typical reactions is given in the text.

mating involving 51-fast. Sonneborn and Schneller (unpublished) have also found a fast mutant which they have called "thin". Thin mated with great difficulty and the trait was found to be controlled by a pair of recessive genes.

In the following discussion of our recent work on behavioral genetics (Kung, 1969; 1971a, b) it will become apparent that it is possible to obtain mutants with altered behavior but with unimpaired motility. For the development of electrophysiology of the mutants see Kung and Eckert (1972).

Using the alkylating agent N-methyl-N-nitro-N'-nitroguanidine as mutagen, we have obtained different types of mutants including some with behavorial abnormalities. Mutagen was applied to populations that were ready to go into autogramy but still rapidly growing and thus synthesizing DNA. After the treatment, the populations were allowed to grow slightly and then autogamy was induced. Following a time-lag to permit genic expression, mutants were screened and isolated 5 to 10 fissions after the autogamy. The success of mutagenesis was shown by the high proportions of exautogamous deaths from lethal mutations – around 50 per cent in our experiments with 75 μg/ml, 1 hr. mutagen treatment.

Four types of mutants will be discussed here.

Fast of the First Type (Fast[1]). Like the 51-fast of Cooper (1965) mutants of this type swim rapidly forward, especially when they are mechanically disturbed. In cleared cerophyl medium (exhausted culture fluid) we have measured the speed at around 1.4 mm/sec as compared to around 0.6 mm/sec for the wild type. It is observed that the rapid forward movement is accompanied by a reduction of spontaneous reversal and reversal induced by the animals' bumping into the wall of the depression slide. Instead of backing up, the cells simply bounce off the wall at a small angle. This makes the animals tend to swim near the periphery of the vessel, as if racing in a circular track. This behavior can be induced in wild type in low $[X^+]/\sqrt{[Ca^{2+}]}$ medium (X^+ can be many cations other than Ca^{2+}, monovalent or not, see Jahn (1962) and Naitoh (1968)), such as pure $CaCl_2$ solution (Golinska 1963) but is not observed in culture media where Ca^{2+} is balanced by Na^+ and other cations. In wild type P. caudatum, both the rapid FLS and high external $[Ca^{2+}]$ are known to correlate with membrane hyperpolarization (Kinosita, Dryl, and Naitoh, 1964b). When the populations are left undisturbed for a long period of time, these mutants do slow down and even stop, but the forward speed, when observed, is still higher than the wild type. Genetic analyses have shown that either of at least two unlinked recessive genes give this phenotype. We have also found a few mutants of this type which, like 51-fast and thin, refuse to mate. Those which do mate do not differ from wild type in that respect and the genes segregate as expected.

Fast of the Second Type (Fast[2]). Like the fast[1], these mutants swim rapidly forward, especially when disturbed. In cleared cerophyl medium their speed was measured at around 1.2 mm/sec. Racing is also observed. There is a definite change in sensitivity to Na^+ stimulation. This can be easily demonstrated by the diagnostic test of introducing a small drop of animals in culture medium into Dryl's solution (4 mM Na^+, 1.5 mM Ca^{2+}). While the wild type or fast[1] would go through avoiding reactions which keep them confined temporarily in the area occupied by the drops introduced, the fast[2] ignores the boundary of the two media and spreads immediately into the Dryl's solution with rapid FLS. This is the same reaction one would see when wild type is introduced into a solution of relatively low $[X^+]/\sqrt{[Ca^{2+}]}$. To date, 5 mutant lines of this kind have been studied. The recessive mutant genes in all 5 cases were at the same locus and may be identical (perhaps even derived from the same induced mutation). At least 5 other lines with the same phenotype, found in different mutagenesis experiments have not yet been genetically examined. Austin (personal communication) has also found a fast mutant of this type, although the genic relationship to the locus found here has not yet been studied.

Pawn. These mutants swim around the periphery of the dish but the forward speed is not markedly different from that of the wild type. Their outstanding characteristic is their virtually complete lack of ciliary reversal. In situations where avoiding reactions are produced in wild type, such as bumping into abstacles, being jabbed at the anterior end or transferred into Dryl's solution, the pawns never avoid. FLS is the only mode of behavior seen. The insensitivity is not just to Na stimulation, as in fast[2], but also to

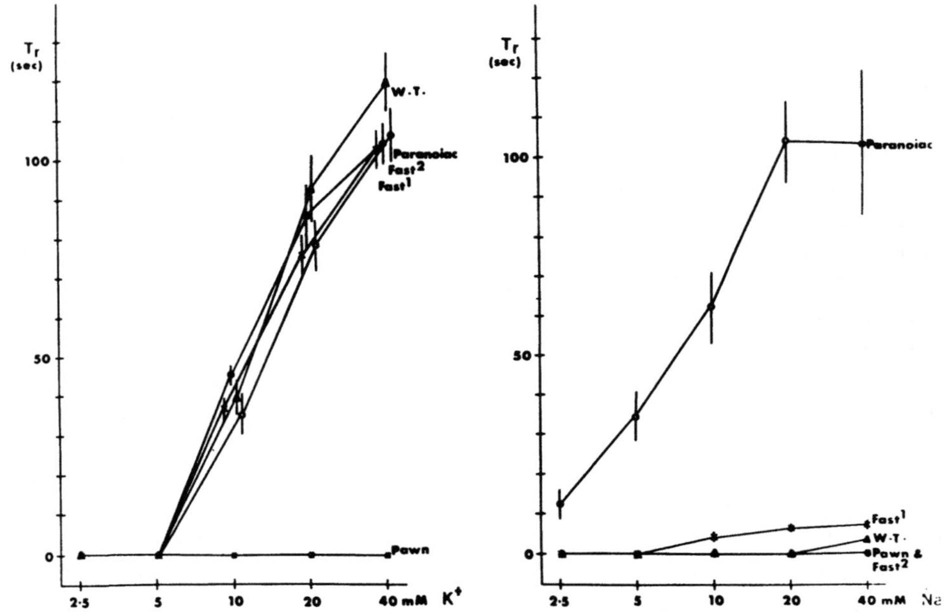

Figure 3. Duration of ciliary reversal (T_r) in relation to the concentrations of the test solution.

The ordinates measure the duration of ciliary reversal (T_r) in seconds upon transfer of the animals from the equilibration medium to the test solutions. The test solutions consist of 1 mM Tris (pH 7.2), 0.3 mM $CaCl_2$ and various amounts of KCl or NaCl. The concentration of K^+ or Na^+ is plotted on a logarithmic scale in the abscissae. Each point represents the mean of 25 measurements (from 5 separate experiments) of the strain of animals marked. The 95 per cent confidence intervals are given together with the means. Some of the points in the K – Ca test are slightly displaced to show clearly the confidence intervals.

K and Ba stimulation. When transferred from culture medium to 8 mM KCl and 0.3 mM $CaCl_2$ for instance, they spread with FLS while wild type, fast^1 and even fast^2 will avoid. In extreme $[X^+]/\sqrt{[Ca^{2+}]}$ jumps, however, very weak avoidance or transient slowing of the FLS can be observed in some cases. All pawns can orient in the electric field and migrate toward the cathode. Reversing the polarity of the field causes 180° turning as in wild type. Increasing current decreases forward velocity and increases the amplitude of the spiral as in wild type, although quantitative measurements have not been carried out. The Ludloff pheomenon of cathodal ciliary reversal probably occurs in the pawns. In starved cultures especially, many more cells which swim in wide spirals are observed. The reason for the wide spiralling is not yet understood.

So far, two unlinked loci for this trait have been identified. The pawn genes at both loci are recessive. One of the loci has at least two detectably different alleles besides the wild type allele. One of these alleles is more "leaky" than the other.

Paranoiac. Instead of being hypo-sensitive or insensitive to stimuli, the paranoiacs over-react. Spontaneous long distance backward swimming

(CCR) is observed sporadically in the culture while normal forward swimming and short avoiding reactions are seen as in the wild type. Mechanical disturbance of the container increases the proportion of backward swimming cells in the culture. Upon transfer to Dryl's solution, the paranoiacs spread immediately into the Dryl's solution by backward swimming (CCR) instead of by the forward movement (FLS) characteristic of fast[2] and pawn under such conditions. This reaction seems to be Na^+ specific, Ethologicall, CCR only appears in wild type under harmful conditions and is never observed in mild disturbances, let alone in the normal environment. Experimentally, CCR can be induced in wild type by transfer to a high $[X^+]/\sqrt{[Ca^{2+}]}$ solution.

Although more than 5 paranoiac lines have been examined, to date only one locus has been found at which the genes produced this interesting phenotype. Other mutant lines which react more strongly to the transfer from culture medium to Dryl's solution but not as strongly as the paranoiac have also been found. One of these was isolated and studied by Austin (personal communication) and was found to be controlled by a recessive gene pair.

The patterns of behavior in culture medium were recorded by the method of Dryl (1958). Figure 1 gives the patterns of the wild type and the 4 types of mutants mentioned.

To test the reactions to K and Na stimulation more carefully, animals are adapted to an equilibration medium of 1 mM KCl, 1 mM $CaCl_2$ 1 mM Tris at pH 7.2 (Naitoh, 1968). Reactions to transfer into test media are observed. The test media are a series of solutions of various amounts of $CaCl_2$ and KCl or NaCl equal to a total concentration of 25 mM besides 1 mM Tris buffer. Four types of immediate reactions can be recognized. They are: Type 1, immediate dispersal with rapid forward movement (FLS); Type 2, repeated short avoiding reactions comparable to PCR although the reactions fade into FLS later; Type 3, dispersal by backward movement (CCR), and Type 4, jerking and whirling in place which lasts for some time with the appearance of PaCR in some cases. CCR can be distinguished very easily from FLS by its much tighter spiral.

Tests on representatives of all 4 mutant types as well as the wild type are summarized in Figure 2. In the K–Ca tests, all strains except the pawn showed the same sequence of transition from type 1 through type 4 with corresponding regions of overlap as the concentration of Ca^{2+} decreases. The regions of overlap in all strains except the pawn are almost the same. The pawn, however, failed to react in any of the ways involving ciliary reversal, giving the type 1 (FLS) response throughout the whole range of K–Ca concentrations tested. In the Na–Ca tests, only type 1 and 2 reactions are observed in wild type, although CCR can be induced with Na–Ca solutions if the cells are adapted differently. Fast[1] gives similar responses although the zone of transition between the types of reaction is shifted slightly. Fast[2] changes from reaction type 1 to type 2 at a region of about 100-fold less Ca^{2+} (with the corresponding increase in Na^+). This means that the threshold for ciliary reversal in terms of stimulation by $[Na^+]/\sqrt{[Ca^{2+}]}$ changes is greatly increased. As in the K–Ca

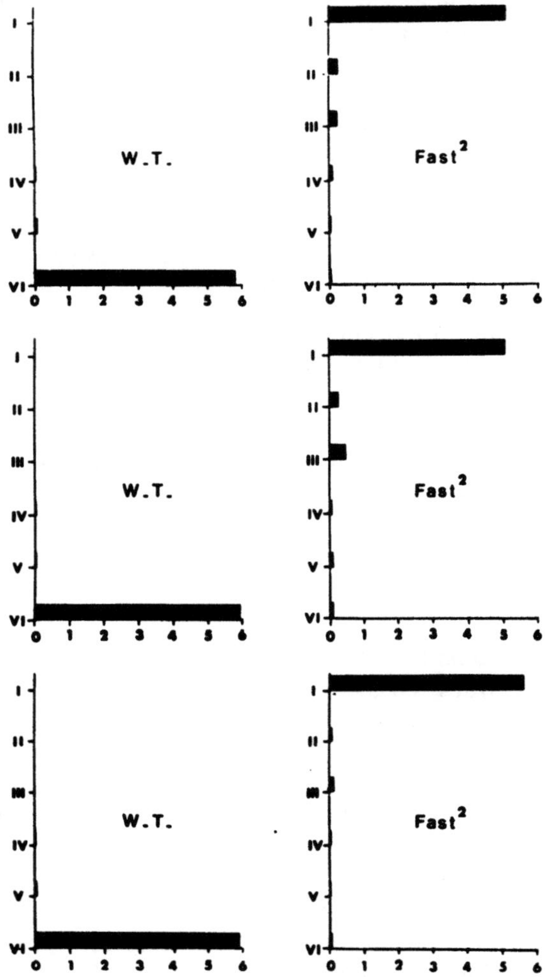

Figure 4. Distributions of animals in vertical column.

Each histogram shows the result of an experiment done with the strain marked (see text). The bars represent the relative densities of animals at 6 different levels, I to VI, from top to bottom, as arranged in the ordinate. A unit in the abscissa represents the average density measured. All bars in each histogram add up to 6 units. For description of the experiments, see the text, and Kung (1971a).

tests, pawn gives only FLS in the Na–Ca tests. The paranoiac begins ciliary reversal at about the same concentration of Na–Ca as the wild type, but instead of short PCR, CCR (type 3 reaction) is induced. This indicates that there is no change in the threshold of induction of ciliary reversal but that the turn off mechanism for the excited state is affected by the genic mutation.

When the ciliary reversal (backing) is induced by transferring the animals from equilibration medium to test media, the duration of backward swimming can be measured by a stop watch (Kamada and Kinosita, 1940; Brebecki, 1964; Naitoh, 1968). Figure 3 summarizes the results of tests on different strains of P. aurelia in a manner similar to Naitoh (1968). The results quantitatively verify the finding noted above. Within the range of K–Ca stimulation tested, the tendency to increase the duration of ciliary reversal with the increase of $[K^+]/\sqrt{[Ca^{2+}]}$ (here the $[Ca^{2+}]$ is fixed at 0.3 mM) is similar in the wild type, the two types of fast and the paranoiac. No reversal is observed in the pawn. The same experiments using Na–Ca test solutions give no reversal for pawn and fast^2, very short durations of ciliary reversal for wild type and fast^1 in high $[Na^+]/\sqrt{[Ca^{2+}]}$. The paranoiac stands out clearly as overreacting to the Na^+ stimulation. The duration of ciliary reversal increases to a plateau with the increase of $[Na^+]/\sqrt{[Ca^{2+}]}$ of the test solutions.

It is also interesting that animals engaged in strong avoiding reactions are unable to orient in space. Depending on the reactions of the strain of paramecia upon transfer from one medium to another, there can be observable differences in their negative geotaxis. This can be tested by injecting the animals into the bottom of a glass manifold filled with test solution and with side-arms at different vertical levels leading to recipient syringes. After a given time, samples at different levels of the liquid column are withdrawn simultaneously into syringes and the contents are examined. Results of representative experiments of the sort are given in Figure 4. Here, samples are taken from 6 levels of the manifold (I to VI, top to bottom) at 30 cm intervals 5 minutes after injecting the animals (in cerophyl medium) into the bottom of the test solution (20 mM NaCl, 0.3 mM $CaCl_2$ and 1 mM Tris, pH 7.2) filled to 2.5 cm above side arm number I. Although there are small differences among tests with the same strain of animals, due mainly to the differences in the disturbances caused by the injections themselves, the results show clearly that the wild type is unable to carry out is upward movement upon such transfer and thus aggregates at the bottom of the liquid column, while fast^2, being unable to react to Na–Ca changes with ciliary reversal, finishes the geotactic migration to the top of the column within 5 minutes. Studies using pawns instead of fast^2 reveal a pattern similar to the fast^2 pattern here.

The difference between certain mutants and the wild type with respect to their ability to migrate upward upon transfer from the culture medium to a solution with high $[Na^+]/\sqrt{[Ca^{2+}]}$ was successfully exploited as a method of screening for mutants. In these screenings the population which is descended from the mutagen treated cells is injected into the bottom of a column of solution, and a small fraction of solution at the top is drawn out after a given time. Single cell isolations are made of all cells which successfully swim upward and appear in this top fraction, and each line derived from such isolations is examined later for its phenotype. In one set of experiments, where the top fractions were collected 6.5 min after cells on the order of 10^5 were injected into a column of 20 mM NaCl, 0.3 mM $CaCl_2$, and 1 mM Tris (pH 7.2), we found 11 fast or pawn mutant lines out of a total of 78 isolations. Control with no selection gave no mutant lines out of 600 isolations. (See Kung (1971b) for a detailed description.) It is therefore clear that we can obtain fractions much enriched with fast and pawn mutants using columns in this manner.

Crossing between mutants of different types reveals a system of epistasis as follows:

$$\text{pawn} > \text{fast}^2 > \text{fast}^1 = \text{paranoiac}$$

That is to say, the double mutants with the genes for both pawn and fast^2 or fast^1 will give the phenotype of pawn in diagnostic tests and the double mutants with the genes for fast^2 and fast^1 give the phenotype of fast^2. This is readily understandable since pawns are more drastically mutated (more insensitive) than fast^2, whereas fast^1 is least affected by mutation as shown in the diagnostic tests. The above sequence also depicts the epistasis of pawn and fast^2 over paranoiac. Why the effect of the gene for paranoiac is masked by the presence of those of pawn or fast^2, though not immediately apparent, can be explained by our previous analysis of the phenotypes (Figure 3). If the above study with one kind of equilibration medium is representative, the defect caused by the genetic lesions in paranoiac is not hyper-sensitivity but over-reaction. In a state of hypo- or insenstivitiy caused by the genes for fast^2 or pawns, reaction (ciliary reversal) to the test solutions simply does not occur. The defect in paranoiac involving the shutting off of excitation that cannot be initiated can therefore not be observed. It is important to point out that the epistatic relations refer only to the reaction to the transfer to a few test solutions and do not necessarily mean the absence of gene action for other possible aspects of the phenotype not expressed in these tests. No epistasis between fast^1 and paranoiac is observed.

Since all the mutants discussed can swim forward at normal or even accerlerated speeds, the structure for motility may have been unimpaired. Preliminary electron microscopic study of sectioned material shows no observable defects in the pellicular and ciliary structure (Dippell and Grimes, personal communication). Thus these mutants are basically different from the motility mutants in Chlamydomonas reinhardi (Randall, 1969). Moreover, most, if not all, mutants can reverse their ciliary beat and exhibit the state of excitation, although the threshold for excitation may be pushed far off the physiological range, as in the case of fast^2. If the correlation between membrane depolarization (excitation) and ciliary reversal and the correlation between hyperpolarization (inhibition) and augmentation of normal beat (rapid FLS) observed in wild type P. caudatum (Kinosita, Dryl, and Naitoh 1964a, b; Kinosita, Murakami, and Yasuda, 1965) are also true in the mutants of P. aurelia, we seem to have here genic mutants with altered membrane structure and excitability. Genic mutations affecting membrane permeability to cations, and thus the resting state, are known in erythrocytes of sheep (Tosteson and Hoffman, 1960), in Neurospora (Slayman and Tatum, 1965) and in Escherichia coli (Damedian and Solomon, 1964). None of these cases, however, has been shown to be directly related to an excitatory function. It is conceivable that the genic mutations in the behavioral mutants in P. aurelia have caused alterations in the macromolecular structure of the cell membrane so that the anionic sites have altered affinities to different cations, or that they have changed the protein structure affecting the permeabilities to various cation species in a more direct way. Recent electrophysiological studies showed that, in the case of a pawn mutant, the crucial membrane component responsible for the voltage-sensitive increase in calcium conductance was impaired by the mutation. For this development and updated discussion, see Kung (1971a, b) and Kung and Eckert (1972).

The convergence of genetical, physiological, and behavioral studies on a unicellular organism with many experimental advantages offers opportunities for understanding the excitable system in this organism as well as the problem of excitation in general.

ACKNOWLEDGMENT

I am grateful to Prof. T. M. Sonneborn for his advice and encouragement during the course of this study and his review of this manuscript.

This work was supported by contract COO-235-69 from the AEC and grant GM-15, 410-03 of USPHS to T. M. Sonneborn, and is contribution No. 844 from the Zoology Department, Indiana University.

REFERENCES

Beale, G. H. (1954). The Genetics of Paramecium aurelia. Cambridge University Press, London.
Cooper, J. (1965). J. Protozool. 12, 381.
Damedian, R. and Soloman, A. K. (1964). Science 145, 1327.
Diller, W. F. (1934). Science 79, 57.
Dryl, S. (1958). Bull. Acad. Polonaise Sci. 6, 429.
Golinska, K. (1963). Acta Protozool. 1, 113.
Grebecki, A. (1964). Acta Protozool. 2, 69.
Grebecki, A. (1965). Acta Protozool. 3, 275.
Jahn, T. L. (1962). J. Cell. Comp. Physiol. 60, 217.
Jennings, H. S. (1906). Behavior of Lower Organisms. Indiana University Press, Bloomington.
Kamada, T. (1934). J. Exp. Biol. 11, 94.
Kamada, T. and Kinosita, H. (1940). Proc. Imp. Acad. (Tokyo) 16, 125.
Kinosita, H., Dryl, S., and Naitoh, Y. (1964a). J. Fac. Sci. U. Tokyo, Section 4. 10, 291.
Kinosita, H., Dryl, S., and Naitoh, Y. (1964b). J. Fac. Sci. U. Tokyo, Section 4. 10, 303.
Kinosita, H., Murakami, A., and Yasuda, M. (1965). J. Fac. Sci. U. Tokyo, Section 4. 10, 421.
Kung, C. (1969). J. Cell Biol. 43, 75a.
Kung, C. (1971a) Z. vergl. Physiologie. 71, 142.
Kung, C. (1971b) Genetics. 69, 29.
Kung, C. and Eckert, R. (1972). Proc. Nat. Acad. Sci., Wash. 69, 93.
Miyake, A. (1968). J. Exp. Zool. 167, 359.
Naitoh, Y. (1968). J. Gen. Physiol. 51, 85.
Naitoh, Y. and Eckert, R. (1968a). Z. vergl. Physiol. 61, 427.
Naitoh, Y. and Eckert, R. (1968b). Z. vergl. Physiol. 61, 453.
Naitoh, Y. and Eckert, R (1969). Science 166. 1633
Naitoh, Y. and Yasumasu, I. (1967). J. Gen. Physiol. 50, 1303.
Preer, J. R., Jr. (1969). In Research in Protozoology, ed. by T. T. Chen, Vol. 3, Pergamon Press, New York, p. 129.
Randall, J. (1969). Proc. Roy. Soc. B173, 31
Slayman, C. W. and Tatum, E. L. (1965). Biochim. biophys. Acta 109, 184.
Sonneborn, T. M. (1937). Proc. Nat. Acad. Sci., Wash. 23, 378.
Sonneborn, T. M. (1939). Anat. Rec. 75, 85.
Sonneborn, T. M. (1959). Adv. Virus Res. 6, 229.
Sonneborn, T. M. (1970). Proc. Roy. Soc. London. B176, 347.
Tosteson, D. C. and Hoffman, J. F. (1960). J. Gen. Physiol. 44, 249.

THE BEHAVIOR OF AMOEBAE

R.D. Allen and M. Haberey
State University of New York at Albany,
Department of Biological Sciences,
Albany,
New York 12203, U.S.A.

The amoeba is said to be one of the simplest organisms to show behavior. By this I mean that its spontaneous activity is modified and modulated by changes in the environment. It responds adaptively to various kinds of physical and chemical stimuli and wages battle with both predators and prey. The behavior of amoebae is a subject about which far too little is known, but I shall try to summarize what knowledge we have and point out some interesting unsolved problems.

It is unfortunate that the heyday of behavioral studies on amoebae occurred in the early days of this century, because many of the observations were reported before it was learned that the cultures used were of mixed species. At that time, too, very little was known about amoeba physiology. Nevertheless, papers of that period are fascinating to read, because biology was changing from a vitalistic phase to a more enlightened era in which physics and chemistry were expected to lead to an understanding of most if not all biological processes.

The fundamental question at the time Jennings (1904) published his monumental work on the behavior of lower organisms was whether phenomena as complex as amoeboid movement and phagocytosis could be explained in terms of physics and chemistry. It was clear even earlier that the behavior of amoebae could not be understood without a knowledge of how pseudopods extend and retract, and how these events are coordinated in the normal locomotion process. The incompleteness of our present knowledge of amoeba behavior is still attributable to uncertainties regarding these fundamental aspects of amoeboid movement.

1. Mechanisms of Pseudopod Extension and Retraction

In the 1870's the physical chemist, Quincke suggested that pseudopodial movements might result from surface tension acting at the surface of cells.

This concept found fertile ground in the minds of several influential German biologists, notably Berthold, Bütschli, and Rhumbler (see De Bruyn, 1947 for an excellent historical review). These authors not only worked out elaborate and plausible theories predicting cytoplasmic streaming patterns resembling those in amoebae, but performed ingenious model experiments with droplets of inanimate fluids demonstrating that such motions could result from surface tension forces.

One of the most remarkable experiments was that of Bernstein (1900), who placed a mercury droplet and a potassium bichromate crystal on opposite sides of a dish containing concentrated nitric acid. For reasons as obvious then as now, the mercury drop migrated across the dish and "phagocytized" the crystal. Brilliant as this model experiment was, it failed to mislead several observant biologists, among them Jennings (1904) and Dellinger (1906), who were more impressed by the fact that the actual patterns of movement in amoebae were not as predicted by surface tension theories. Nevertheless, surface tension theories were still discussed almost a generation after the evidence was on hand to lay them to rest (Cf. Tiegs, 1925).

Almost every case of flow encountered in the inanimate world results from a gradient in hydrostatic pressure. It was therefore natural that pressure gradients would be invoked as an explanation for cytoplasmic streaming in the amoeba. In fact, the suggestion first came from Ecker (1849) and was the "accepted" explanation of amoeboid movement when the surface tension theories were proposed. The pressure gradient theory passed out of vogue to return cloaked in the terminology of colloid chemistry as the "sol–gel theory".

Pantin (1923) and Mast (1926) presented in slightly different forms the idea that a pressure gradient arose by contraction of the ectoplasmic tube in the tail (and retracting pseudopods) of an amoeba. Mast in particular described and interpreted the details of amoeboid movement in Amoeba proteus in terms of this model. Unfortunately, he neglected to describe several interesting facets of amoeba behavior which invalidated his model!

The pressure gradient theory (also called the sol–gel–, tail contraction–, and "toothpaste tube" theories) became untenable when it failed to account for the behavioral pattern of Amoeba proteus and Chaoss carolinensis (Allen, 1961 a, 1961 b) and for the behavior of cytoplasm removed from amoebae (Allen, Cooledge, and Hall, 1960). It is interesting to note that Rinaldi and Jahn (1963) and Jahn (1964) have revived the pressure gradient theory under a new name ("the contraction-hydraulic theory"). These authors have simply disregarded a large body of behavioral and experimental evidence invalidating the pressure gradient model, in whatever form it may appear.

In 1961 I proposed a radically different model to account for pseudopod extension in the Amoeba–Chaos group of large, free-living amoebae, based on the well-known contractile properties of amoeba cytoplasm (Allen, 1961 b). Contraction was postulated to occur continuously at pseudopod tips, pulling the viscoelastic endoplasm forward, where each portion of it would in turn contract and gelate while everting to form the ectoplasmic tube.

Whether or not it was substantially correct, the frontal contraction model considerably simplified the understanding of many facets of amoeba behavior. The functional independence of individual pseudopodia in polypodial specimens, for example, became readily understandable. So did the tendency of all reversals (and re-reversals) to be initiated at the new pseudopodial tip. These and other basic aspects of amoeba behavior had been so troublesome to proponents of various versions of the pressure gradient theory that they tended to be disregarded or explained by complicated assumptions, such as the passage of invisible waves of contraction over the ectoplasmic tube.

The only value of a model is that it has predictions that can be tested. The most important predictions of the frontal contraction model have been tested and confirmed. For example, a cycle of birefringence changes has been recorded in advancing pseudopod tips. In this experiment, the amoeba's own cytoplasm has been used as a photoelastic strain transducer to detect tensile and compressive forces acting in just the regions predicted by the model (Allen, Francis, and Nakjima, 1965). The hyaline cap has been shown to consist of a low-refractive index syneretic fluid (Allen, Cowden, and Hall, 1962), squeezed from the region where the cytoplasm contracts into the hyaline cap (Allen and Francis, 1965). The endoplasm shows strong birefringence when stretched by sucking it with a micropipette, showing that it has sufficient viscoelastic "structure" to transmit forces (Francis and Allen, 1971). Taken together, these experimental data and the behavioral complexity of amoebae constitute strong evidence that pseudopods extend (and cytoplasm streams into them) due to forces generated by contraction near their tips.

The preciding statement does not, however, eliminate the possibility that pressure might play an auxilliary role in amoeboid movement by forcing endoplasm out of retracting pseudopodia. Seravin (1967) has suggested that at least two mechanisms might be operating: contraction at pseudopod tips for pseudopod extension, and contraction in the tail and in retracting pseudopodia to empty them of endoplasm.

The only way to test this hypothesis is to apply a reverse pressure gradient and find out whether the direction of streaming reverses. Early attempts at influencing streaming inside the cell by externally applied pressure were not designed to measure the pressure difference required to reverse the entire column of cytoplasm from a retracting to an advancing pseudopod (Allen and Roslansky, 1959; Kamiya, 1964). A way to approach this question was suggested in an experiment of Kanno reported by Professor Tohru Abé (Allen and Kamiya 1964, p. 457). Kanno inserted a micropipette into the tail of an Amoeba proteus and sucked a significant volume of cytoplasm from the tail without reversing the direction of movement. Allen, Francis and Zeh (1971) applied pressure reductions of 30-35 cm of water by placing a glass capillary around a retracting Chaos pseudopod and found no reversal of the streaming of cytoplasm into advancing pseudopodia. Cytoplasmic streaming thus cannot be the result of a positive pressure gradient. No advantage is seen at this time of invoking hydrostatic pressure, even as an auxilliary mechanism, until some valid evidence is offered in its support (see review by Allen, 1972).

It is necessary at this point to introduce a word of caution: at the beginning we spoke of "the amoeba" as if amoebae differed only in insignificant detail. As far as mechanisms of movement and behavior are concerned, the situation is not so simple. Significant differences exist. For example, the giant herbivorous amoeba, Pelomyxa palustris behaves as if tailored to the specifications of a proponent of the pressure gradient theory (Griffin, 1964). Its behavior is correspondingly simple, and entirely unlike that found in the carnivorous giant amoebae, which we refer to as the Amoeba–Chaos group. The testacean (shelled amoeba), Difflugia appears to extend pseudopodia in the same manner as the carnivorous amoebae, but in addition has a striking mechanism for rapid and forcible pseudopod refraction. It lays down bundles of microfilaments in the cytoplasm parallel to the pseudopod axis. These contract rapidly and perform considerable mechanical work in transporting the heavy shell (Wohlman and Allen, 1968). The numerous smaller genera of amoebae are so diverse as to their structure, movement, and behavior (Cf. Bovee, 1964) that it is unprofitable to generalize about the mechanisms or even the details of amoeboid behavior. Because of the apparent diversity in mechanisms of amoeboid movement (Cf. Allen, 1968), my comments on the behavior of amoebae will be limited to some generalizations about the Amoeba –Chaos group.

2. Basic Behavior Patterns

The amoeba changes its form so actively that it is sometimes difficult to distinguish response patterns from "spontaneous" activity. Perhaps the most interesting attempt to ascertain what is really basic about amoeboid movement is that of Seravin (1966), who inhibited movement by both physical and chemical means, and then allowed amoebae to reorganize under continuous observation. The stages in progressive resumption of normal movement were almost the exact reverse of the stages of progressive disorganization observed in the cytoplasm of broken cells by Allen et al. (1960). Seravin observed first movement of individual particles, then streamlets, then larger streams forming pseudopods, and finally coordinated locomotion.

Considerable progress has been made recently in linking observed events in intact and broken cells to processes at the molecular level. Thompson and Wolpert's (1963) method of preparing bulk cytoplasm capable of streaming on the addition of ATP has recently been improved and extended by Pollard and Ito (1970) who, by fractionation, have managed to purify partially the fraction capable of streaming. In it they have found two sets of filaments, both of which are apparently necessary for streaming. Bulk cytoplasm preparations have a limited self-organizing capacity that requires ATP and has the same temperature dependence as the ability of streaming to self-organize in the intact amoeba (Seravin, 1966).

The formation of pseudopodia and their coordination in locomotion is dependent on the presence of a nucleus. Anucleate cells show cytoplasmic streaming, but pseudopod formation is abortive and there is no response to light (Willis, 1916; Cohen, 1956). During cell division in Amoeba proteus normal locomotion ceases. Jeon (1968) has found that transplanting a resting nucleus to a dividing amoeba restores locomotion. This may be interpreted to mean that the dividing nucleus loses temporarily its influence on the organization of streaming and pseudopod formation required for locomotion.

The plasmalemma apparently plays little if any role in cytoplasmic streaming and its organization into loop and fountain patterns (Allen, Cooledge, and Hall, 1960). The membrane seems chiefly involved in locomotion and behaviour, as we shall see later.

3. Responses to Light

It is important to know how light affects amoeboid movement and behavior, because light microscopy is required to study these processes. Intense light, e.g. from an unfiltered mercury or xenon arc source, is highly damaging to amoebae of the Amoeba–Chaos group. They stop moving, round up, show uncoordinated streaming, become vacuolated, and eventually die. It was shown very early that light damage can be avoided by the use of filters limiting irradiation from the shorter wavelengths (Harrington and Leaming, 1900). According to Hitchcock (1961), the maximum effect is found at approximately 515 nm.

The direction in which amoebae move can be controlled by shining blue light from the side. Cohen (1956) found this response useful in separating nucleate and anucleate fragments.

Amoebae irradiated by white light stop streaming temporarily, then increases their locomotion velocity (Mast and Stahler, 1937). The maximum effect is at about 15,000 meter candles. If amoebae are irradiated partially by a microbeam of white or blue light through the microscope, the effects are complicated (Mast, 1932). The rate of streaming out of retracting pseudopodia can be increased. Irradiation of pseudopod tips causes immediate cessation of streaming into that pseudopod but no effect in other pseudopodia. The sensitive region of the pseudopod is just behind the hyaline cap in the granular cytoplasm nearest the pseudopod tip. Effects of light on the rest of the cell are less obvious; if the main body of cytoplasm is irradiated, there is subsequently an increase in the relative thickness of the ectoplasmic layer formed by the irradiated endoplasm when it becomes everted to form the ectoplasmic tube.

The responses of amoebae to light are not yet subject to unique interpretation. The effects may be on the contractile mechanism, the mitochondrial bioenergetic pathways, or the consistency of the cytoplasm. Further investigation will be required.

4. Responses to Mechanical Stimulation

The reaction of A. proteus to generalized mechanical shock was described by Folger (1926). The shock of jarring a slide with a stimulus of standard intensity causes a cessation of streaming that lasts 5-12 seconds after a latent period of 0.8 to 1.8 seconds. Both times depend on the strength of stimulus, and a second complete response can occur only after a substantial recovery time.

The characteristic avoidance response of amoebae to localized mechanical stimulation was described by Jennings (1904). Pseudopodia stop or change direction when prodded with a microneedle. Goldacre (1952) observed that amoebae responded only when the microneedle has forced the cell membrane across the hyaline region into the granular cytoplasm. He suggested that membrane-plasmagel contact might be an essential feature of the amoeba's response mechanism. It seems more likely that some gelated regions of the cytoplasm react directly when disturbed, because gold spheres falling through the endoplasm of A. dubia have been observed to elicit the characteristic reaction of the cell on bumping into the inner wall of the ectoplasmic tube (Allen, 1961 a).

There is very little reliable quantitative information about the responses of amoebae to mechanical stimuli beyond what was known to Jennings (1904). With modern piezoelectric micromanipulators and delicate control of magnetic particles implanted in the cell, it should not be difficult to systematically study the response of amoebae to external and internal stimuli.

5. Responses to Food and Chemical Stimuli

The older literature on feeding reactions and responses to chemical stimuli contains most of our present knowledge mixed with considerable anecdotal information of doubtful scientific value. Taxonomic uncertainties and the doubtful purity of chemicals combined with poor experimental design in many of the earlier reports to render them nearly worthless. Early authors could not agree on whether amoebae had a chemical sense. Schaeffer (1917 a) showed that amoebae would respond to isolated proteins, yet believed (1917 b) that their response to food was largely mechanical. Schaeffer (1916) placed particles of "inert" substances (glass, India ink, carmine etc.) "in the probable path of" amoebae and then concluded that amoebae could somehow "sense" and seek our particles up to 60 microns away. On the other hand, Jeon and Bell (1965) demonstrated what appears to be chemotaxis and associated food cup formation initiated from 800 microns away.

Proving the existence of chemotaxis in amoebae requires more than the simple anecdotal evidence of the type that Schaeffer and others produced. Mr. M. Haberey in my laboratory has applied the dark-field streak method of Dryl (1963) to the detection of chemotaxis in amoebae. Haberey places food amongst amoebae in culture, then records movements as interrupted streaks showing the velocity and direction of movement in each amoeba in the culture. He has shown that A. proteus does not respond chemotactically to Tetrahymena. This supports the similar finding of Chrisiansen and Marshall (1965), who found no evidence of chemotaxis in Chaos toward Paramecium.

Bell (1963) has described a most interesting reaction of amoebae to homogenates of Hydra. A. proteus respond chemotactically and form food cups in response to intact hydra, extracts of Hydra, and to heparin (Bell and Jeon, 1962; Jeon and Bell, 1965). Seravin (1968) has reported that food cups may be induced locally without any locomotor chemotactic response. Boiled egg yolk or activated carbon incubated with boiled yolk extract can elicit such a response. On the basis of such experiments, Seravin has concluded that amoebae will eat "inert" particles if they have absorbed the "smell" of food. However, the probability that such particles will be actually ingested is increased if the particle is agitated. Thus Seravin believes that feeding often results from a combination of chemical and mechanical stimuli.

Haberey (unpublished) has recently studied the behavioral pattern of Amoeba proteus in the presence of Tetrahymena. When prey are introduced, the amoebae stop streaming temporarily and assume what we have come to call an "attitude of expectation". They form short, blunt pseudopodia which are easily converted to food cups. Amoebae respond within one second to contact with prey by an almost explosive hyaline cap formation. Soon the granular endoplasm rushes into the hyaline cap and the newly laid down ectoplasmic gel takes the form of a food-cup. On glass surfaces one dorsal and two lateral pseudopodia encircle the prey from the top and fuse. Closure on the side next to the glass occurs when a thin and flat pseudopod with a broad hyaline front forms in contact with the glass. Finally, the food cup is subdivided internally by a pseudopod bisecting it and confining the prey to a smaller compartment. According to Salt (1961), A. proteus feed voraciously on Tetrahymena for the first few hours of their cell cycle, consuming over thirty prey in that time. As they fill with food vacuoles, they become sluggish and resume active movement only shortly before the next cell division.

In nature amoebae have an enormous choice of potential food and other objects to ingest. Schaeffer (1917 a) showed that they prefer prey to inert objects nearby, but will ingest glass, carbon, India ink, carmine, etc. Allen (1961 a) found that A. dubia would ingest spheres of iron, mercury, or gold. In a culture of mixed ciliates, they show definite food preferences (Mast and Hahnert, 1935). A. proteus seem to thrive on Tetrahymena cultured separately (Prescott and James, 1955), a technique that has proven invaluable to amoeba physiologists.

It is in collections from the wild that some of the most fascinating amoeba behavior is observed. I have watched and photographed A. proteus "plucking" Vorticella from their contractile stalks so gently that their response mechanism was not triggered. Mast and Root (1961) observed that A. proteus food cup pseudopodia can cleave a paramecium in two. By duplicating this feat with a calibrated glass needle, they showed that pseudopodia are of such rigidity, and exert such a force, that surface tension could not be responsible. Mast and Root also described the ingestion of active nematodes and rotifers.

Liquid nutrients induce another type of response: pinocytosis (or cell drinking). While it seems likely that the motile machinery of the cell is mobilized in some way to deform the cell surface into channels through which pinocytosis takes place, pinocytosis differs from phagocytosis in an important way: pinocytosis inhibits locomotion and streaming (Nachmias, 1968; Seravin, 1968). In phagocytosis, on the other hand, locomotion and streaming are increased in intensity, and are merely directed toward food.

6. Response to Electrical Stimulation

Nearly all authors agree on the details of the response of Amoeba proteus to electric current (Mast, 1931; Hahnert, 1932; Jahn, 1964). There is little agreement, however, on how electric current produces its response. Some authors interpret the effect to be on membranes, others have postulated gelating or solating effects, an enhancement or inhibition of contraction, etc.

Electrically induced pseudopod formation imitates very closely the details of normal pseudopod formation. Within one second of stimulation, a hyaline cap forms which is soon invaded by particles. The resulting pseudopod is usually normal in shape and behavior, unless the strength of stimulus is too high. Stopping the stimulus may or may not lead to cessation of induced streaming once it has begun.

Electrically induced streaming always is directed toward the cathode and begins at the tip of the forming pseudopod, exactly as in spontaneous pseudopod formation. Amoebae initially moving toward the anode will quickly reverse direction when stimulated. Here again, the first motion in the new direction occurs where the new pseudopod tip will form.

Electrical stimulation will probably prove to be the method of choice for analyzing the behavior and electrophysiology of amoebae. A start in this direction has already been made by Kamiya (1964) and Tasaki and Kamiya (1964). Unfortunately, several technical problems remain, not the least of which is the mechanical stimulation from microelectrodes and the effects of the light required to observe cells under experimental conditions.

7. Mechanisms of Response in the Amoeba

Despite disagreements about the localization of the motive force for pseudopod formation and retraction (Seravin, 1964 for a review), no one doubts that the amoeba contains a contractile system. Amoeba cytoplasm is contractile (Allen, Cooledge, and Hall, 1960). Whole amoebae can be glycerinated and contract on the addition of ATP (Simard-Duquesne and Couillard, 1962). Pollard and Ito (1970) have found two filament fractions in isolated bulk cytoplasm, one of which is apparently an amoeba actin.

Given a contractile cytoplasm, it is possible to understand the mechanism of amoeba responses to stimuli if a common, direct effect of stimuli on the contractile system can be found. Such a suggestion was made by Heilbrunn (1952), who visualized nearly all excitation phenomena as the result of the release of calcium from one region of the cell to occupy new and physiologically more important binding sites. Allen, Cooledge, and Hall (1960) pointed out the extreme sensitivity of amoeba cytoplasm to calcium ions, which cause contraction and vacuolization. Spirostomum and Physarum have recently been shown to have calcium-containing vesicles which evidently store and release calcium ions as a way of controlling the state of contraction (Ettienne, 1970 and unpublished). It is important to find out whether calcium ions play a direct role in the amoeba's response mechanism. Because of the lability of amoeba cytoplasm in fixatives, this will not be easy to determine.

There are a number of indications that the plasmalemma plays a role in responses to stimuli. Although the electrophysiological approach will undoubtedly be valuable in the long run, the results so far obtained by various workers are not consistent with one another. Bingley and Thompson (1962) obtained different membrane potentials varying from −21 to −100 mV. Successive punctures in different regions of the same amoeba convinced them of an anterio-posterior potential gradient of almost 1V/cm magnitude. Batyev (1964) very carefully reinvestigated the matter and found variations in membrane potential according to how deeply the electrodes were inserted. Neither result leads to a complete understanding of the electrophysiology of amoebae, but Batyev's result suggests that gel potentials may be superimposed upon membrane potentials proper. The matter is resolvable by experiments using programmed piezoelectric placement of electrodes in known regions of the amoeba. Considering the foregoing uncertainties, we do not know how properly to interpret the results of Bingley, Bell, and Jeon (1962) that extracts of food organisms and heparin lower the membrane potential of amoebae. The authors extrapolated from their work and that of Bingley and Thompson (1962) to postulate that substances capable of depolarizing the amoeba's membrane (locally) could induce pseudopod formation. This may be quite true, but it should be ascertained by microelectrode experiments on amoebae exposed to the local action of chemical stimulators.

The electrophysiology of amoebae is still in its infancy, but available methods should permit us to clarify the role of the plasmalemma in excitation and in the coordination of pseudopodial activity. There was hope that progress in this direction had been made by the recording of what appeared to be "spike potentials" in Chaos during movement inside a special double-chamber (Tasaki and Kamiya, 1964). Bruce and Marshall (1965), however, were unable to repeat these results with unconfined amoebae.

It should be apparent that much of the classical work on amoeboid behavior falls short of giving us an understanding of the processes involved. Clearly much needs to be done to extend our present knowledge of how pseudopods extend and retract to an understanding of how these processes are coordinated and controlled by the organism.

REFERENCES

Allen, R. D. (1961 a). "Amoeboid Movement" in The Cell 2, 135. Academic Press. N. Y.

Allen, R. D. (1961 b). Exp. Cell Res. Suppl. 8, 17.

Allen, R. D. (1968). Soc. Exp. Biol. Symp. 22, 151.

Allen, R. D. "Biophysical Aspects of Pseudopod Formation and Refraction" in Biology of the Amoeba. (K. Jeon, ed.) Academic Press, in press 1972.

Allen, R. D., Cooledge, J. W., and Hall, P. J. (1960). Nature 187, 896.

Allen, R. D., Cowden, R. R., and Hall, P. J. (1962). J. Cell Biol. 12, 185.

Allen, R. D. and Francis, D. W. (1965). Soc. Exp. Biol. Symp. 19, 259.

Allen, R. D., Francis, D. W., and Nakajima, H. (1965). Proc. Natl. Acad. Sci. 54, 1153.

Allen, R. D., Francis, D. W. and Zeh, R. (1971). Science, 174, 1237.

Allen, R. D. and Kamiya, N. (Eds.) (1964). Primitive Motile Systems in Cell Biology. Academic Press, N. Y.

Allen, R. D. and Roslansky, J. (1959). J. Biophys. Biochem. Cytol. 6, 437.
Batyev, N. V. (1964). Tsitologiya 6, 209.
Bell, L. G. E. (1963). Int. Soc. for Cell Biol. 2, 215.
Bell, L. G. E. and Jeon, K. W. (1962). Nature 195, 400.
Bernstein, J. (1900). Pflugers Arch. 80, 628.
Bingley, M., Bell, L. G. E., and Jeon, K. W. (1962). Exp. Cell Res. 28, 208.
Bingley, M. and Thompson, C. M. (1962). J. Theor. Biol. 2, 16.
Bovee, E. C. (1964). In Primitive Motile Systems in Cell Biology (R. D. Allen and N. Kamiya, Eds.) Academic Press, N. Y. 189.
Bruce, D. L. and Marshall, J. M., Jr. (1965). J. Gen. Physiol. 49, 151.
Christiansen, R. G. and Marshall, J. M., Jr. (1965). J. Cell Biol. 25, 443.
Cohen, A. L. (1956). J. Biophys. Biochem. Cytol. 2, 15.
De Bruyn, P. P. H. (1947). Quart. Rev. Biol. 22, 1.
Dellinger, O. P. (1906). J. Exp. Zool. 3, 337.
Dryl, S. (1963). Animal Behavior 1, 393.
Ecker, A. (1849). Zeits. Wiss. Zool. Abt. A. 1, 218.
Ettienne, E. (1970). J. Gen. Physiol. 56, 168.
Folger, H. T. (1926). J. Morph. and Physiol. 42, 359.
Francis, D. W. and Allen, R. D. (1971). J. Mechanochem. Cell Motility. 1, 1.
Goldacre, R. J. (1952). Symp. Soc. Exp. Biol. 6, 128.
Griffin, J. L. (1960). Exp. Cell Res. 21, 170.
Griffin, J. L. (1964). In Primitive Motile Systems in Cell Biology (R. D. Allen and N. Kamiya, Eds.) Academic Press, N. Y. 303.
Hahnert, W. J. (1932). Physiol. Zool. 5, 491.
Harrington, N. R. and Leaming, E. (1900). Am. J. Physiol. 3, 9.
Heilbrunn, L. V. (1952). An Outline of General Physiology, 3rd Ed. W. B. Saunders and Co. Phila.
Hitchcock, L., Jr. (1961). Protozool. 8, 322.
Jahn, T. L. (1964). In Primitive Motile Systems in Cell Biology (R. D. Allen and N. Kamiya, Eds.) Academic Press, N. Y. 279.
Jennings, H. S. (1904). Carnegie Inst. Wash. Publ. 16, 129.
Jeon, K. W. (1968). Exp. Cell Res. 50, 467.
Jeon, K. W. and Bell, L. G. E. (1962). Exp. Cell Res. 27, 350.
Jeon, K. W. and Bell, L. G. E. (1965). Exp. Cell Res. 38, 536.
Kamiya, N. (1964). In Primitive Motile Systems in Cell Biology (R. D. Allen and N. Kamiya, Eds.) Academic Press, N. Y. 257.
Mast, S. O. (1926). J. Morph. and Physiol. 41, 347.
Mast, S. O. (1931 a). Zeits. f. Vergleich. Physiol. 15, 309.
Mast, S. O. (1931 b). Biol. Bull. 61, 223.
Mast, S. O. (1932). Physiol. Zool. 5, 1.
Mast, S. O. and Hahnert, W. F. (1935). Physiol. Zool. 8, 255.
Mast, S. O. and Root, F. M. (1916). J. Exp. Zool. 21, 33.
Mast, S. O. and Stahler, N. (1937). Biol. Bull. 73, 126.
Nachmias, V. (1968). Exp. Cell Res. 51, 347.
Pantin, C. F. S. (1923). J. Mar. Biol. Assoc. U.K. 13, 24.
Pollard, T. D. and Ito, S. (1970). J. Cell Biol. (in press).
Prescott, D. M. and James, T. W. (1955). Exp. Cell Res. 8, 256.
Rinaldi, R. A. and Jahn, T. L. (1963). J. Protozool. 10, 344.
Salt, G. W. (1961). Exp. Cell Res. 24, 618.
Schaeffer, A. A. (1916 a). J. Exp. Zool. 20, 529.
Schaeffer, A. A. (1917 a). J. Exp. Zool. 22, 53.
Schaeffer, A. A. (1917 b). J. Anim. Behav. 7, 220.
Seravin, L. N. (1964). Tsitologiya 6, 653.
Seravin, L. N. (1966). Zoological Journal (Russian) 45, 334.
Seravin, L. N. (1967). Herald of Leningrad University 3, 41.

Seravin, L. N. (1968 a). Tsitologiya 10, 506.
Seravin, L. N. (1968 b). Acta Protozool. 6, 97.
Simard-Duquesne, N. and Couillard, P. (1962). Exp. Cell Res. 28, 85.
Tasaki, I. and Kamiya, N. (1964). Jour. Cell Comp. Physiol. 63.
Thompson, C. M. and Wolpert, L. (1963). Exp. Cell Res. 32, 156.
Tiegs, O. W. (1928). Protoplasma 4, 88.
Willis, H. S. (1916). Biol. Bull. 30, 253.
Wohlman, A. and Allen, R. D. (1968). J. Cell Sci. 3, 105.

FLAGELLA AND CILIA

BIOCHEMISTRY OF BACTERIAL FLAGELLA

K. Dimmitt, S. Emerson, K. Tokuyasu and M. Simon
University of California at San Diego,
Department of Biology,
La Jolla,
California 92057, U. S. A.

1. INTRODUCTION

Flagella are the organelles responsible for motility in bacteria. Since they are relatively simple in structure particularly when compared to the flagella of eucaryotic cells, they offer an opportunity to study the basic mechanisms of biological movement as well as the mechanisms involved in the assembly of subcellular organelles and the regulation of their biosynthesis.

Much of the work that has been done in these areas has been summarized in recent articles on flagellar chemistry (Iino, 1969) and motility (Doetsch and Hageage, 1968). We will, therefore, not attempt a comprehensive review in this paper. We will introduce some relevant background information in order to facilitate the discussion of the structure and function of bacterial flagella.

When flagella are examined by electron microscopy (Abram, Koffler, and Vatter, 1965, 1966; Cohen-Bazire and London, 1967; Vaituzis and Doetsch, 1969) they are found to be composed of three morphologically distinct sections: (a) The filament which is generally about 10-15 microns long, (b) the filament ends in a short "hook" region which is about 100 mμ long; and, (c) the hook in turn is attached to a cap-like basal structure which is bound to the cell membrane.

Figure 1 shows B. subtilis which has flagella arranged laterally over its surface. The filaments have a regular helical shape with a characteristic wavelength and amplitude. They can be easily removed from the bacteria by shearing (Stocker, 1957). They can then be purified by differential centrifugation (Koffler, 1970) or ion-exchange chromatography (Martinez, 1963). The purified filaments can be disaggregated by treatment with heat, urea, low pH or a variety of other denaturing agents. These treatments yield flagellin (Koffler and Kobayashi, 1957; Weibull, 1950) which is a single protein subunit

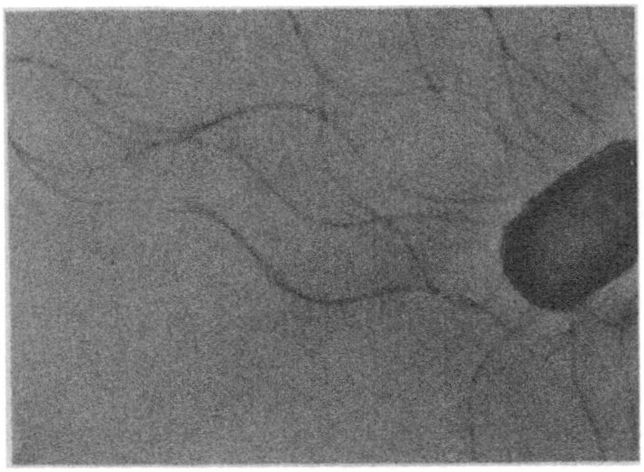

Figure 1. B. subtilis stained with 1 per cent phosphotungstic acid. This photograph and all the others in this paper were taken with a Philips 200 Electron Microscope operated at 60kV.

with a monomeric molecular weight of 40,000 daltons in most bacterial species. The electrophoretic and hydrodynamic properties of disaggregated filaments (Ada et al. 1963; Kobayashi, Rinker and Koffler, 1959; Martinez, Brown and Glazer, 1967) all indicate that flagellin is homogeneous. Furthermore, highly purified preparations of flagellin can be reaggregated to form filaments which are morphologically identical to the flagella filaments on the bacterium (Abram and Koffler, 1964; Asakura, Eguchi and Iino, 1964). These observations suggest that flagellin is the only major protein component of the filament.

The relative ease with which flagellin can be purified and reaggregated has allowed its use in studying the requirements for the formation of specific structures. Under certain conditions flagellin subunits will only reaggregate in the presence of small "seed fragments". The nature of the subunit can be varied by choosing appropriate flagellin mutants, the conditions for reassembly and the structure of the seed can also be varied independently (Asakura, Eguchi and Iino, 1964, 1966, 1968) and the effect of these variables on reaggregation can be measured. While these studies have led to interesting data concerning polymorphism and the nature of filament formation, they have shed little light on the mechanism of motility.

The problem of motility in bacteria is further complicated since all of the present evidence indicates that there is no specific enzymatic activity associated with the filament. A variety of questions arise, e.g., what kind of chemical transformations are involved? where does the transduction of chemical energy into a physical change take place? and how is flagellar activity controlled and integrated? It has been suggested that these functions might be carried out by a specific basal structure ". . . the basal granule (might act as) the required signal box and periodic source of energy. . . " (Weibull, 1960). Genetic studies in Salmonella suggest that flagellation is controlled by at least eight cistrons. In B. subtilis there is evidence for at least five structural genes. The proteins that represent these cistrons may be part of the basal

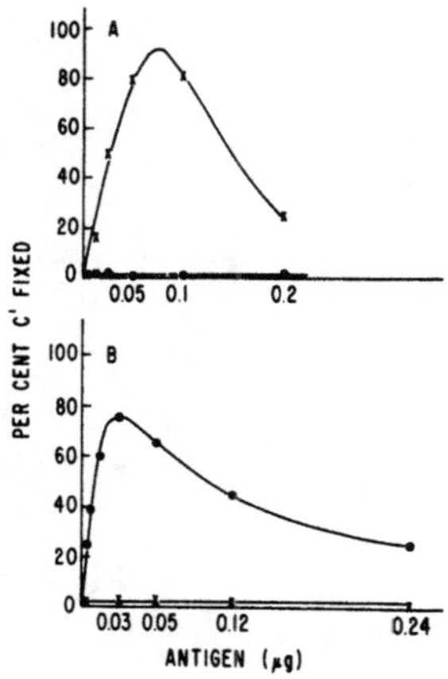

Figure 2. The immunochemical reaction of flagella and flagellin. (A) the complement fixation reaction of antiflagellin antiflagellin antibody diluted 1/2000 with flagellin (X — X) and flagella (—●—●). Complement fixation was carried out according to the methods of Wasserman and Levine (1965). (B) The complement fixation reaction of antiflagellar antibody with flagella (—●—●) and flagellin (X — X).

structure and could be involved in regulating both the synthesis and function of flagella. Koffler and his co-workers (Abram et al., 1970; Mitchen and Koffler, 1969; Mitchen, Koffler, and Smith, 1970) have shown that the hook structure differs from the filament in its susceptibility to denaturing agents and suggested that it might be composed of different proteins. It is therefore, important to isolate and characterize the basal structures and their components and to determine the relationship between these structures and the filament. The approach taken in our laboratory has been to isolate flagella in as intact a form as possible and then to use standard biochemical, immunochemical and genetic procedures to analyze their components.

2. Measurement of Flagella and Flagellin

One of the major difficulties encountered in studying structural proteins is that they usually lack enzymatic activity and consequently cannot be easily measured. Flagella, however, can be followed by preparing specific antisera and measuring the antigen—antibody reaction. Ichiki and Martinez (1969) showed that antisera may contain antibodies directed toward determinants that are unique to the flagellar filament and others unique to the flagellin subunit, as well as determinants that are common to both the subunit and the filament. By varying the means of immunization and the conditions of reaction, antisera that measure only the filament and do not react appreciably with the subunit (Figure 2B) and other antisera that react only with the subunit but do not show reaction with the filament (Figure 2A) can be obtained. These antisera can then be used to specifically measure both flagellar filaments and

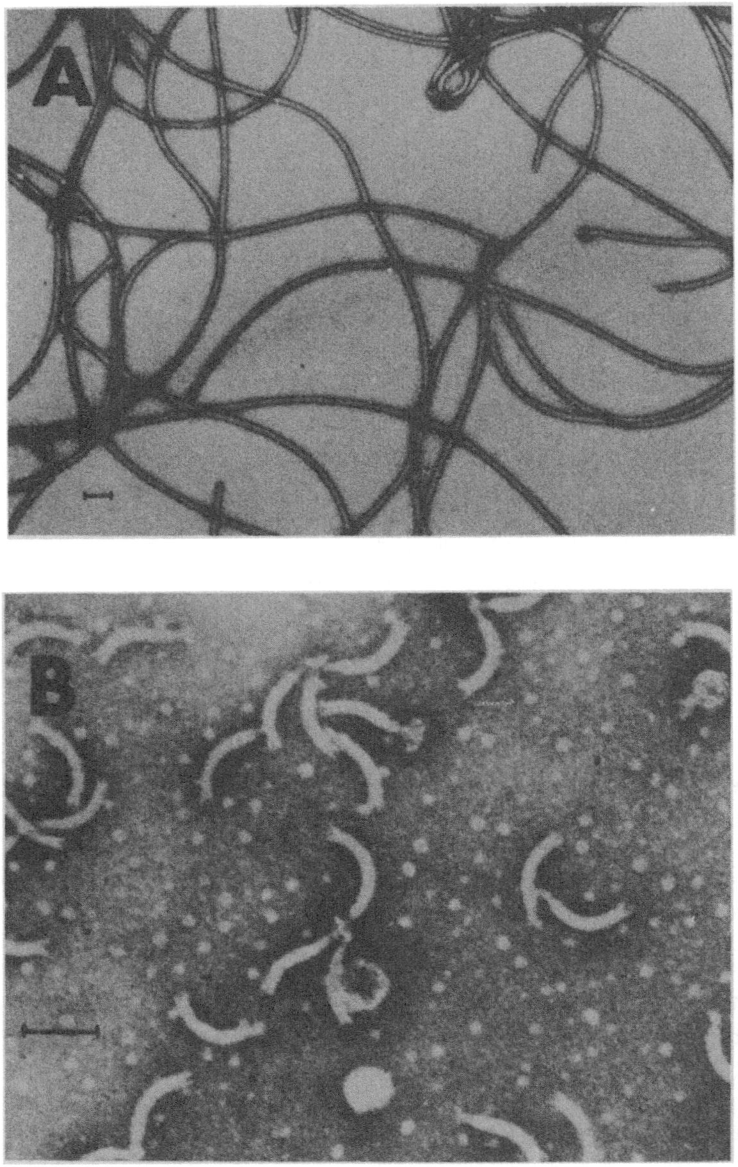

Figure 3. Electron micrographs of intact flagella and isolated hook. (A) intact flagella stained with 1 per cent uranyl acetate pH 4.5. (B) hooks obtained after shearing and heating thermolabile flagella stained with 1 per cent phosphotungstic acid. The bar is 100 nanometers.

flagellin. A variety of relatively simple assays are available that allow the rapid and precise quantitation of these antigens.

3. Isolation and Properties of Intact Flagella

Instead of removing the flagella from the bacteria, intact flagella were isolated by dissolving the bacteria with lysozyme–DNase and detergent. The

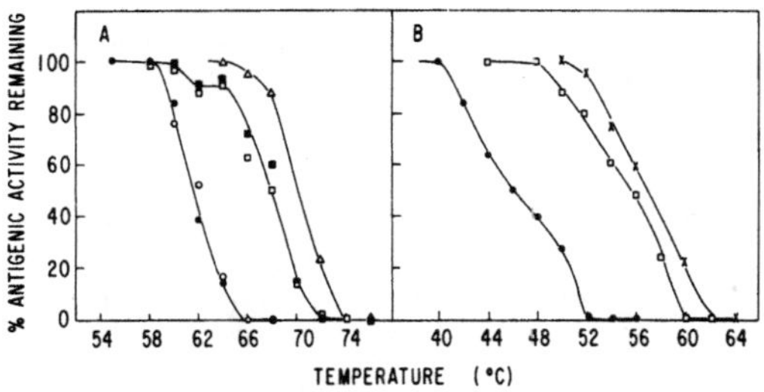

Figure 4. Thermal stability profile of sheared and intact flagella. Appropriate samples of flagella were heated in 0.01 M Tris – HCl buffer pH 7.3 and 0.05 M sodium chloride at the desired temperature for 15 minutes. A sample was removed and diluted with cold buffer and its antigenic activity was measured with antiflagellar anti-serum (Dimmitt and Simon, J. Bact, (1971) 105, 369. (A) flagella from wild type bacteria (●) sheared flagella obtained by shearing washed bacteria (16,000 rpm in Virtis omnimixer 30 seconds) and removing bacteria by centrifugation (○) sheared flagella were purified by ammonium sulfate fractionation and cesium chloride density centrifugation. (□) Intact flagella obtained by lysis and centrifugation. (■) Intact flagella after ammonium sulfate and cesium chloride gradient purification. (△) Whole bacteria washed once in buffer. (B) Flagella from thermolabile mutant GID. (●) sheared flagella, (X) whole bacteria, (□) intact flagella.

flagellar filaments were then collected by ammonium sulfate precipitation and finally purified by isopycnic gradient centrifugation. Figure 3A shows some purified flagella with intact hooks and basal structures. More then 95 per cent of the protein in these preparations is flagellar antigen and most of the filaments were found to end in hook and basal structures.

In order to further characterize the purified flagella their thermal stability was compared to that of flagella obtained by shearing the bacteria under conditions that leave most of the hooks with the bacteria. Flagella disaggregate over a narrow temperature range (Martinez and Rosenberg, 1964) and the transition from flagellar filament to subunit can be followed immunochemically (Dimmitt and Simon, J. Bact., (1971) 105, 369. Figure 4A shows that flagella obtained by lysing the bacteria are more stable than sheared flagella and their thermal stability profile is similar to that of flagella on intact bacteria. This increased stability does not result from the purification procedure since it is observed with crude lysates of bacteria before CsCl or ammonium sulfate treatment. It is not a function of the presence of extraneous material or cells since there is no stabilization of sheared flagella when they are measured in the presence of cell extracts. The same thermal stability profiles are also found after sheared flagella are purified by ammonium sulfate and CsCl treatment.

The difference in thermal stability is even more dramatically observed with a flagellar mutant GD1 (Figure 4B). Its flagellin differs from wild type in a single peptide and this difference results in destabilization of the flagellar

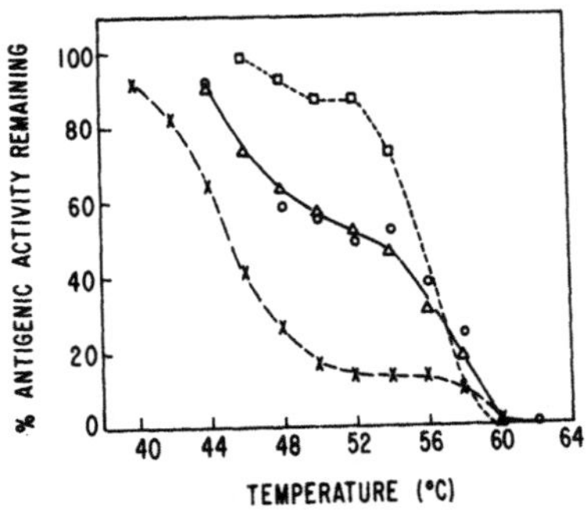

Figure 5. Thermal stability of GID flagella after shearing. (□) Thermal stability of intact flagella. (X) Intact flagella after shearing by passing through 24 gauge needle ten times. (O) A mixture of intact and sheared flagella. (Δ) Curve calculated for thermal stability of mixture of sheared and intact flagella.

filament (Grant dissertation, Emerson and Simon, unpublished data). The sheared flagella disaggregate at temperatures that are 10°C lower (Td, 46°C) than flagella purified from lysed bacteria (Td, 56°C).

There are a variety of possible explanations for the relative stability of the flagella obtained by the lysis procedure. Some of the explanations that we have considered are: (a) the stability may be a function of the length of the filament and sheared filaments might be shorter than those obtained by lysis, (b) the shearing process could damage or distort the filament structure and thus destabilize it, (c) the presence of the hook structure could stabilize the filament; the sheared flagella for the most part lack the hook structure and would therefore disaggregate more readily. In order to distinguish among these possibilities flagella obtained by the lysis procedure were sheared by passing them through a 24 gauge needle ten times. The flagella were broken into relatively short pieces. When these flagella were heated they showed a biphasic thermal stability profile (Figure 5). Eighty-five per cent of the flagellar antigen showed a thermal stability profile characteristic of sheared flagella and the temperature stability of 15 per cent of the antigen was similar to the original intact flagella. On the basis of the first two proposed explanations we would predict that the 15 per cent of the flagellar antigen that remains relatively stable, represents flagella that have escaped shearing and are therefore long or intact. On the other hand if the hook structure stabilizes the adjacent filament we would expect the residual fraction to be enriched in filaments carrying the hook structure. Direct observation in the electron microscope confirmed the latter hypothesis. The ratio of flagellar fragments without hooks to those with hooks goes from 9.4 after incubation at 30°C to 0.34 after incubation at 52°C. There was also no apparent enrichment for relatively long fragments. Furthermore when flagellin was prepared and then reaggregated into long

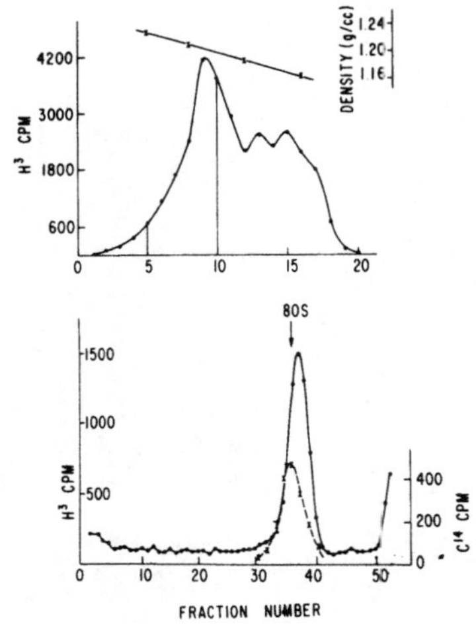

Figure 6. Purification of hooks from intact GID flagella. B. subtilis GID was grown in minimal media supplemented with 0.08 mc/ml of ^{3}H-labeled leucine and histidine. The cells were harvested and intact flagella were prepared by the usual procedures. These were then sheared by passing them through a 24 gauge needle ten times and then heated to 65°C for 15 min. The solution was layered on a gradient formed of three layers of sucrose 38 per cent, 45 per cent, and 53 per cent in Tris 0.01 M pH 8.0 and 0.5 per cent Brij 58 after centrifugation at 100 kg for 5 hr (TB buffer). A band was formed at the interface between the 38 per cent and 45 per cent sucrose. The band was removed, dialyzed against TB buffer and then applied to a linear, preformed, renographin gradient and spun 12 hr at 144 kg. Top, shows the pattern obtained after the renographin run. Bottom, fraction 9 from the renographin gradient was concentrated and run on a 15 per cent to 30 per cent sucrose density gradient for 90 min at 180,000 × g at 5°C. The dotted line shows the ^{14}C-labeled MS-2 RNA which was used as a marker.

filaments which lacked hook structures they showed exactly the same thermal stability as sheared flagella. On the basis of the evidence we conclude that the presence of the hook stabilizes the adjacent filament.

If one of the mechanisms for thermal dissociation of the flagella involved the preferential denaturation of flagellin on the proximal end of the filament then the presence of the hook and its connection to that end would protect it, thus stabilizing the filament structure. On the other hand the hook may be able to influence the overall structure of the filament in some subtle way thus selecting a more thermostable structure.

4. Isolation and Properties of Hook Structures

While a clear explanation of the stabilizing effect of the hook structure is not presently available we could nonetheless make use of this fact in devising

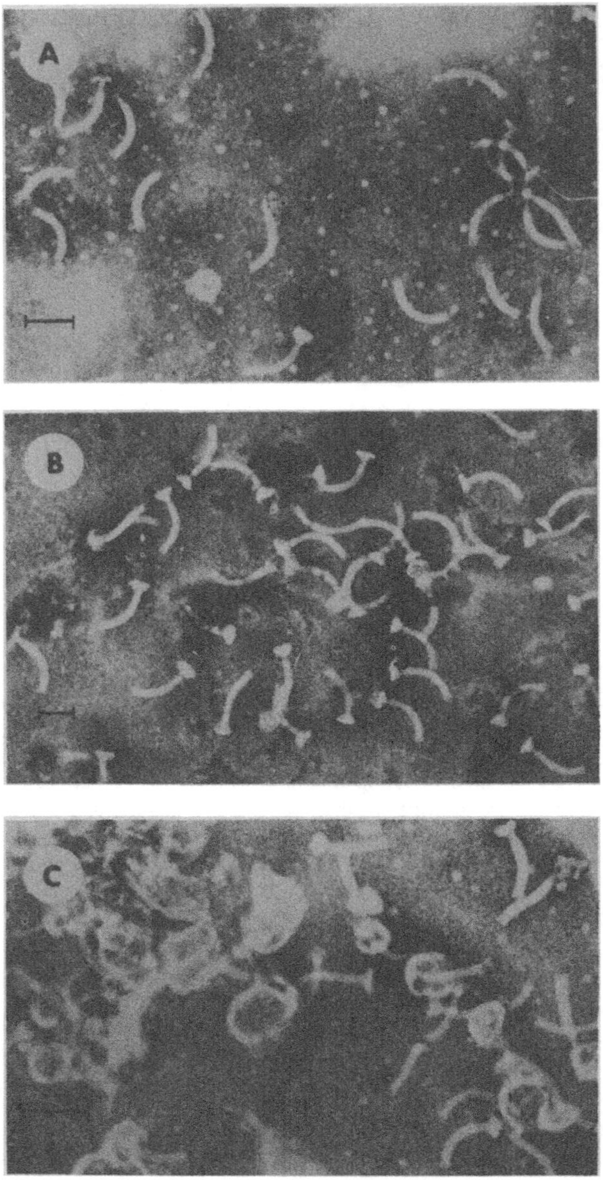

Figure 7. Electrón micrographs of samples were diluted and placed on grids and stained with 1 per cent PTA. (A) Sample taken from fraction 6, (B) taken from fraction 10, (C) taken from fraction 15 (see Figure 6).

procedures to prepare intact hooks. Shearing and then heating flagella resulted in a mixture of hooks, flagellin, and some membrane fragments. These were layered on a preformed sucrose gradient and centrifuged to separate the hooks from most of the flagellin. The hook band was then further purified by isopycnic gradient centrifugation in renographin (Figure 6). When fractions

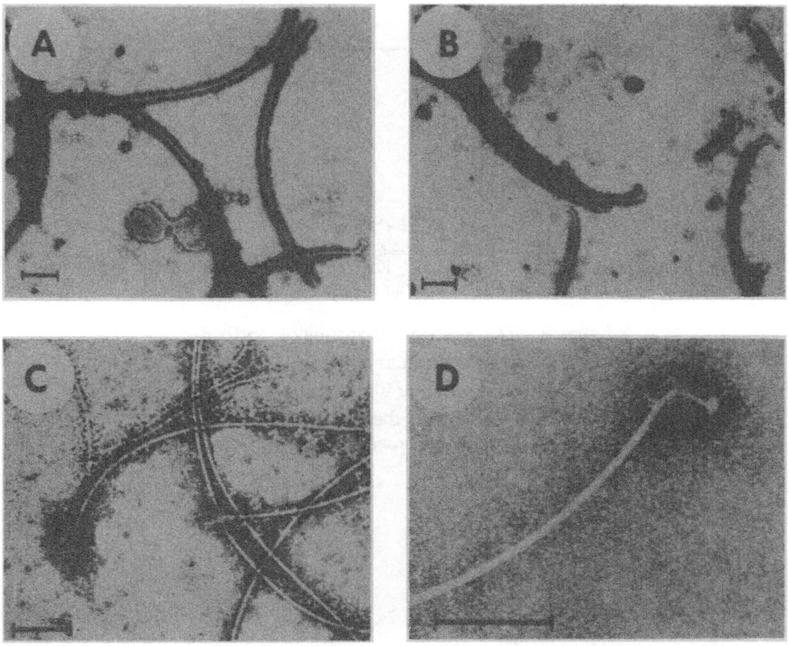

Figure 8. Direct observation of the binding of antiflagella and anti-hook antibody (Dimmitt and Simon, 1970). (A) flagella were put on a formavar carbon coated grid then an appropriate dilution of the antibody was washed away by washing the grid with 0.1 N sodium chloride 0.01 M Tris pH 8.0 and finally distilled water. (A) and (B) antiflagellar antibody, (C) and (D) anti-hook antibody.

were removed from the gradient and observed by electron microscopy it was found that the material banding at the highest density was mostly bare hooks without basal structures (Figures 7A, B, C). At intermediate densities hooks bearing the basal structures were most abundant and finally in the least dense fractions most of the hooks were attached to relatively large pieces of membrane.

The relative sedimentation velocity of the hooks was determined by sucrose gradient centrifugation of the partially purified hooks (Figure 6). The material had an S value of about 77S.

The hooks were also used as antigen to prepare specific antisera. Lawn (1967) showed that when antiflagella filament antibody was used to stain flagella it covered the filament but did not attach to or cover the hook, (Figure 8A, B, Dimmitt and Simon, 1970). Figure 8C, D shows the reaction of anti-hook antibody with intact flagella. The anti-hook serum coats only the hook region and not the filament. The specificity of this serum is more quantitatively demonstrated by complement fixation tests. Figure 9 shows that intact flagella react strongly with the antibody, sheared flagella react weakly since they lack the hook structures, and reaggregated flagellar filaments and flagellin do not react at all. The antibody can also be used to measure the thermal denaturation of the hook structure (Figure 10). Thus it is clear that the hook is antigenically

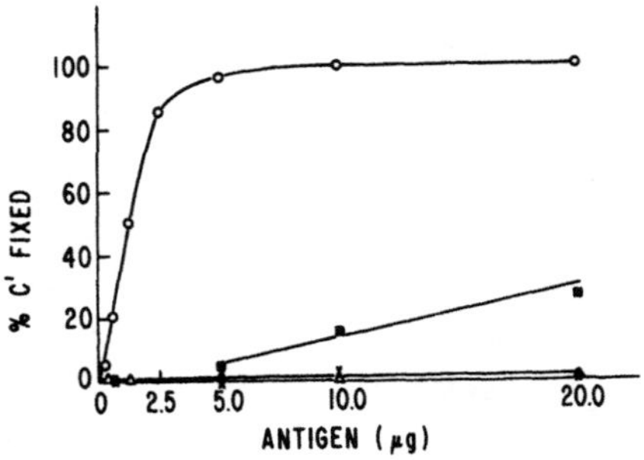

Figure 9. The reaction of anti-hook antibody measured by complement fixation. Anti-hook antibody was used at 1/4000 dilution (—O—O) intact flagella, (—■—) sheared flagella, (—Δ—) reaggregated flagella, (—X—) flagellin.

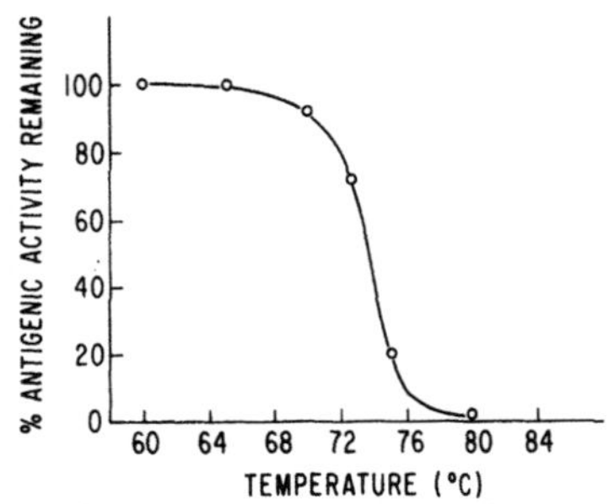

Figure 10. The thermal stability of the purified hooks. Thermal stability was determined as described in the legend to Figure 4. Anti-hook anti-serum was used and residual antigenic activity was measured by complement fixation.

distinct from the filament. We can further begin to examine the hook components. Figure 11 shows the pattern obtained on polyacrylamide gel electrophoresis in sodium dodecyl sulfate. This procedure separates proteins according to molecular weight. The hooks apparently contain one major protein and a number of minor components. The major protein is clearly differentiated from flagellin. It is 20 per cent smaller than flagellin and does not co-run with flagellin. The major hook protein could result from some enzymatic modification of flagellin or it may be an entirely different protein. The minor bands may correspond to other hook components. Further work is required to resolve these questions. It is clear, however, that the hook is made up of proteins that can be clearly distinguished from flagellin.

5. Assembly of Flagella

These data raise the question of how flagellin is assembled into flagellar filaments. Since the hook structure is not made of flagellin, the subunits have

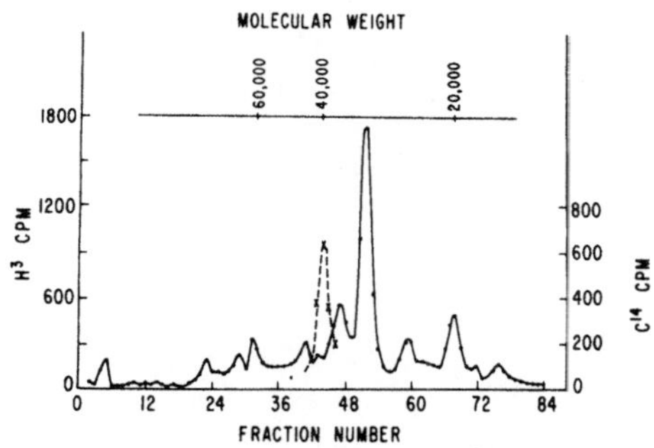

Figure 11. SDS-acrylamide gel electrophoresis of purified hooks. From the graident shown in Figure 6 top, fractions 5-10 were pooled and collected by high speed centrifugation. The pellet was resuspended in 1 per cent SDS, 1 per cent β-mercaptoethanol and 0.01 M Tris pH 9.1. It was then heated at 100°C for three minutes, chilled and diluted, and then applied to the 7 per cent cross-linked gels. ^{14}C-labeled flagellin was co-run as a marker.

to be transported out of the cell past the hook before they can be assimilated into the filament. Thus the subunits must either intercalate near the base at the end of the hook or throughout the filament or they might be added at the distal tip of the filament. Studies by Iino (1969) suggested that the subunits were transported to the tip of the filament. He showed that fluorophenylalanine incorporation into flagellin causes flagella to become curly, i.e., to have half the normal wavelength. He sheared bacteria and allowed them to partially regenerate flagella in minimal medium, he then shifted the bacteria to medium containing fluorophenylalanine. He subsequently examined the shape of the flagella and found that the curly region appeared at the distal end of the filament suggesting that the elongation of the filament occurred at the tip. We repeated these experiments with B. subtilis and obtained similar results. However, we could not do the reciprocal experiment, i.e., label first with fluorophenylalanine and then phenylalanine and find the curly region at the base. This raised the possibility that the curly region did not represent the position of the fluorophenylalanine containing flagellin but might result from conformational changes in the filament induced at other places. We (Emerson, Tokuyasu and Simon, 1970) therefore sought a more direct approach and this was provided by radiography. B. subtilis were grown and then sheared and allowed to regrow flagella for a short time. They were then transferred to radioactive media and allowed to continue regeneration. These bacteria were then lysed and their flagella purified and tested by radioautography. Some of the radioautographs are seen in Figures 12A and B. It is clear that the labeling is most dense near the tip of the flagella. We have counted over 200 flagella and measured the frequency of developed silver-grains per wave. All of the labeling was found to be consistent with growth of the flagellar filament from the distal tip.

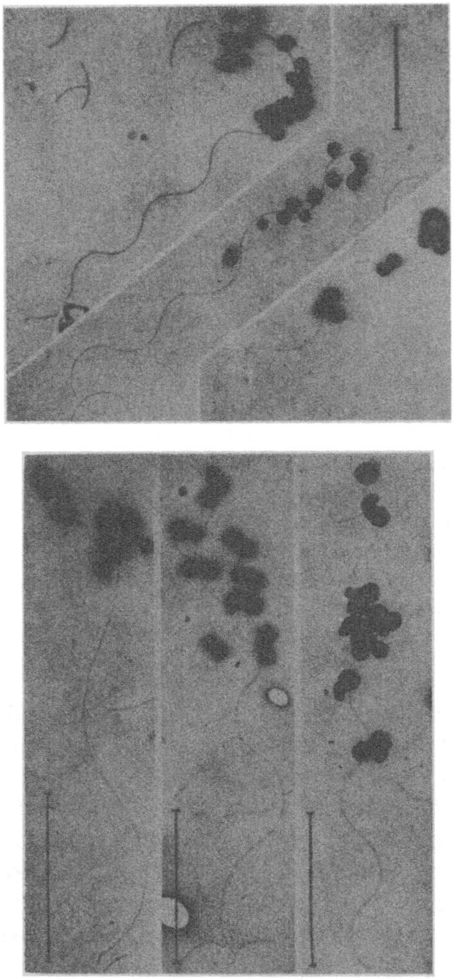

Figure 12. (A and B) Radioautographs of flagella partially regenerated in medium containing radioactive leucine. These results were obtained by methods that have been described previously (Emerson, Tokuyasu and Simon, 1970). The bar is 1 micron.

SUMMARY

In order to understand how bacterial flagella function and how they are assembled, it is necessary to describe the flagellar components, to measure them and to understand their relationship to each other. Using a variety of procedures, it has been possible to isolate intact bacterial flagella, including the flagellar filament, the hook structure and the basal region. The intact filaments are different with respect to their thermal stability when compared to flagellar filaments that have been sheared from the bacteria and are not contiguous with the hook structure. The increased stability conferred on the filament by the presence of the hook may result from protection of one end of the flagellar filament from heat denaturation or the hook may be involved in stabilizing the overall structure of the filament. The isolation of intact flagella has provided material for the preparation of hook and basal cap structures. An analysis of these structures shows that the hook contains one major protein subunit which is approximately 20% smaller than flagellin (i.e., 34,000 daltons). The basal region also contains a variety of other proteins that are distinguished from the flagellin subunit protein. We have been further able to show that in vivo the flagellar filament structure is assembled by a step-wise addition of flagellin subunits to the distal tip of the filament. These results raise further questions about both the structure and function of flagella. For example, what is the mechanism that is involved in the transport of flagellin subunits to the tip of the growing filament? What determines the length of the flagellar hook structure? The answers to these questions as well as others that arise in connection with the mechanism of motility in bacteria seem to lie in a clearer understanding of the basal structure and its relationship to the cell membrane. This will obviously be the focus of future biochemical studies on the flagellar organelle.

ACKNOWLEDGEMENTS

This work was supported by grants from the National Science Foundation.

REFERENCES

Abram, D. and Koffler, H. (1964). J. Mol. Biol. 9, 168.

Abram, D., Koffler, H., and Vatter, A. E. (1965). J. Bact. 90, 1337.

Abram, D., Koffler, H., and Vatter, A. E. (1966). J. Gen. Microbiol. 44, v.

Abram, D., Mitchen, J. R., Koffler, H., and Vatter, A. E. (1970). J. Bact. 101, 250.

Ada, G. L., Nossal, G. J. V., Pye, J., and Abbot, A. (1963). Nature (London) 199, 1257.

Asakura, S., Eguchi, G., and Iino, T. (1964). J. Mol. Biol. 10, 42.

Asakura, S., Eguchi, G., and Iino, T. (1966). J. Mol. Biol. 16, 302.

Cohen-Bazire, G. and London, J. (1967). J. Bact. 94, 458.

Dimmitt, K. and Simon, M. (1970). Infec. Immunity. 1, 212.

Dimmitt, K. and Simon, M. (1971). J. Bact. 105, 369.

Dimmitt, K. and Simon, M. (1971). J. Bact. 108, 282.

Doetsch, R. N. and Hageage, G. J. (1968). Biol. Rev. 43, 317.

Emerson, S., Tokuyasu, K., and Simon, M. (1970). Science 169, 190.

Ichiki, A. T. and Martinez, R. J. (1969). J. Bact. 98, 481.

Iino, T. (1969). J. Gen. Microbiol. 56, 227.

Iino, T. (1969). Bact. Rev. 33, 460.

Kobayashi, T., Rinker, J. N., and Koffler, H. (1959). Arch. Biochem. Biophys. 84, 342.

Koffler, H. (1970). In Methods in microbiology, J. R. Norris and D. W. Ribbons (ed). Academic Press Inc., New York, in press.

Koffler, H. and Kobayashi, T. (1957). Arch. Biochem. Biophys. 67, 246.

Lawn, A. M. (1967). Nature (London) 214, 1151.

Martinez, R. J. (1963). J. Gen. Microbiol. 33, 115.

Martinez, R. J. and Rosenberg, E. (1964). J. Mol. Biol. 8, 702.

Martinez, R. J., Brown, D. M., and Glazer, A. N. (1967). J. Mol. Biol. 28, 45.

Mitchen, J. R. and Koffler, H. (1969). Bact. Proc. 1970, 29.

Mitchen, J. R., Koffler, H., and Smith, R. W. (1970). Bact. Proc. 1970, 22.

Stocker, B. A. D. (1957). J. Pathol. Bact. 73, 314.

Vaituzis, A. and Doetsch, R. (1969). J. Bact. 100, 512.

Wasserman, E. and Levine, L. (1961). J. Immunol. 87, 290.

Weibull, C. (1950). Acta Chem. Scand. 4, 268.

Weibull, C. (1960). In The Bacteria, Vol. 1., I. C. Gunsalus and R. Y. Stanier (ed), Academic Press Inc., New York, 153.

Also see Silverman, M. R. and Simon, M. I. (1972). Flagellar assembly mutants in Escherickia coli. J. Bacteriol. in press. (Polyhook mutants.) — J. Adler.

THE BASAL BODY OF BACTERIAL FLAGELLA

M.L. DePamphilis
Stanford University Medical Center,
Department of Biochemistry,
Palo Alto,
California 94305, U.S.A.

1. INTRODUCTION

The bacterial flagellum is composed of three structurally defined parts: the filament, the hook, and the basal body. The filament is a long, narrow helical structure composed of the protein flagellin, and comprises approximately 98 per cent of the flagellum's length. At the proximal end of the filament is a hook-shaped structure whose morphological, chemical, and serological properties are distinct from the filament (Abram et al., 1970; Dimmit and Simon, 1970a; Lawn, 1967). This "hook" enters the cell wall where it is attached to a complex structure called the basal body. The basal body is firmly bound into the cell envelope and is the only part of the flagellum inside the cell wall.

Although our knowledge of flagellar filaments is extensive (Iino, 1969), studies of flagellar basal bodies in various gram negative bacteria such as Rhodospirillum (Cohen-Bazire and London, 1967), Spirillum (Abram, 1969; Murray and Birch-Andersen, 1963), Proteus (Abram, 1965; Hoeniger et al., 1966; van Iterson et al., 1966), Vibrio (Glauert et al., (1963); Ritchie et al., 1966; Tawara, 1965; Vaituzis and Doetsch, 1969), and Ectothiorhodospira (Remsen et al., 1968), and in Gram positive cells such as Bacillus (Abram et al., 1966; Abram et al., 1970) have met with varying degrees of success. Electron microscopy of thin sections of whole or partially degraded cells, as well as negatively stained flagella released during cell lysis, demonstrated that the basal body is a 15 to 50 nm structure closely associated with the cell envelope. However, the reported structures and dimensions of the basal body vary widely both within and between the genera. The variation in these data probably results from the presence of cell wall and membrane material which either masks the basal body structure or forms artifacts with it, in addition to real generic differences.

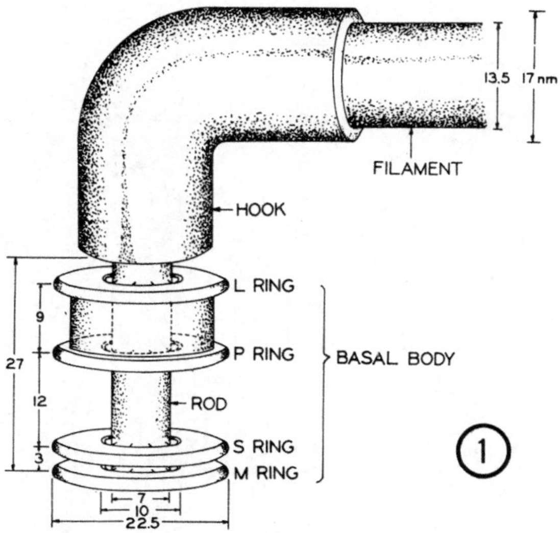

Figure 1. Model of the basal end of an E. coli flagellum. Dimensions are in nanometers.

One approach to understanding the structure, chemistry and function of the base of the flagellum is the development of suitable purification techniques. The object of this paper is to discuss (1) the purification of filament-hook-basal body complexes (referred to as "intact flagella"), (2) the structure of the basal body, and finally (3) the relationship between the basal body and the cell envelope.

2. Purification of Intact Flagella

The following procedure was recently reported by DePamphilis and Adler (1971a). Escherichia coli were harvested just after exponential growth on tryptone broth and converted to spheroplasts by incubating the cells in lysozyme and EDTA buffered at pH 7.8 with Tris. The presence of 12 per cent sucrose prevented osmotic rupture of the spheroplasts. Immediate lysis occurred on addition of the nonionic detergent, Triton X-100. $MgCl_2$ and Mg^{2+} activated deoxyribonuclease were added to reduce the viscosity by degrading DNA which also adhered to basal bodies in the extracts. Flagella could then be removed from the lysate within 25 min of lysis by precipitating them in 25 per cent $(NH_4)_2SO_4$ at 5°C. In order to completely free basal bodies from adhering cellular material, it was necessary to dialyze the precipitated flagella for at least 24 hr at 5°C against a Tris–EDTA buffer (0.1 M Tris, 0.5 mM EDTA, pH 7.8) containing 0.1 per cent Triton X-100. This treatment was particularly necessary to dissociate fragments of outer (lipopolysaccharide) membrane which is stabilized by divalent metal ions such as Mg^{2+}. Following dialysis, the flagella were sedimented at 58,000 × g for 1 hr into a layer of 60 per cent sucrose. The sucrose prevented tightly packed pellets from forming which were difficult to resuspend without breaking off about 70 per cent of the basal bodies. The sucrose was then removed by dialysis and this was

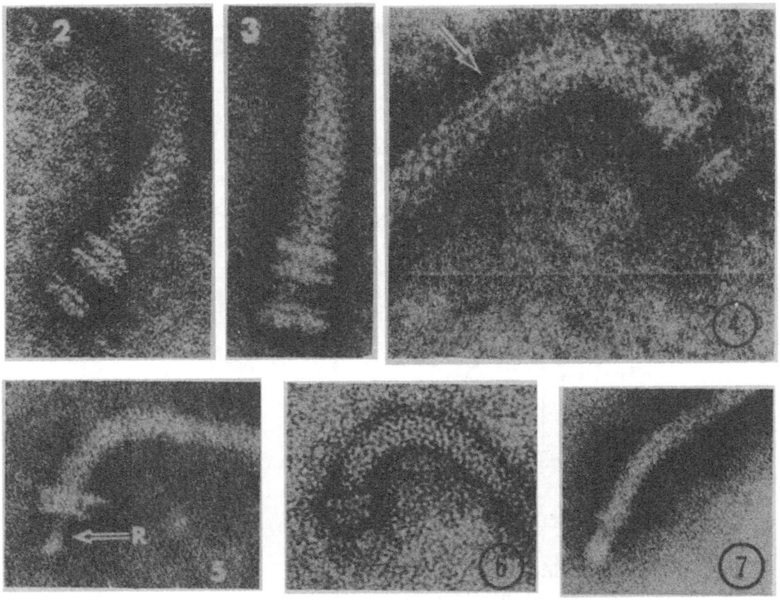

Figure 2. Basal end of intact flagellum from E. coli. Note the circular appearance of the rings. Uranyl acetate. ×445,000.

Figure 3. Basal end of intact flagellum from E. coli. Rings appear thicker. Stain has not penetrated the top rings. Uranyl acetate. ×520,000.

Figure 4. Basal end of E. coli flagellum with only one ring at bottom of basal body. Junction between hook and filament is marked by arrow. Uranyl acetate. ×620,000.

Figure 5. Flagellar end from E. coli with only L and P rings attached and rod visible. S and M rings are missing. Uranyl acetate. ×400,000.

Figure 6. Flagellar end from E. coli with only L and P rings of the basal body still attached. Uranyl acetate. ×300,000.

Figure 7. Flagellar filament-hook complex with part of the rod still attached to the hook. Uranyl acetate. ×290,000.

followed by a low speed centrifugation to remove unlysed cells and large aggregates. The intact flagella were then banded at their equilibrium density of 1.30 gm/ml in CsCl. The flagella were collected, dialyzed against Tris –EDTA buffer and examined.

3. Properties of Purified Intact Flagella Preparations

Electron microscopy showed only the presence of flagella, most of which still had their basal body-hook complex. About 1 basal body was found per 6 μm of filaments present. Since the average length of flagella in vivo was about 5 μm, very little loss of basal bodies occurred during the purification. The basal bodies had a uniform appearance with no debris attached to them.

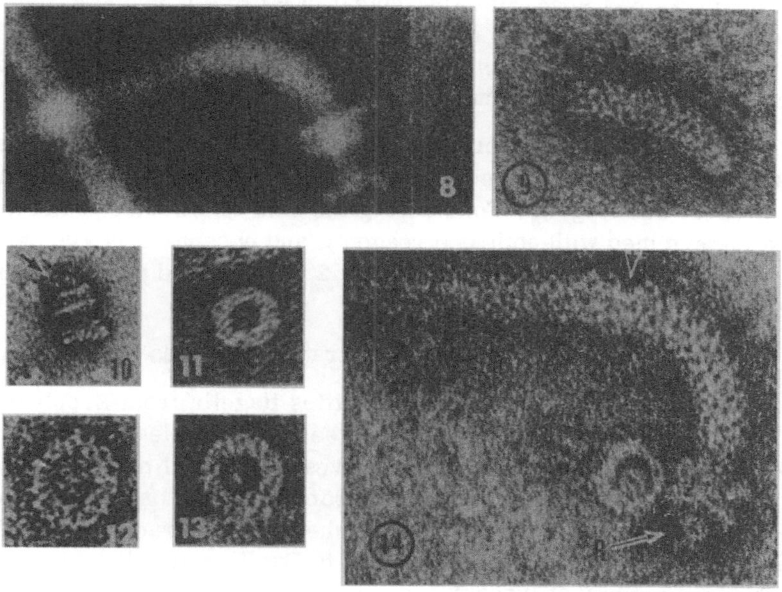

Figure 8. Basal end of an intact flagellum from E. coli with rod visible between L and P rings. Compare with similar appearance of the stain where two filaments have crossed, preventing stain penetration at the point of cross over. Phosphotungstic acid. ×520,000.

Figure 9. Isolated hook from E. coli. Uranyl acetate. ×445,000.

Figure 10. E. coli flagellar basal body detached from hook. Connection to the hook is visible (arrow). Uranyl acetate. ×356,000.

Figure 11. A detached ring found after damaging intact flagella from E. coli. The center appears empty. Uranyl actate. ×520,000.

Figure 12. A picture of a detached ring with a core in its center underfocused for contrast. Uranyl acetate. ×735,000.

Figure 13. Detached ring with a core remaining in its center. Uranyl acetate. ×670,000.

Figure 14. Flagellar basal end from E. coli missing the bottom rings. The rod is visible (arrow) and a detached ring containing a core is associated with the top rings of the basal body. The junction between the hook and the filament is marked by a large arrow. Uranyl acetate. ×620,000.

Polyacrylamide gel electrophoresis showed no detectable (<1 per cent) acidic or basic proteins of M.W. 100,000 or less. Treatment with either heat, acid or urea under conditions which dissociate flagellar filaments produced only one band corresponding to flagellin. The basal body-hook complexes either did not dissociate under these conditions, or any bands resulting from them were to faint to detect since 98% of the protein present is flagellin.

The ultraviolet spectrum was typical of a protein having a maximum at 278 nm and a minimum at 255 nm with a 280/260 ratio of 1.35-1.40. The spectrum of intact flagella was identical to that obtained from purified flagellar filaments that had been mechanically removed from cells.

Measurements of total protein using the Lowry method and flagellar protein using ^{125}I labeled flagellar antibody showed that 94-99 per cent of the protin present was flagella. Considering the sum of the total protein, carbohydrate (determined with anthrone reagent), and phosphate as 100 per cent, carbohydrate accounted for approximately 2 per cent and phosphate for less than 0.15 per cent.

The yields of flagella in these preparations were as high as 40 per cent.

Therefore, the above procedure purifies flagella from E. coli in the form of a filament-hook-basal body complex, free of detectable cell wall, membrane and cytoplasmic material. The method gives substantial product recovery and is adaptable to large scale preparations from which the basal body and hook could be isolated and their structure and chemistry characterized. The procedure has also been successfully applied to Bacillus subtilis and is probably applicable to a variety of lysozyme-sensitive bacteria despite strikingly different cell envelopes. A similar procedure has been independently developed by Dimmit and Simon (1971) for B. subtilis.

4. The Structure of Flagellar Basal Bodies

The following data, schematically summarized in Figure 1, deals with the structural details of falgellar basal bodies from E. coli (DePamphilis and Adler, 1971b). E. coli flagella have a basal body which consists of five primary components: a rod and four rings. The two rings proximal to the hook (the "top rings") were 22.5 nm in diameter and spaced 9 nm apart. These were connected by the rod to two similar rings distal to the hook (the "bottom rings"), 22.5 nm in diameter and 3 nm apart. The rod was approximately 27 nm in length.

Electron micrographs of undamaged flagellar basal bodies from E. coli (Figures 2, 3) were clearly consistent with the model in Figure 1. Each ring is 1.5 nm thick based on measurements of pictures such as Figure 2 in which the top and bottom edges of the rings are resolved. Penetration of the stain between the top rings was always substantially less than its penetration into the gap between the top and bottom rings (Figures 2-5, 8). This fact, together with evidence presented later, suggests the existence of a structure connecting the top rings near their periphery to form a cylinder.

Further support for the model in Figure 1 comes from studies of damaged basal ends. Damage was brought about by centrifuging intact flagella, or collecting them on a Gelman cellulose actate filter, and then abruptly resuspending them. Basal bodies were found that had apparently lost one of their bottom rings (Figure 4). Some basal bodies were missing both bottom rings although the rod remained (Figure 5). More commonly, however, the rod had broken off at its junction with the P ring (Figure 6). Sometimes part of the rod

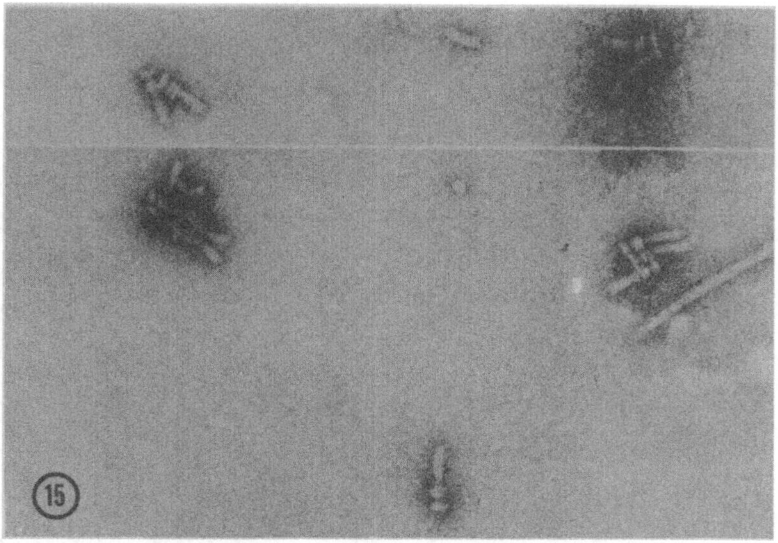

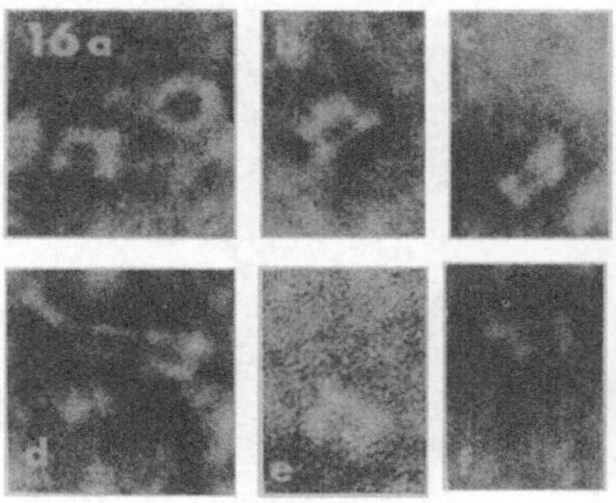

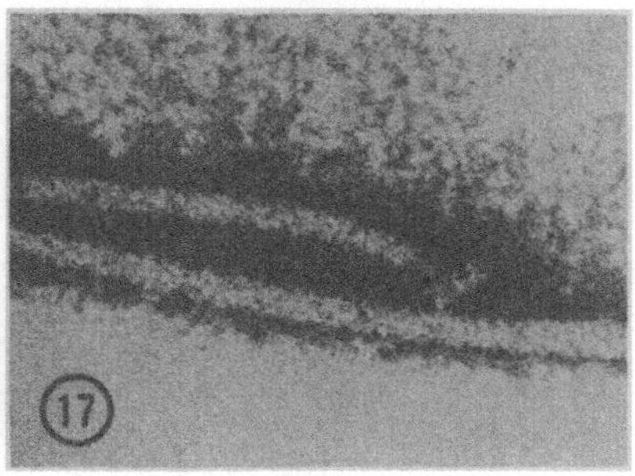

Figure 15. Basal body-hook complexes found after treatment of intact flagella from E. coli at pH 3.4. Uranyl acetate. ×150,000.

Figure 16. Rectangular shaped structures seen after treatment of intact flagella from E. coli at pH 2.7. A ring is also visible in Figure 16a. Uranyl acetate. ×310,000.

Figure 17. Basal end of an intact flagellum from B. subtilis. Uranyl acetate. ×380,000.

remained on the hook after the other components of the basal body were gone (Figure 7). This part of the rod evidently mounted the top rings (Figure 8), and extended only as far as the P ring. Isolated hooks (Figure 9), and basal bodies (Figure 10) were also found.

Isolated rings were found (Figures 11-13), 22.5 nm in diameter, which had evidently broken off of basal bodies. Some of the isolated rings appeared to have empty centers (Figure 11), 10 nm in diameter, and some contained a core (Figures 12-14), 7 nm in diameter which did not completely fill the opening. In a damaged basal body with the bottom rings missing (Figure 14), part of the rod was seen and it appeared that stain had entered the end, suggesting

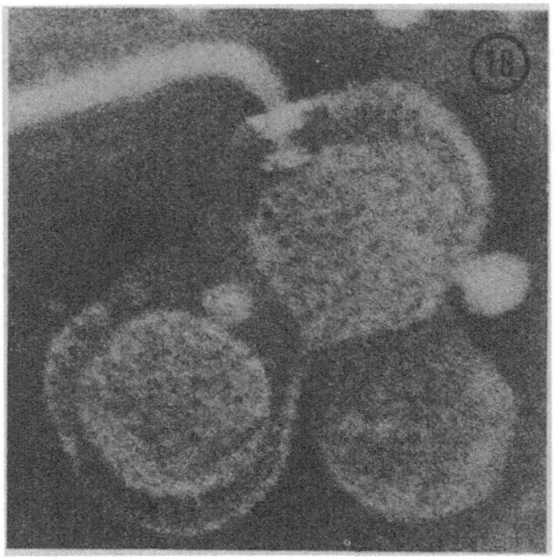

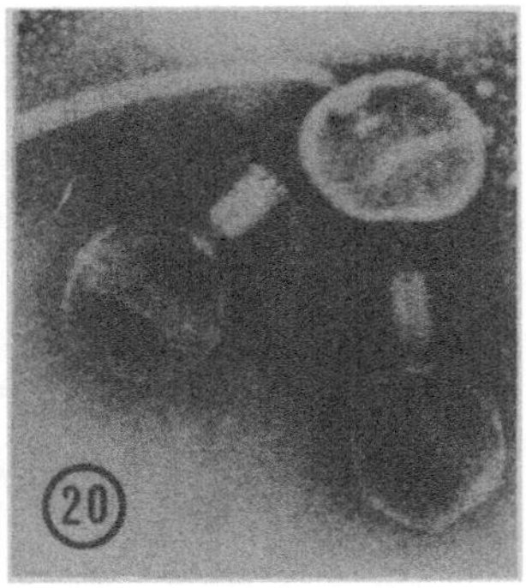

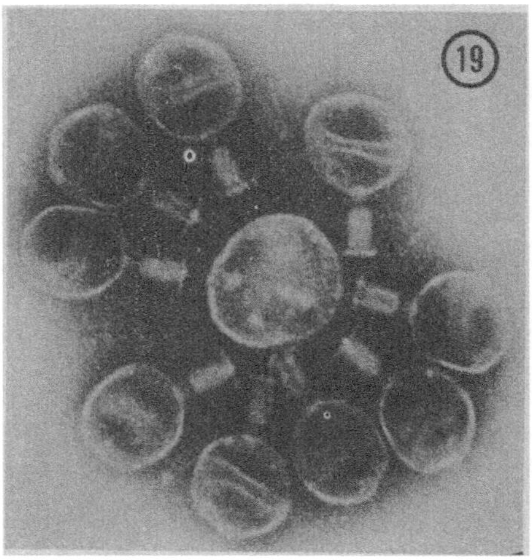

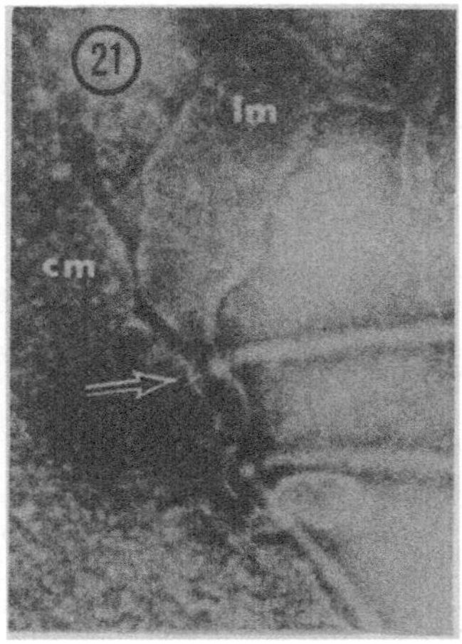

Figure 18. Basal body of E. coli flagellum attached to L membrane vesicle at L ring. Phosphotungstic acid. ×154,000.

Figure 19. Nine T2 phages attached to a single L membrane vesicle, 124 nm in diameter. Phosphotungstic acid. ×154,000.

Figure 20. Basal body of an E. coli flagellum enclosed in an L membrane vesicle with T2 phage attached to the vesicle. Phosphotungstic acid. ×160,000.

Figure 21. Cytoplasmic membrane prepared from osmotically shocked E. coli spheroplasts. Note the flagellar basal bodies attached to both cytoplasmic membrane (CM) and L membrane (LM). Only the basal body's M ring is attached to the cytoplasmic membrane (arrow). Phosphotungstic acid. ×133,000.

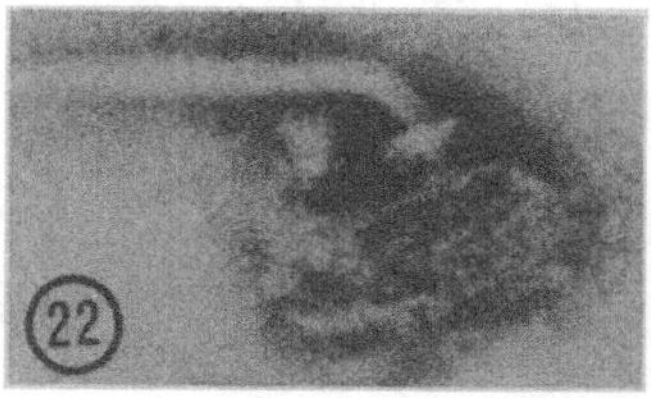

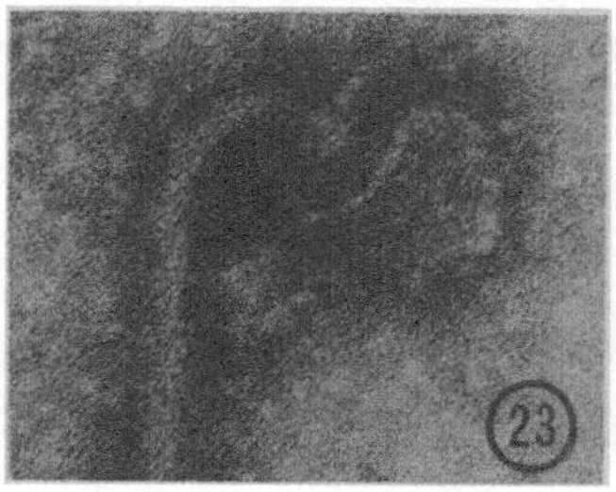

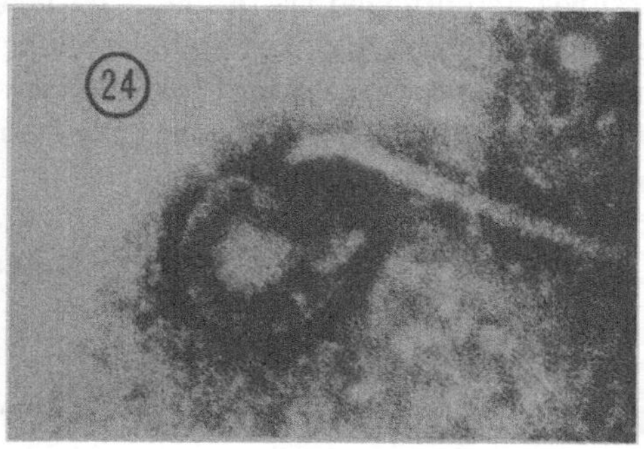

Figure 22. Basal body of an E. coli flagellium attached to a fragment of cytoplasmic membrane. Phosphotungstic acid. ×265,000.

Figure 23. Basal body of an E. coli flagellum attached to a fragment of cytoplasmic membrane. Phosphotungstic acid. ×265,000.

Figure 24. Basal body of an E. coli flagellum attached to both an L membrane vesicle and a spherical cytoplasmic membrane fragment. Phosphotungstic acid. ×185,000.

the rod was hollow. The core seen in the detached ring had the same diameter as the rod and was evidently part of a rod.

5. Isolation of Basal Body-Hook Complexes from Intact Flagella

Flagella filaments are known to dissociate under various conditions such as low pH or high temperature in which the hooks are relatively stable (Abram et al., 1970). Viscometry measurements showed that purified flagellar filaments from E. coli were completely dissociated at 30°C after 30 min in either 4.5 M urea or at pH 3.4, or at 55°C for 10 min in 0.05 M KCl. Under these conditions the basal body-hook complexes remained intact and the basal bodies appeared undamaged (Figure 15).

Basal body-hook complexes were degraded when the pH was lowered to 2.8 for 30 min at room temperature. The filaments, hooks, and rods dissociated and only isolated rings and hollow rectangular structures were found (Figure 16). These rectangular structures had the dimensions and appearance expected of the top rings if connected near their periphery. The existence of these structures further supports the concept that the top rings are attached to form a cylinder through which the rod passes.

6. Flagellar Basal Bodies from Bacillus subtilis

Using the same purification methods described for E. coli, intact flagella were prepared from Bacillus subtilis. The flagellar basal end from B. subtilis consists of a hook and a rod with only two rings present (Figure 17). The structures and dimensions of the basal body are similar to those of E. coli except that the top pair of rings is missing. The rings were 21 nm wide and 3.5 nm apart and were mounted on the bottom of a rod 7.8 nm in diameter. As with E. coli flagella, the basal body-hook complexes could be isolated by dissolving the filaments at pH 3.2.

7. Attachment of Flagellar Basal Bodies to the Cell Envelope

a) Specific Attachment to the Outer Membrane

In order to determine what specific attachments existed between basal body and cell envelope structures, the two membrane components from the cell envelope of E. coli were isolated with flagellar basal bodies still attached.

The procedure for purifying intact flagella from E. coli was changed (DePamphilis and Adler, 1971c) by incubating spheroplasts in 40 mM $MgCl_2$ prior to lysis and then maintaining an environment of 10 mM $MgCl_2$ instead of 0.5 mM EDTA. This resulted in the purification of flagella still attached to fragments of outer, lipopolysaccharide, membrane (the L membrane). L membrane fragments had a vescicular configuration. Only the L ring on flagellar basal bodies was attached to the L membrane vesicles (Figure 18).

Infrequently basal bodies were seen with an enlarged or extended L ring which was probably due to the presence of L membrane. Neither variation in ring diameter nor attachments to L membrane vesicles were seen with the other rings.

These isolated vesicles were not cytoplasmic membranes because: (1) cytoplasmic membranes are rapidly solubilized by Triton X-100 (Birdsell and Cota-Robles, 1968), and (2) intact cytoplasmic membranes have a density approximately 1.1-1.2 g/ml (Morowitz and Terry, 1969). L membrane vesicles have a density in CsCl of 1.34 g/ml.

These vesicles were identified as the outer lipopolysaccharide membranes based on the following criteria: (a) Purified lipopolysaccharide also has a vesicular configuration in the presence of Mg^{2+}. (2) Thin sections of L membrane vesicles showed the trilaminar structure characteristic of the outer membrane in E. coli cell walls (DePetris, 1967). (3) Chemical analysis of L membrane preparations and lipopolysaccharide purified from the same E. coli strain had similar molar ratios of heptose, glucose, 7-keto-3-deoxy-octonate, and phosphate. These compounds are characteristic of lipopolysaccharide (Osborn, 1969). (4) Both L membrane vesicles and lipopolysaccharide vesicles will dissociate when dialyzed against EDTA and then reassemble into a vesicular configuration when dialyzed against Mg^{2+} (DePamphilis, 1971a). (5) Reassembly of L membrane or lipopolysaccharide in the presence of intact

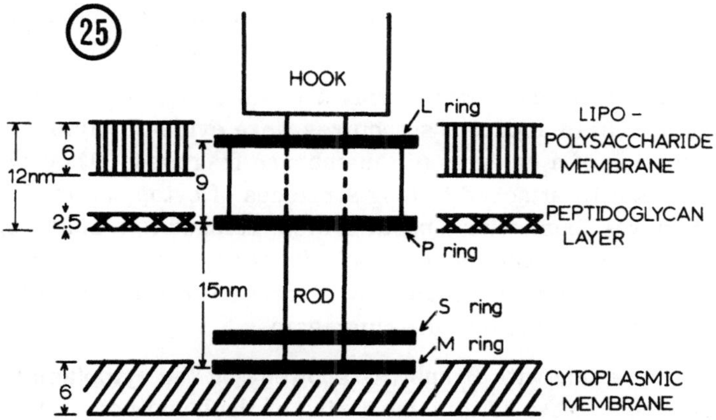

Figure 25. A model of the attachment of flagellar basal bodies from E. coli to the cell envelope. Dimensions are in nanometers. Dimensions for cell envelope are from thin sections of E. coli by DePetris, 1967.

flagella results in the attachment of flagellar basal bodies by their L rings to the reconstituted vesicles. (6) Following T2 or T4 phage adsorption to cells prior to spheroplast formation, L membrane was isolated with phage attached to the outside. About 80 per cent of the vesicles had one or more phage attached (Figure 19). The phage were oriented perpendicular to the surface of the vesicle, and had contracted sheaths and empty heads. This indentifies the vesicles as originating from the outer membrane of the cell envelope which contains the T2 and T4 phage receptor sites (DePamphilis, 1971b).

In a preparation of flagella-L membrane complexes, some basal bodies were found encapsulated by small vesicles with a diameter of 60-70 nm and looked very similar to basal body structures frequently reported (Abram, 1969; Abram et al., 1965; Hoeniger et al., 1966; van Iterson et al., 1966; Tawara, 1965). This raised the question of whether such vesicles attached to basal bodies represent a true structure of the basal body, or artifacts resulting from vesiculation of L membrane fragments. When T2 was adsorbed to cells prior to L membrane purification, phage were found adsorbed to the outside surface of such small basal body-vesicle complexes (Figure 20). This proves that these vesicles originated from the surface of the cell and are not true structures of the basal body.

b) Specific Attachment to the Cytoplasmic Membrane

In order to examine the association of flagellar basal bodies with the cytoplasmic membrane, E. coli spheroplasts were lysed osmotically rather than with Triton X-100 and the resulting membranes isolated by differential centrifugation. Flagellar basal bodies were found still attached to isolated membranes (Figure 21). This association resulted from the cytoplasmic membrane's attachment to the basal body ring farthest from the hook (the "M" ring, for membrane), as well as the L membrane's attachment to the L ring. Flagella were also found that had apparently pulled free from a cytoplasmic membrane, leaving a fragment of the membrane still attached to the basal body (Figures 22, 23). The "S" ring ("supramembrane") is visible just above the cytoplasmic membrane. These membrane fragments could be removed by addition of Triton X-100, thereby exposing the M ring.

Some flagellar basal bodies were found with spherical structures attached to the bottom. These apparent structures were evidently artifacts resulting from vesiculation of a cytoplasmic membrane fragment. They were never seen on basal bodies still attached to long stretches of cytoplasmic membranes and one specimen was found with 8 basal bodies attached to a single sphere. Figure 24 shows both artifacts derived both from vesiculation of cytoplasmic and L membranes. We have not found any evidence for a part of the basal body extending past the M ring into the cytoplasm.

A similar study with B. subtilis showed that the cytoplasmic membrane was attached only to the bottom-most ring of the basal body. Therefore, the rings on B. subtilis basal bodies are analogous to the S and M rings of E. coli basal bodies on the basis of their position at the bottom of the rod, their size and proximity, and particularly their relationship to the cell membrane.

8. Discussion

Figure 25 diagramatically illustrates the relationship between E. coli basal body and cell envelope structures. The L ring of flagellar basal bodies specifically attaches to the cell envelope's outer membrane, a lipopolysaccharide–protein–phospholipid complex referred to as the L membrane. The evidence is that (1) purified L membrane vesicles are attached to flagellar basal bodies via the L ring, (2) purified L membrane or purified lipopolysaccharide vesicles can be dissociated and then reassembled onto flagellar basal bodies via attachment to their L ring, (3) preparations of membranes from osmotically shocked spheroplasts contain some L membrane still attached to basal bodies via the L ring.

The M ring specifically attaches to the cell envelope's inner membrane, a lipopolysaccharide lipoprotein complex referred to as the cytoplasmic membrane. The evidence is that preparations of membranes from osmotically shocked spheroplasts contain cytoplasmic membrane attached to the bottom ring of flagellar basal bodies.

The S ring is visible in these preparations just above the cytoplasmic membrane. The S ring has no obvious associations with any of the cell envelope components visible in thin sections and appears to be unattached.

Given the locations of the L and M rings in the cell envelope, the second ring from the top would be in register with the peptidoglycan layer to which it (the "P" ring for peptidoglycan) is presumably attached. Consistent with this is the fact that the P ring was always free of any attached material after lysozyme treatment. However, the space between the peptidoglycan layer and the L membrane contains a lipoprotein (Braun and Schwarz, 1969) covalently bound to the peptidoglycan and apparently attached to the lipopolysaccharide membrane. The P ring could be associated with the lipoprotein component.

The spherical capsules attached to E. coli basal bodies under certain conditions were artifacts resulting from vesiculation of fragments of L membranes or cytoplasmic membranes and their specific attachment to L and M rings respectively. Reports in the liberature of spherical basal body structures probably resulted from the same artifacts. Flagella apparently do not penetrate the cytoplasm but terminate at the junction of their M ring with the cytoplasmic membrane.

The structural model of the basal body described for E. coli is apparently a general structure found in flagellated Gram negative bacteria that have cell envelopes comparable in structure to that of E. coli. Electron micrographs of basal bodies on flagella from Rhodospirillum (Cohen-Bazire and London, 1967), and on axial filaments from Leptospira (Nauman et al., 1969) show structures strikingly similar to E. coli. Data from Proteus (Abram et al., 1965; Hoeniger et al., 1966; van Iterson et al., 1966), Ectothiorhodospira (Remsen et al., 1968), and Vibrio (Vaituzis and Doetsch, 1969) sugges the same structure.

The basal body from B. subtilis lacks the top set of rings found on the E. coli basal body. The data of Abram (Abram et al., 1970; Abram et al., 1966) on five other strains of Bacillus appear consistent with this description. These top rings interact specifically with the complex multilayered cell wall of E. coli. Apparently the top rings are not needed with the dense single layered wall of B. subtilis. This indicates that the top rings per se are not involved in motility but only serve an attachment function in Gram negative bacteria. Therefore, it appears that the structure of the basal body directly reflects the structure of the cell envelope, and one would then expect two major classes of flagellar basal bodies as exemplified by E. coli and B. subtilis.

The complexity of the basal end of the flagellum may explain the results of genetic analysis of flagella synthesis. In Salmonella, mutations in 10 genes, besides the gene for flagellin synthesis, have been recognized as responsible for the nonflagellated phenotype (Iino, 1969). The basal body-hook complex may account for as many as 7 structural genes.

REFERENCES

Abram, D. (1969). Bacteriol. Proc., p. 29.
Abram, D., Koffler, H., and Vatter, A. E. (1965). J. Bacteriol. 90, 1337.
Abram, D., Mitchen, J. R., Koffler, H., and Vatter, A. E. (1970). J. Bacteriol. 101, 250.
Abram, D., Vatter, A. E., and Koffler, H. (1966). J. Bacteriol. 91, 2045.
Birdsell, D. and Cota-Robles, E. (1968). Biochem. Biophys. Res. Comm. 31, 438.
Braun, V. and Schwarz, U. (1969). Soc. Gen. Microbiol. Proc. in J. Gen. Microbiol. 57, iii.
Cohen-Bazire, G. and London, J. (1967). J. Bacteriol. 94, 458.
DePamphilis, M. L. (1971a). J. Bacteriol. 105, 1184.
DePamphilis, M. L. (1971b). J. Virology. 7, 683.
DePamphilis, M. L. and Adler, J. (1971a). J. Bacteriol., 105, 376.
DePamphilis, M. L. and Adler, J. (1971b). J. Bacteriol. 105, 384.
DePamphilis, M. L. and Adler, J. (1971c). J. Bacteriol. 105, 396.
DePetris, S. (1967). J. Ultrastruct. Res. 19, 45.
Dimmit, K. and Simon, M. (1970a). Immunity 1, 212.
Dimmit, K. and Simon, M. (1971). J. Bacteriol., 105, 369.
Glauert, A. M., Kerridge, D., and Horne, R. W. (1963). J. Cell Biol. 18, 327.
Glauert, A. M. and Thornley, M. J. (1969). Ann. Rev. Microbiol. 23, 159.
Hoeniger, J. F. M., van Iterson, W., and van Zanten, E. N. (1966). J. Cell Biol. 31, 603.
Iino, T. (1969). Bacteriol. Rev. 33, 454.
Iterson, W. van, Hoeniger, J. F. M., and van Zanten, E. N. (1966). J. Cell Biol. 31, 585.

Lawn. A.M. (1967). Nature 214, 1151.
Morowitz, H. and Terry, T. (1969). Biochim. Biophys. Acta 183, 276.
Murray, R. G. E. and Birch-Andersen, A. (1963). Can. J. Microbiol. 9, 393.
Nauman, R. K., Holt, S. C., and Cox, C. D. (1969). J. Bacteriol. 98, 264.
Osborn, M. J. (1969). Ann. Rev. Biochem. 38, 501.
Remsen, C. C., Watson, S. W., Waterbury, J. B., and Truper, H. G. (1968). J. Bacteriol. 95, 2374.
Ritchie, A. E., Keeler, R. F., and Bryner, J. H. (1966). J. Gen. Microbiol. 43, 427.
Tawara, J. (1965). Jap. J. Microbiol. 9, 49.
Vaituzis, Z. and Doetsch, R. N. (1969). J. Bacteriol. 100, 512.

THE NATURE OF THE FLAGELLAR HOOK AND THE LIKELY INVOLVEMENT OF SURFACE STRUCTURES IN THE FORMATION OF BACTERIAL FLAGELLUM

H. Koffler, R.W. Smith, J.R. Mitchen and E. McGroarty
Purdue University,
Department of Biological Sciences,
Lafayette,
Indiana 47907, U.S.A.

The bacterial flagellum is differentiated into three morphologically distinct regions: an extracellular spiral microtubular filament, which constitutes over 90 per cent of the organelle, a hook, and a basal region that appears to be closely associated with the cytoplasmic membrane and the cell wall. If bacteria have any "sensory" receptors at all, it would be functionally plausible if such devices were located within or near surface structures. Probably this is true also for the machinery necessary to accomplish the transformation of chemical to kinetic energy and to coordinate the motion of individual flagella. Apparently the integrity of the cell surface is required for motility, since protoplasts of bacteria retain their original number of flagella, but are no longer motile (Weibull, 1953). More recently there have been indications that the prior formation of an intact cell wall is necessary for the synthesis of flagellin (Vaituzis and Doetsch, 1965) and that inhibitors capable of preventing the incorporation of diaminopimelic acid into the wall of Bacillus cereus also prevent the formation of flagella (Mendel et al., 1965). Since a relationship between the membrane-wall complex and the bacterial flagellum is implicated, it is regrettable that the nature of the basal structures and the flagellar hook, the components of the flagellum nearest to the surface structures, is only little understood. This paper attempts to contribute towards understanding this complex relationship in two respects, namely regarding the nature of the hook protein and the involvement of the cell wall or the wall-membrane complex in the formation of flagella.

1. The Nature of the Flagellar Hook

The filamentous portion of the organelle can be easily purified and consists of flagellin, a protein capable of assembling by itself to form flagellar filaments (Abram and Koffler, 1964; Ada et al., 1964; Asakura et al., 1964). The hook differs from the filament not only in morphology, but also in fine structure (Abram et al., 1965, 1966), stability (Abram et al., 1970), and, as will be shown in the first part of this report, in its constituent protein. Since

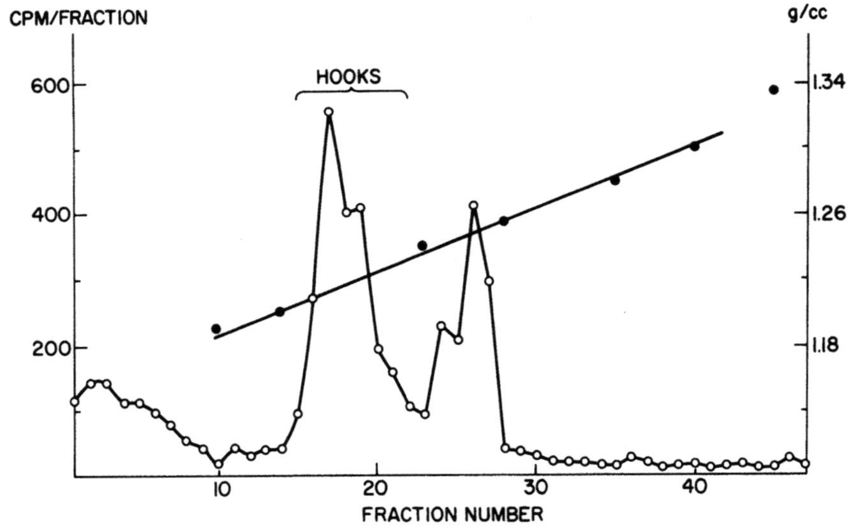

Figure 1. Purification of flagellar hooks on a renografin density gradient.

the hook represents only a minute fraction of the total organelle and therefore is difficult to isolate in amounts sufficient for analysis, knowledge regarding its nature has come only slowly. The following recent improvements (Mitchen et al., 1970) in the procedures for isolating hooks (Abram et al., 1967, 1970; Mitchen and Koffler, 1969) have been helpful: Flagella are broken off cells of Bacillus pumilus suspended in phosphate buffer, pH 7, by shaking with a commercial paint shaker for 10 minutes. Cell bodies are separated from the flagella by centrifugation at 13,200 × g at 4° for 25 minutes; the flagella are then precipitated by centrifugation at 40,000 × g at 4° for 120 minutes. Forty per cent of the hooks remain with the filaments, while the other 60 per cent remain attached to the cells, as determined by electron microscopy (for preparation of samples and other techniques see Abram, 1965, and Abram et al., 1970). Further purification of hooks involves three critical steps: The first is the selective disintegration of filaments by treatment with HCl at pH 3 for 30 minutes at 37°, a condition that has no effect on hooks. Since native filaments are not completely dissolved by this treatment, either filaments fragmented by slow freezing and thawing are used or the disintegration process is repeated until complete solubilization is achieved. The hooks together with contaminant cell debris are collected by centrifugation at 5,000 × g, 4°, for 15 minutes, as observed by electron microscopic examination. The next step involves addition to the pellet of one-fifth of the original volume of four per cent Triton X100. This solubilizes most of the non-hook material after incubation at 37° for 60 minutes, and crude hook preparations can be obtained by centrifugation at 100,000 × g for 60 minutes. This treatment also makes it possible to resuspend an otherwise fairly insoluble precipitate. Thirdly, further purification of the hooks is achieved by density gradient centrifugation in renografin (1.16 to 1.34 g per ml renografin-76, Squibb, in 0.1 N Tris–HCl, pH 8) for eight hours at 200,000 × g and 15°. To increase the sensitivity of our analysis ^{14}C-labeled hooks were used isolated from cells grown in a

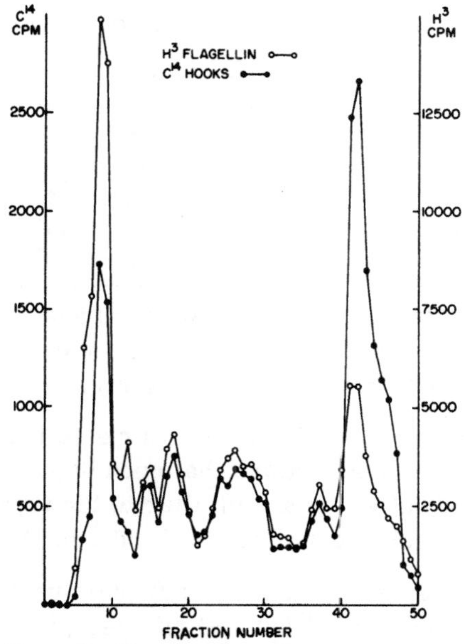

Figure 2. Eluation of tryptic peptides from a Dowex-50 ion exchange column (first 50 1.5 ml fractions).

defined medium containing biotin (2×10^{-7} M), ammonium sulfate (1.5×10^{-2} M), magnesium sulfate (10^{-3} M), calcium chloride (10^{-4} M), potassium phosphate buffer (0.15 M, pH 7), and uniformly ^{14}C-labeled glucose (2.2×10^{-3} M, 46 c per M) as the sole source of carbon. The ^{14}C-cells were mixed with non-radioactive carrier cells inthe ratio of 1 to 2000 (w per w) before isolation of the hooks. In Figure 1 the appearance of two radioactive peaks upon density gradient centrifugation is shown. The fractions containing radioactivity were pooled, diluted five times, centrifuged at 100,000 × g for one hour at 4°, and examined electron microscopically. The hooks sediment uniformly when centrifuged again in a renografin density gradient. Under these conditions the proteins of the filament do not enter more than a few fractions of the gradient.

The final yields are shown in Table 1. Since both the filaments and hooks are uniformly ^{14}C-labeled, it is convenient to use assays for radioactivity to determine recovery. The isolated flagellar filaments constitute 0.127 per cent of the total radioactivity incorporated into cells, and the hooks represent about one-half a percent of the filaments isolated.

Aside from differences in morphology, fine structure, and stability, there have been other indications that hooks differ from filaments. In 1967 Lawn showed electron microscopically that anti-H sera (antisera against whole cells absorbed with somatic antigens) react with flagellar filaments but not with hooks. Since then McGroarty and Oiler in this laboratory have shown that filaments and hooks react differently to antisera prepared against purified flagellin. The different antigenic nature of hooks was further confirmed by

TABLE 1. Recovery of Radioactivity from Cells Grown on ^{14}C-Glucose

Isolate	C^{14}; CPM	Percent of cell	Percent of flagella
Cells.	8.60×10^9	1.00×10^2	–
Flagella	1.06×10^7	1.27×10^{-1}	1.00×10^2
Hooks	5.25×10^4	6.00×10^{-4}	4.95×10^{-1}

Dimmitt and Simon (1970) who found that antisera against hooks do not react with flagellar filaments. While these experiments suggest a different composition for hooks, they do not prove this conclusively.

What then is the nature of the hooks? Our data indicate that the hooks consist mostly of one or more proteins that upon digestion with trypsin yield peptides most but not all of which are similar to the tryptic peptides released upon digestion by the flagellin contained in the filament.

When radioactive hooks from cells of B. pumilus are precipitated with hot 10 per cent trichloracetic acid (90°, 30 minutes), virtually all counts become insoluble. This observation eliminates numerous compounds as likely constituents and suggests the protein nature of the hook.

Upon electrophoresis on 10 per cent acrylamide–sodium lauryl sulfate (SLS) gels (0.05 per cent w per v SLS, pH 7.2, 8 ma per tube, 2.5 hours), flagella pretreated with one per cent SLS and one per cent mercaptoethanol at 37° for one hour give two bands, one for flagellin A and the other for flagellin B (Sullivan et al., 1969). Hooks are not disintegrated by such a pretreatment and do not enter the gels. When hooks are layered on such gels no flagellin bands can be demonstrated. Furthermore, as mentioned before, the proteins in the filament do not enter more than a few fractions isolated during the separation involving renografin density gradient centrifugation.

In order to learn more about the nature of the hook material, ^{14}C-hooks and ^{3}H-flagellin from filaments were isolated from cells grown as mentioned previously on uniformly labeled ^{14}C- and ^{3}H-glucose (specific activity of ^{3}H-glucose in the medium was 92 c per M), respectively. The ^{14}C-hooks purified on renografin gradients were mixed with ^{3}H-filaments, and after having been heated at 100° for 30 minutes, pH 2.5, the mixture was digested with trypsin (10 μg per mg protein), at pH 8, 37°, for 10 hours. After removal of the undigested material by centrifugation at 100,000 × g for one hour, the resulting peptides were separated on a Dowex-50 type ion exchange column using the elution system of Benson et al. (1960), and 1.5 ml fractions were assayed for ^{14}C- and ^{3}H-radioactivity by differential counting in a scintillation spectrometer. Eighty-five per cent of the hooks and 90 per cent of the filaments were solubilized by trypsin under the conditions used. As shown in Figure 2 the first 50 fractions from hook protein are similar or perhaps identical to those released from the flagellin contained in the filament, with the possible exception

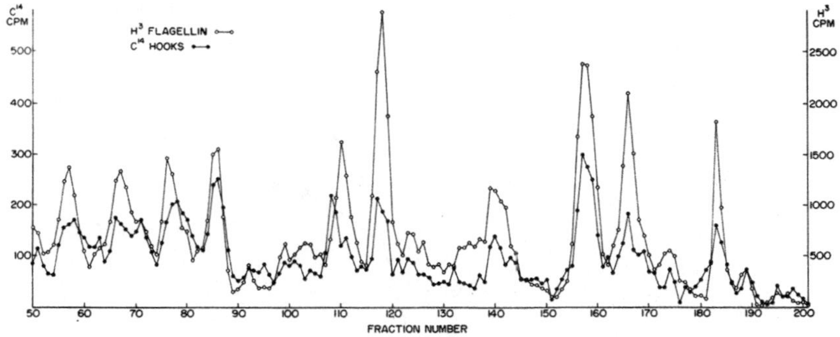

Figure 3. Elution of tryptic peptides (fractions 50 to 200).

of two (i.e., those shown as fractions 12 and 40 to 48). At least two differences are also seen in the next 150 fractions (Figure 3). These are found in fractions number 108 to 114 and 133 to 138.

Apparently, hooks contain one or more proteins that are similar but not identical to the flagellins contained in the filamentous portion of the organelle. While this finding simplifies hypotheses regarding the assembly of the flagellum, it does not yet explain how apparently few differences in the primary structure have such profound consequences on the morphology, fine structure, and the relative stability of the hooks.

2. Essential Relationship between the Cell Surface and the Formation of the Bacterial Flagellum

The second part of this paper deals with data that strongly suggest an essential interaction between the cell surface and the flagellum in the formation of the organelle (McGroarty et al., 1970).

It has been previously reported by Quadling and Stocker (1956, 1962), Bisset and Pease (1957), and Kerridge (1963) that cells of Salmonella typhimurium when grown at 44° do not form flagellar filaments. The filaments already synthesized before temperature shift up appear to be diluted out by cell division. Similar effects of temperature on flagellation were reported for a strain of Escherichia coli by Morrison (1961) Morrison and McCapra (1961), and for Proteus vulgaris by Bisset and Pease (1957). When cultures of nonflagellated cells of Salmonella grown at 44° are transferred to a lower temperature, flagellar filaments regenerate either without a time lag or after only a short interval. Dimmit et al. (1968) found in Bacillus subtilis that either leucine or uracil starvation or inhibition by chloramphenicol or actinomycin prevented regeneration of filaments from deflagellated cells. Aamodt and Eisenstadt (1968) found in Salmonella typhimurium that a mixture of actinomycin and ethylenediamine tetraacetic acid (EDTA) inhibited filament formation. Apparently the synthesis of both nucleic acid and protein is required for filament formation.

Since the turning "off" and "on" of flagellation represents an experimental situation that might lend itself to analyze the morphogenesis of the flagellum,

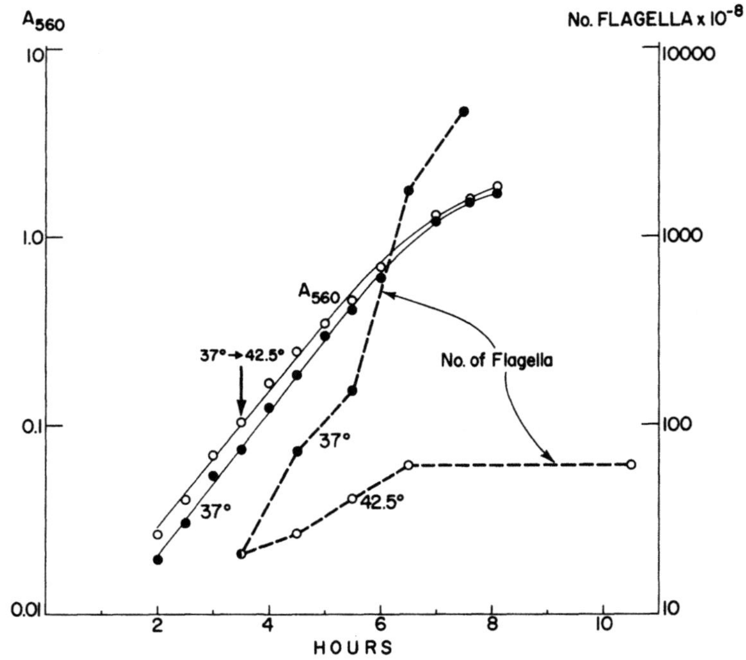

Figure 4. Effect of temperature shift from 37° to 42.5° on cell growth and formation of flagella. Solid lines indicate absorption at 569 mμ (A_{560}). The arrow indicates the time of temperature shift from 37° to 42.5°. The broken lines represent the number of flagella in the culture either growing at 37° or after shift up to 42.5°. Cells were grown in 100 ml of the following medium contained in 500 ml Erlenmeyer flasks (g per liter): trypticase, 10 and yeast extract, 2. Aeration was provided by agitation of the culture on a New Brunswick Gyratory Shaker Model G-25 at a speed of 240 rpm and a rotation of a one inch circle. Ten-ml samples of the culture were used to measure A_{560} values. To determine the total number of flagella in the culture 10 ml samples were centrifuged at 15,000 × g at 4° for 15 minutes after the addition of potassium cyanide to 0.1 N. The cells were resuspended in 0.01 M potassium phosphate buffer, pH 7, or distilled water. The cell suspension was applied to carbon coated collodion grids and the total number of flagella per cell was counted on 200 to 300 cells. This was multiplied by the total number of cells in the culture as determined by direct counting with the Petroff-Hauser counter.

we studied the effects of temperature on flagellation and flagellin synthesis further. When grown at 37° in nutrient broth, cells of Proteus vulgaris are peritrichously flagellated with about seven flagella per cell. These cells grow with a generation time of 50 to 60 minutes, which does not appreciably change as the temperature is raised up to 43°. In Figure 4 the growth curves of cells grown at 37° is compared to that of cells transferred from 37° to 42.5°. Also shown is the total number of flagella present in the culture. Apparently, as noted by others, the flagellar filaments are diluted out as the cells multiply, since at high temperatures the total number of flagella after

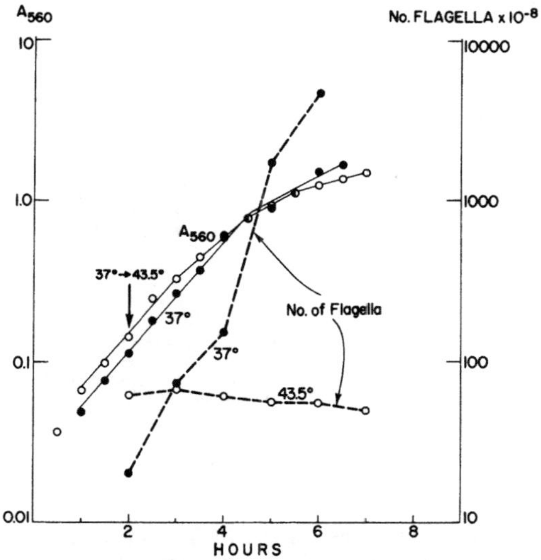

Figure 5. Effect of temperature shift from 37° to 43.5° on cell growth and formation of flagella. Conditions as in Figure 4.

transfer to 42.5° seems to remain constant after an interval of 2 to 2.5 hours. Except for flagellation, cells grown at 42.5° appear to be normal in all other morphological characteristics, as examined by electron microscopy. However, if the cells are grown between 43° and 44°, the cell morphology becomes markedly changed. Enlarged bulbous cells occur which appear to suffer from inpaired cross-wall formation. At this higher temperature range cells grow with a generation time between 80 and 110 minutes, as shown in Figure 5. Upon shift up to this higher temperature there is no further net increase in the number of flagella. As mentioned previously, the existing flagellar filaments appear to be diluted out with cell division.

While there is not net increase in the number of flagella at 42° to 44°, is the net synthesis of flagellin also inhibited at these temperatures? To answer this question the total flagellin concentration at these two temperatures was assayed immunologically. First, spheroplasts were prepared by treatment of 500 to 900 mg dry weight of exponentially growing cells with lysozyme (0.1 per cent, 0.02 M tris buffer, pH 8, in the presence of 20 mg per ml EDTA and 20 per cent lactose) at 37° for one hour, followed by centrifugation at 15,000 × g for 30 minutes. The spheroplasts were then lysed in 0.01 M KCl at 23° for 30 minutes in the presence of 20 μg per ml DNase. Secondly, polymerized flagellin was solubilized by acid treatment. The pH of the suspension was adjusted to 2, and the precipitate was washed with 0.01 M KCl at pH 2 by centrifugation at 15,000 × g for 25 minutes. Thirdly, after dialysis against 0.01 N HCl followed by dialysis against potassium phosphate buffer, pH 7.0, the supernatant liquid was concentrated by ultrafiltration to 1/50 of the original volume and the amount of flagellin was determined by radial immunodiffusion according to the procedure of Ryan (1967). No flagellin (<0.004 per cent) can be detected in cultures grown at 42° to 44°.

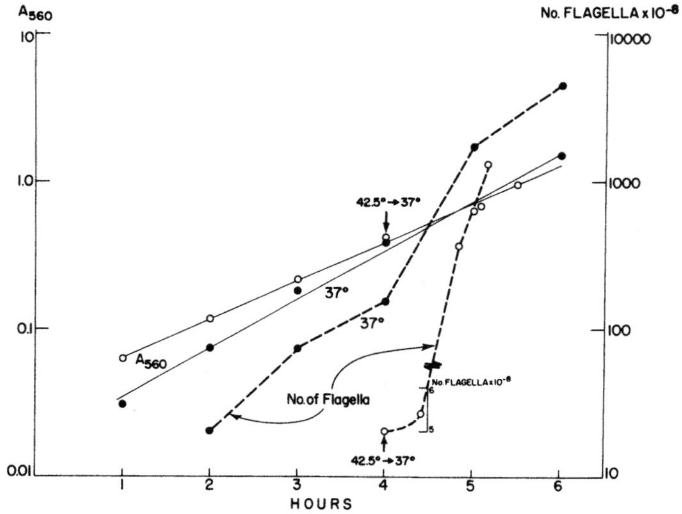

Figure 6. Effect of temperatures shift from 42.5° to 37°. Conditions as in Figures 4 and 5. To determine flagellin cells were grown in two to four 500-ml a liquots of tryplicase yeast extract broth contained in two-liter flasks, and the cultures were pooled before flagellin was analyzed by a radial diffusion method. The inoculum for the experimental cultures at 42.5° was cultured for 10 to 20 generations at that temperature in each of three successive transfers.

Regeneration of flagella after prolonged growth at the two high temperatures was studied next. The results of a temperature shift down experiment are shown in Figure 6. On cells grown at 42.5° and shifted down to 37° flagella first can be observed electron microscopically 45 to 50 minutes after transfer. Total flagellin, assayed immunologically, is also first detectable after 45 minutes after transfer.

When preparations of membranes isolated from cells that had been transferred from 42.5° to 37° are examined in the electron microscope, numerous regenerating flagella often are seen to arise together from small areas of membrane as if they arose in localized regions. On ghosts of whole cells, however, flagella are seen to be regenerating fairly uniformly over the entire cell surface. Therefore, this observation may be due to an artifact brought about by the aggregation of basal materials with themselves and/or with membrane-cell wall complexes.

The regeneration of flagella by cells grown between 43° and 44° and then shifted down to 37° requires from 120 to 150 minutes as shown in Figure 7. As indicated in the inset, flagellin, on the other hand, can be detected as early as 80 minutes after temperature shift down. The reason for this lag is not known. Probably, the synthesis of some other cell structure is impaired by growth at the high temperature and must be restored before flagellin can again be normally assembled.

Some clues regarding the nature of the critical lesion imposed by high temperatures can be obtained by studying the effect of such inhibitors as chloramphenicol and penicillin.

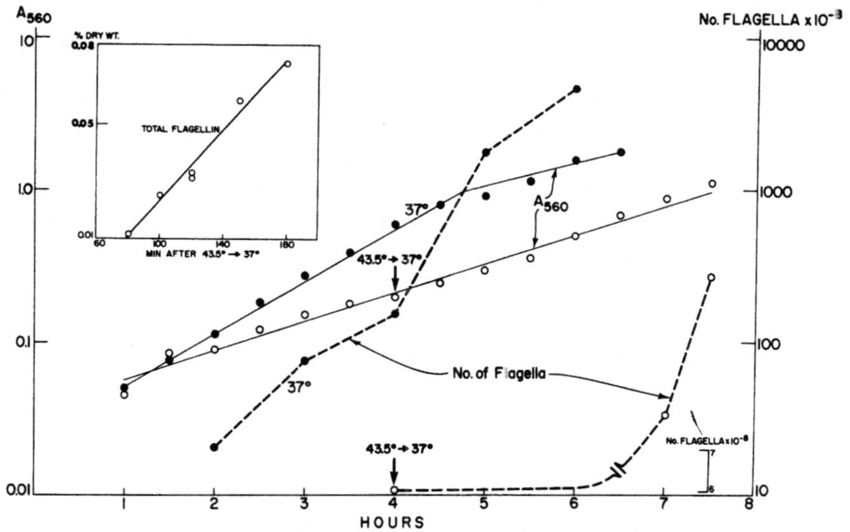

Figure 7. Effect of temperature shift from 43.5° to 37°. Inset shows the net synthesis of intracellular flagellin after temperature shift. Conditions as in Figures 4 and 6. To determine flagellin in this or other experiments cells were grown in two to four 500-ml aliquots of trypticase yeast extract broth contained in two-liter flasks, and the cultures were then pooled before flagellin was analyzed by a radial diffusion method. The inoculum for the experimental cultures at 43.5° were cultured for 10 to 20 generations at that temperature in each of three successive transfers.

Cells were grown through three transfers in 100-ml trypticase-yeast extract broth in 500-ml Erlenmeyer flasks at 42.5°. The experimental cultures were grown at 42.5° to approximately the midpoint of the logarithmic growth phase (A_{560} about 0.6), and then transferred to 37°. After various periods of time 5-ml aliquot were added to sterile test tubes containing in one set of experiments one ml of chloramphenicol (Sigma; 20 μg per ml) and in another set one ml of penicillin (Squibb; 6000 units per ml) and 0.2 g lactose. In either case the samples were then incubated at 37° for two hours on a gyratory shaking machine. During this time a drop of each sample was analyzed at 10 minute intervals for the presence of motile cells by the hanging drop technique. The remainder of each sample was fixed with potassium cyanide at a final concentration of 0.1 N, centrifuged at 15,000 × g, 4°, 30 minutes, and washed once with distilled water. The cells were then resuspended in distilled water and examined electron microscopically; the number of flagella was determined on 100 to 200 cells in each sample.

If chloramphenicol is added within 20 minutes after transfer from 42.5° to 37° and within 30 minutes after shift down from 43.5° neither motility nor flagellation can be observed. When chloramphenicol is added after these times flagella regenerate and motility is restored. Since chloramphenicol when added to "normal" cells does not completely inhibit the formation of flagella, it is probable that the inhibitory effect of chloramphenicol on the regeneration of flagella within 20 or 30 minutes after shift down is exerted through preventing the synthesis of one or more non-flagellar structures. A likely candidate for this is the membrane-wall complex, as is shown by the effect of pencillin on the regeneration of flagella. If penicillin is added during any time before motility and flagella reappear after shift down to 37° (within 45 minutes in the case of cells grown at 42.5° and 150 minutes for cells grown at 43.5°) flagella are not regenerated. In fact, additions of penicillin after these times reduce but do not prevent the increase in the number of new flagella. These data strongly suggest that the presence of cell wall or the concomitant synthesis of cell wall is required for the regeneration of flagella. At the moment it is not clear whether the observed effect is brought about directly by damage to the wall or indirectly by alterations in the condition of the membrane brought about by abnormalities of the wall.

REFERENCES

Aamodt, L. W. and Eisenstadt, J. M. (1968). J. Bact. 96, 1079.

Abram, D. (1965). J. Bact. 89, 855.

Abram, D. and Koffler, H. (1964). J. Mol. Biol. 9, 168.

Abram, D., Koffler, H., and Vatter, A. E. (1965). J. Bact. 90, 1337.

Abram, D., Vatter, A. E., and Koffler, H. (1966). J. Bact. 91, 2045.

Abram, D., Koffler, H., Mitchen, J. R., and Vatter, A. E. (1967). Bact. Proc. 1967, 39.

Abram, D., Mitchen, J. R., Koffler, H., and Vatter, A. E. (1970). J. Bact. 191, 250.

Ada, G. L., Nossal, G. J. V., Pye, J., and Abbot, A. (1964). Austral. J. Exp. Biol. Med. Sci. 42, 267.

Asakura, S., Eguchi, G., and Iino, T. (1964). J. Mol. Biol. 10, 42.

Benson, J. V., Jones, R. T., Cormick, J., and Patterson, J. A. (1966). Anal. Biochem. 16, 91.

Bisset, K. A. and Pease, P. (1957). J. Gen. Microbiol. 16, 382.

Dimmitt, K. and Simon, M. (1970). Infec. Immunity. 1, 212.

Dimmitt, K., Bradford, S., and Simon, M. (1968). J. Bact. 95, 801.

Kerridge, D. (1963). J. Gen. Microbiol. 33, 63.

Lawn, A. M. (1967). Nature, Lond. 214, 1151.

Mandel, H. G., Latimer, R. G., and Riis, M. (1965). Biochem. Pharmacol. 14, 661.

McGroarty, E., Koffler, H., and Smith, R. W. (1970). Bact. Proc. 1970, 22.

Mitchen, J. R. and Koffler, H. (1969). Bact. Proc. 1970, 29.

Mitchen, J. R., Koffler, H., and Smith, R. W. (1970). Bact. Proc. 1970, 22.

Morrison, R. B. (1961). J. Path. Bact. 82, 189.

Morrison, R. B. and McCapra, J. (1961). Nature, Lond. 192, 774.

Quadling, C. and Stocker, B. A. D. (1956). J. Gen. Microbiol. 15, i.

Quadling, C. and Stocker, B. A. D. (1962). J. Gen. Microbiol. 28, 257.

Ryan, C. A. (1967). Anal. Biochem. 19, 434.

Sullivan, A., Bui, J., Suzuki, H., Smith, R. W., and Koffler, H. (1969). Bact. Proc. 1969, 30.

Vaituzis, Z. and Doetsch, R. N. (1965). J. Bact. 89, 1586.

Vaituzis, Z. and Doetsch, R. N. (1966). J. Bact. 91, 2103.

Weibull, C. (1953). J. Bact. 66, 688.

GENETICS OF BACTERIAL FLAGELLA IN SPECIAL REFERENCE TO MOTILITY

T. Iion
University of Tokyo,
Laboratory of Genetics,
Faculty of Science,
Hongo,
Tokyo, Japan.

Bacterial flagella are locomotive organelles which consist of protein fibers 120 to 180 Å in diameter and 15 μ in maximum length, extending outward from the cell body. An end of a flagellar fiber is connected with a basal body under the cell membrane. A flagellar fiber is a tubular polymer of a single kind of acidic globular protein called flagellin. Its arrangement in a flagellum and its biochemical characteristics were discussed by Drs. H. Koffler and M. Simon in the preceding sections of this symposium.

According to the topic of this symposium, "behavior of microorganisms", I would like to focus the discussion on the contribution of the genetical studies of mutants in flagellar characters to the understanding of motility behavior of flagellate bacteria. I shall leave out the chemotactic mutants presented in an excellent report by Dr. J. Adler in this symposium. An advantage of the use of flagellar mutants is that they permit us to examine the effect of an alteration in a specific flagellar character on motility under the condition of least interference with other cellular structures or biochemical processes.

1. Gene System Controlling Flagellar Characters

The genetic analysis of bacterial flagella was initiated with Salmonella (Stocker et al., 1953), and later extended to Escherichia coli (Armstrong and Adler, 1967), Bacillus subtilis (Stocker, 1963; Joys and Frankel, 1967) and Proteus mirabilis (Coetzee, 1963). The discussion here will be necessarily confirned to these peritrichoulsy flagellate eubacteria. These organisms were found to have in common the following genes controlling the flagellar characters.

H : structural genes of flagellin. A mutation in H causes a change of amino acid composition of flagellin resulting in an alteration either of antigenicity, shape, physicochemical stability, or flagellotropic phage-receptor of flagella. Bacteria other than Salmonella possess only one H gene while

*Present address: Laboratory of Genetics, Faculty of Science, University of Tokyo, Hongo, Tokyo, Japan.

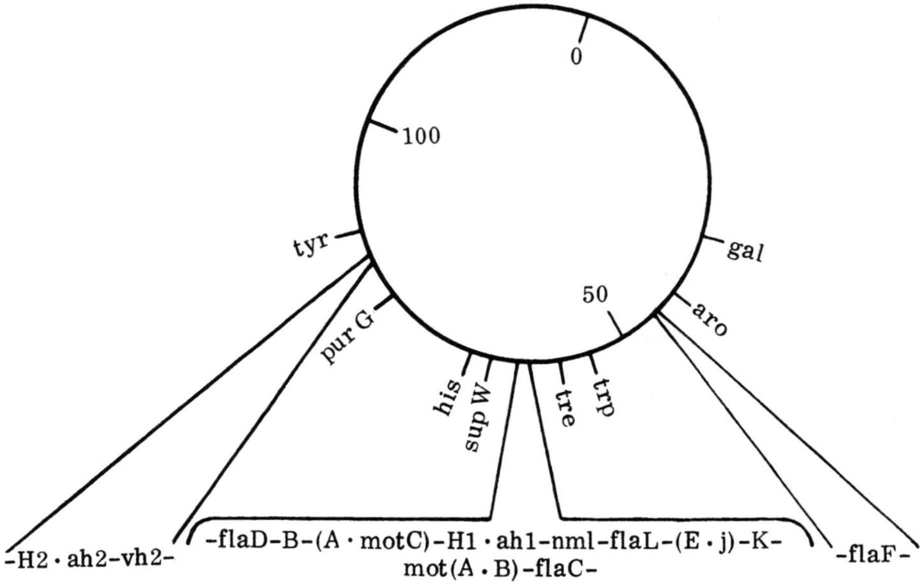

Figure 1. Linkage map of the genes controlling flagellar characters in Salmonella typhimurium.

many serotypes of Salmonella possess two non-allelic structural genes for flagellin, H1 and H2. These two structural genes are expressed alternatively in a clone (Lederberg and Iino, 1956). When the flagella produced under the control of each of these structural genes manifest distinct characteristics, the alternative expression appears as flagellar phase variation. A bacterial strain showing flagellar phase variation is called diphasic. The alternative expression of H1 and H2 occurs due to epistasis of H2 over H1 and frequent changes in activity of spistatic H2. In Salmonella, activity controllers ah1 and ah2 are present for H1 and H2 respectively, adjoining to the corresponding structural genes (Iino, 1961, 1962).

fla: regulator genes of flagellation. The number of cistrons belonging to this group so far disclosed ranges from two to eight among different bacterial species (Joys and Stocker, 1965; Iino and Enomoto, 1966; Matsumoto and Tazaki 1967; Joys and Frankel, 1967). A mutation in any one of fla cistrons causes a change in the number of flagella per bacterium without a change in their length. An extreme type of mutation, i.e. mutation from fla^+ to fla^-, results in the entire loss of flagellar formation. fla^+ is dominant over fla^-. Test of immunogenicity of the fla^- cells of Salmonella indicated that the fla^- cells, except $flaG^-$, do not synthesize a detectable amount of flagellin (Iino and Enomoto, 1966). In order to explain both decrease of flagellar number in the leaky mutants and absence of flagellin synthesis in fla^-, as a hypothesis it was proposed that a flagellin synthesizing system and a flagellar forming apparatus are functionally, and probably structurally, coupled at the base of a flagellum and that each fla cistron controls a component of this complexed flagella forming apparatus (Iino, 1969).

mot :genes controlling motility of flagella. One to three mot cistrons are known among different bacterial species (Enomoto, 1966a; Armstrong and Adler, 1967; Joys and Frankel, 1967). A mutation in a cell of any one of the mot cistrons from mot^+ to mot^- results in paralysis of the cell without affecting the structure of flagellar fibers. mot^+ is dominant over mot^-.

Mapping of these genes on the chromosome was carried out for Salmonella (Smith and Stocker, 1962; Enomoto 1966) and E.coli (Armstrong et al., 1967). In these bacteria most of the genes controlling structure and function of flagella were found to cluster in a chromosome region (Figure 1).

2. Flagellation and Motility

Indispensability of flagella for the locomotion of flagellate bacteria is definitely shown by the intimate correlation between the loss of flagella by mutation and the loss of cellular motility. A genetic defect of flagellar formation occurs either by mutation of fla^+ to fla^-, ah^+ to ah^-, or nonsense mutation of H. In motile diphasic strains, such as many Salmonella serotypes, the later two types of mutation in phase-1 result in a repeated dissociation of non-flagellate and flagellate cells in a clone, which clearly shows the prerequistite of flagellation for motility; the alternation between flagellate and non-flagellate always accompanies the change between motile and non-motile (Iino, 1961). As will be discussed later, the presence of flagella does not fulfil the condition of conferring motility on bacteria.

3. Flagellar Shape and Motility

For the locomotion of flagellate bacteria, the spiral shape of a flagellum seems to be essential. Flagella-shape mutants which produce straight flagella were found to be entirely non-motile. Genetic analysis in Salmonella (Iino and Mitani, 1967) and chemical analysis in Bacillus (Martinez et al., 1968) of those mutants indicated that the mutation occurred in a structural gene of flagellin, H1, and that the mutants differed from the wild type only in a single amino acid of flagellin. In contrast to a mot^- mutation, a straight mutation in a diphasic bacteria results in the repeated dissociation of motile (i.e. normal flagellar) and non-motile (i.e. straight flagellar) cells. The straight flagellar mutant is only one exception among non-motile bacteria in regard to the response to flagellotropic phage. Generally, non-motile bacteria are resistant to flagellotropic phage, even though they are flagellated (Meynell, 1961), while straight flagellar mutants are sensitive to the phage. This phenomenon is explained by assuming that cellular locomotion is not a prerequisite for infection by flagellotropic phage but that the presence of motile flagella rather is. Thus, in straight flagellar mutants, the flagella per se may have retained motility but, because of loss of spiral structure, their movement may not effect the locomotion of the bacterial bodies.

In addition to straight flagellar mutants several flagella-shape mutants, namely curly, para-curly, hooked-curly, and small-amplitude, have been obtained in Salmonella (Iino and Mitani, 1966). All of them occurred by mutation

TABLE 1. Characteristics of the Flagella-Shape Mutants Obtained from Salmonella Abortusequi SL23

Strain	Flagellar shape		Shape of flagellar bundle		A · sin 2θ†	Spreading ability†	Cell aggregation
			pitch (μ)	amplitude (μ)			
SL23	Normal		2.20 ± 0.09	0.53 ± 0.06	0.51 ± 0.08	1.00	−
SJ712	Small-amplitude	form 1	1.69 ± 0.14	0.32 ± 0.02	0.28 ± 0.04	0.53	−
		form 2	0.95 ± 0.10	0.45 ± 0.09	0.41 ± 0.13		
SJ715	Hooked-curly		0.98 ± 0.06	0.42 ± 0.03	0.40 ± 0.05	0.08	+
SJ713	Para-curly		1.08 ± 0.06	0.31 ± 0.04	0.30 ± 0.05	0.15	−
SJ30	Curly		0.91 ± 0.06	0.29 ± 0.08	0.28 ± 0.08	0.00	+

† Relative efficiency of locomotion as expressed by A × sin 2θ, where A indicates amplitude and θ the angle of spiral of flagellar bundle to equatorial plane of the spiral axis.

‡ Diameter of a swarm grown on semisolid medium after 8 hr incubation at 37° C; the value of SL23 was taken as 1.00.

TABLE 2. Cellular Motility of the Flagella-Shape Mutants Obtained from Salmonella Abortusequi SL23

Strain	Flagellar shape	Representative type of movement	Frequency of translationally moving cells (%)	Maximum speed (μ/sec)
SL23	Normal	Translation	71.8	36
SJ712	Small-amplitude	Wobble and translation	19.8	19
SJ715	Hooked-curly	Wobble and wriggle	8.5	17
SJ713	Para-curly	Wobble and wriggle	11.0	17
SJ30	Curly	Wobble	4.8	13

Bacteria were suspended in broth at 20° C, and observed by the motility track method of Vaituzis and Doetsch (1969) on 400 cells for each strain.

either in H1 or H2. Both pitch and amplitude of flagellar spiral in these mutants are smaller than those of normal flagella (Table 1). Observations of these mutants indicated that the difference in the spiral shape of flagella is decisively reflected in the efficiency of cellular locomotion: movement of these mutant cells is less efficient than that of normal and they show the tendency of wriggling or wobbling. In other words, the spiral shape of normal flagella is most efficient for cellular locomotion among the known flagellar shapes. Among the mutants, cellular motility is best in small-amplitude and worst in curly (Table 2).

Flagella of each bacterial strain manifest specific antigenicity. In Salmonella, a considerable number of flagellar antigen types has been identified in natural isolates. Pairs of their antigenically unrelated flagellins show a minimum amino acid substitution from 11 to 38 of approximately 380 residues of the polypeoptide chain (McDonohgh, 1965); that is, the difference in amino acid compostion among them is far greater than among flagella-shape mutants. However, so far as the flagellar shapes are identical and the strains are isogenic except for H, no significant difference in the moving speed was observed among the antigen types b, i, gp, enx and 1.2 at the pH range of 6 to 7 when the speed was measured by the motility track method of Vaituzis and Deotsch (1969): the maximum speed was 34 to 38 μ/sec with the mode at 22 to 26 μ/sec under aerobic condition in broth at 20°C.

In peritrichously flagellate bacteria such as Salmonella, several flagella appear from all over the surface of a cell. When a bacterium moves, peritrichous flagella are bundled winding around each other (Mitani and Iino, 1965, 1968). Under a dark field microscope, rotation of a flagellar bundle is seen at the posterior end of the swimming bacterial body (Pijper et al., 1956). Pijper and his collaborators (1956) observed by dark field microscopy of moving cells of Sarcina, Salmonella, and Bacillus that the spiral of flagellar bundles shows a dimorphic change between normal and curly. They called this phenomenon biplicity. An active role of biplicity for the locomotion has been considered by some investigators (Jarosch, 1964). However, observations of the flagella-shape mutants mentioned above indicated that the biplicity occurs only in a particular flagellar type, namely the small-smplitude type, as a result of bundle formation, and not necessarily associated with the bacterial movement (Iino and Mitani, 1966; Mitani and Iino 1968). Rather, flagella seem to be semi-rigid fibers generally holding their specific spiral shape while bacteria move. Of course, this does not exclude the possibility that some conformational changes of flagellin without gross change in flagellar spiral are associated with the locomotive activity of flagella.

The morphological uniformity of flagellar spiral in moving bacteria, together with the biochemical informations such as absence of SH-containing amino acids in flagellin molecules and failure of ATP to cause observable contraction in the flagellar fibers, strongly support the hypothesis that flagella are inert semi-rigid fibers and their movement is exerted not by their own undulation but by their rotation operated by their basal apparatus (Doetsch, 1966). The synchronized movement of flagellar fibers in a bundle is possible even for peritrichous flagella as far as speed and direction of the rotation of each flagellar fiber are the same.

Are the differences in the efficiency of translational movement among various flagellar shape mutants explained from the above viewpoint? According to the above hypothesis, the translational movement of a bacterium is expected to result from the axial moment of the force conferred from the environmental liquid to its flagellar bundle as a reaction to its rotation. The geometrical proportion in a spiral expected to influence the translational movement are amplitude (A) and angle (θ) of spiral to equatorial plane of spiral axis: the longitudinal force must be in proportion to A and sin 2θ when speed of the rotation and length of the flagellar bundle are the same. The value A times $\sin 2\theta$ in various flagellar shape strains is shown in Table 1. In parallel to the motility observed under microscope, the value for a normal bacterium is larger than for any flagellar shape mutants, and the value for curly is the smallest. The two distinct values in the two forms of the small-amplitude mutant may correspond respectively to translationally moving and wobbling cells. Wriggling or wobbling of bacteria may appear when the rotation of the flagellar bundle cannot elicit enough force for translational movement of the bacterial body. $A \times \sin 2\theta$ value of the hooked-curly mutant is as high as that of the type-2 flagella of the small-amplitude, but spreading ability of the hooked-curly cultures in semisolid medium is considerably lower as compared with that of the small-amplitude culture. This may be due to the tendency of cell to cell aggregation by linkage of flagellar bundles in dense cultures of the former.

4. Number of Flagella and Motility

It is very difficult to count the number of flagella and measure the speed of movement of the same bacterial cell. However, it is possible to estimate the correlation between the two from comparison of the distribution of moving speed between two bacterial populations differing in flagellar number per bacterium. The experiment was carried out on a wild strain of <u>S. typhimurium</u>,

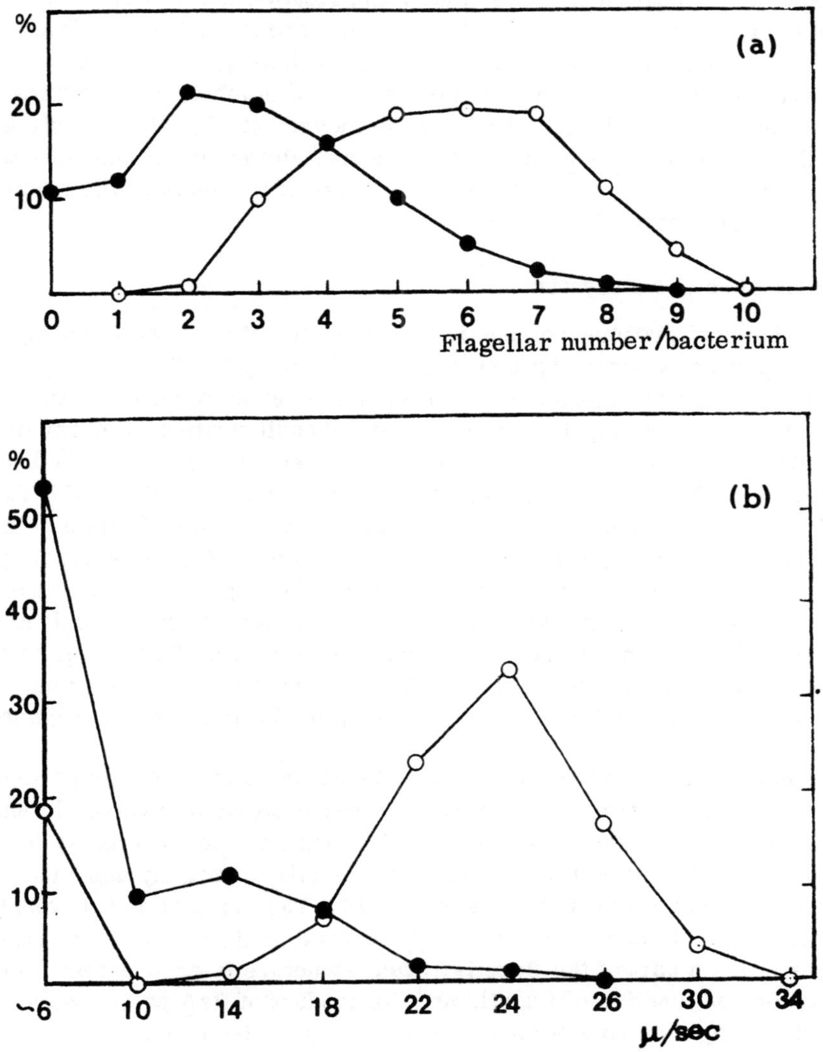

Figure 2. Distribution of flagellar number per bacterium (a) and speed of bacterial movement (b) in a wild strain TM2 (○) of Salmonella typhimurium and its leaky fla mutant SJ772 (●). Ordinate: per cent cell fraction.

TM2, and its leaky fla mutant, SJ772, which produces about half the number of flagella per cell generation as compared with the wild strain. As shown in Figure 2, the decrease in the number of flagella was parallel to the decrease in the speed of cellular locomotion. It is also shown that the fraction of cells showing no-translational movement exceeds the cell fraction having less than three flagella in both strains. Of the cells showing no translational movement, one third to one fourth of them wobble. These results may mean that a flagellar bundle must be composed of more than three flagella for a peritrichously flagellate cell to move and that the increase in the number of flagellar filaments in a bundle enhances the speed of bacterial movement. When the number of flagella per bacterium is less than four, rotation exerted by the flagellar bundle may not be strong enough to drive forward the cell body. It may be worth noting here that Pseudomonas and the related genera, which are characterized by the presence of a single or a small number of polar flagella, can move translationally as efficiently as the movement of peritrichously multiflagellate cells of Salmonella in liquid media. However, the movements of the former fall off more steeply with the increase of viscosity of the media than the movements of the latter.

5. Genetic Paralysis

The most pronounced genetic defect in motility is genetic paralysis. Genetic paralysis occurs by mutation of mot^+ to mot^-. The mot^- mutants produce flagella indistinguishable from wild ones as to shape, antigenicity, number per bacterium, (Enomoto, 1966a), or configuration by X-ray diffraction (Beighton et al., 1958). Although it has been suggested that the bound energy of ATP is involved in motility (Derobertis and Peluffo, 1951; Sherris et al., 1957), ATP and ATPase activity are not detected in flagella detached from both wild-type and paralyzed cells (Enomoto, 1962). In addition, paralysis occurs in diphasic strains regardless of the flagellar phase. From these observations it has been concluded that the mutation affects some factors responsible for the functioning of the flagellum other than flagellin (Enomoto, 1966a; Armstrong and Adler, 1967). The dominancy of mot^+ over mot^- excludes the possibility that mot^- produces an inhibitor of flagellar motion.

Recently, a group of mutants was found which are not only paralyzed but also have a decreased number of flagella per bacterium (Yamaguchi and Iino, details will be published elsewhere). Differing from the ordinarily leaky fla mutants, even a cell with more than four flagella is entirely non-motile. The mutant sites are mapped in a region of flaA. The mutants do not complement or weakly complement with other flaA mutants. This phenomenon strongly suggests that a part of the flagellar basal structure is responsible both for formation and function of flagella and the product of flaA participates as a component or plays the role of an activator. For the disclosure of the motive apparatus at the base of flagella, more intensive biochemical and ultrastructural studies on fla and mot mutants are required.

REFERENCES

Armstrong, J. R. and Adler, J. (1967). Genetics 56, 363.
Armstrong, J. B., Adler, J., and Dahl, M. M. (1967). J. Bacteriol. 93, 390.
Beighton, E., Porter, A. M., and Stocker, B. A. D. (1958). Biochim. Biophys. Acta 29, 8.
Coetzee, J. N. (1963). J. Gen. Microbiol. 33, 1.
Derobertis, E. and Peluffo, C. A. (1951). Proc. Soc. Exp. Biol. 78, 584.
Doetsch, R. N. (1966). J. Theoret. Biol. 11, 411.
Enomoto, M. (1962). Ann. Rep. Nat. Inst. Genet. (Japan) 13, 75.
Enomoto, M. (1966a). Genetics 54, 715.
Enomoto, M. (1966b). Genetics 54, 1069.
Iino, T. (1961). Jap. J. Genet. 36, 268.
Iino, T. (1962). Ann. Rep. Nat. Inst. Genet. (Japan). 13, 72.
Iino, T. (1969). Bacteriol. Rev. 33, 454.

Iino, T. and Enomoto, M. (1966). J. Gen. Microbiol. 43, 315.
Iino, T. and Mitani, M. (1966). J. Gen. Microbiol. 44, 27.
Iino, T. and Mitani, M. (1967). J. Gen. Microbiol. 49, 81.
Jarosch, R. (1964). Ost. Bot. Z. 111, 173.
Joys, T. M. and Frankel, R. W. (1967). J. Bacteriol. 94, 32.
Joys, T. M. and Stocker, B. A. D. (1965). J. Gen. Microbiol. 43, 439.
Lederberg, J. and Iino, T. (1956). Genetics, 41, 744.
Martinez, R. J., Ichiki, A. T., Lundh, N. P., and Tronick, S. R. (1968). J. Bacteriol. 91, 870.
Matsumoto, H. and Tazaki, T. (1967). Jap. J. Microbiol. 11, 13.
McDonough, M. W. (1965). J. Mol. Biol. 12, 342.
Meynell, E. W. (1961). J. Gen. Microbiol. 25, 253.
Mitani, M. and Iino, T. (1965). J. Bacteriol. 90, 1096.
Mitani, M. and Iino, T. (1968). J. Gen. Microbiol. 50, 459.
Pijper, A., Neser, M. L., and Abraham, G. (1956). J. Gen. Microbiol. 14, 371.
Sherris, J. C., Preston, N. W., and Shoesmith, J. G. (1957). J. Gen. Microbiol. 16, 86.
Smith, S. M. and Stocker, B. A. D. (1962). Brit. Med. Bull. 18, 46.
Stocker, B. A. D. (1963). J. Bacteriol. 86, 797.
Stocker, B. A. D., Zinder, N. D., and Lederberg, J. (1953). J. Gen. Microbiol. 9, 410.
Vaituzis, Z. and Doetsch, R. N. (1969). Appl. Microbiol. 17, 584.

STRUCTURAL BASIS OF CILIARY ACTIVITY

P. Satir
University of California,
Department of Physiology-Anatomy,
Berkeley,
California, 94720, U.S.A.

The overt behavior of many single celled eukaryotic organisms, as well as most sperm cells and some multicellular organisms, is, in large measure, swimming behavior determined by the physiological parameters controlling a single cell organelle, the cilium.[1] The eukaryotic cilium is considerably more complex than the prokaryotic flagellum, both biochemically and structurally, but the larger diameter of the cilium permits the single living organelle to be used in physiological experiments.

The swimming cilium is a system with a low Reynolds number which implies that the swimming is done against viscous forces, inertial forces and turbulence being negligible. It is well known that increasing the viscosity of the medium usually slows down the movement of microorganisms. Energy must also be expended to overcome elastic forces within the cilium. Since the wave forms travel up the axoneme with constant amplitude, energy is apparently expended along the entire length of the cilium (cf. Holwill, 1967). Ultimately, ciliary structure and activity has a genetic base. Ciliary morphopoiesis apparently begins with nuclear gene initiated protein synthesis. There are independent pathways of synthesis of the main structural elements of the axoneme and certain of these elements, including the ciliary microtubules, may self-assemble in the cell cytoplasm. The further steps in assembly are sequential and of increasing complexity, with morphopoietic controls at various levels of the process (cf. Wade and Satir, 1968; Randall, 1969). It is remarkable that the long evolutionary history of the eukaryotes has produced very little diversity in the structural organization of the cilium. The identical arrangement of microtubules in all motile cilia, excepting only a few gametes, has come to be known as the 9 + 2 pattern (Figure 1). The range of ciliary activity that governs swimming of ciliated cells includes (Figure 2) (1) the initiation and propagation of bending, (2) ciliary coordination or "metachrony"

[1] In this article I do not distinguish between eukaryotic cilia and flagella.

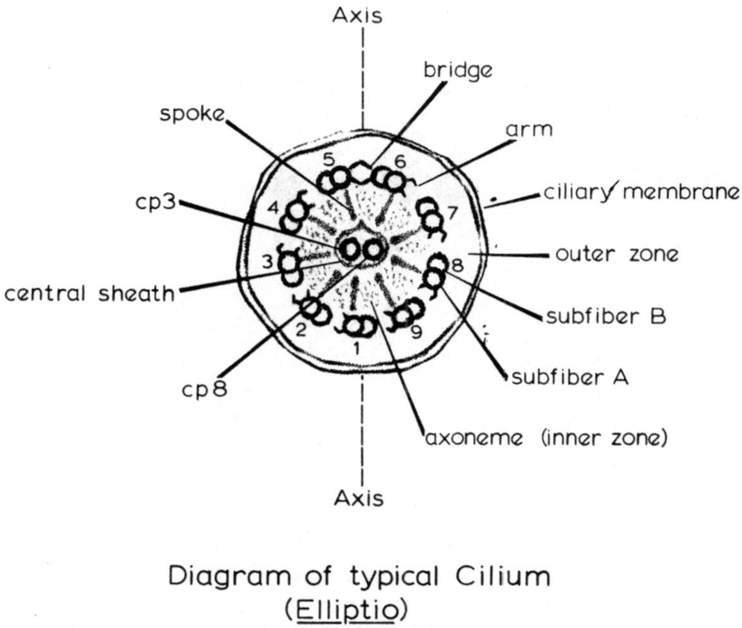

Figure 1. Diagram of axonemal cross-section of a typical cilium viewed base to tip.

(3) the direction of bend propagation, (4) the timing of the ciliary stroke, and (5) ciliary reversal or the spatial orientation of the ciliary stroke. Complex behavioral patterns are produced by temporary changes in some or all of these properties and different microorganisms achieve the same net behavioral result in various ways. For example, the "avoiding reaction" can be produced by alteration of any one of the last three properties without any change in the other two.

There have been a number of increasingly elegant demonstrations that within the cilium alone lies the structural basis of motion, and perhaps even certain controls of motion that produce swimming behavior. Models of ciliary axonemes devoid of ciliary membranes initiate and propagate bends and may swim when re-activated with ATP in the presence of appropriate cations, but there remains some dispute about the ability of such models to exhibit more complex ciliary behavior. (Goldstein, Holwill, and Sylvester, 1970) have been able to sever selected Crithidia cilia from the cell bodies by laser microsurgery. The severed cilia swim, often for a number of beats.

In addition, they can reverse direction so that bending waves can be propagated base to tip or tip to base along the same isolated organelle. In this case, even the avoiding reaction seems to be a property of the membrane-bound ciliary axoneme.

The swimming stroke of a few types of cilia has been analyzed in detail. Even if we disregard behavioral complication such as reversal, for different cilia the basic strokes at first appear far from identical. For example, there

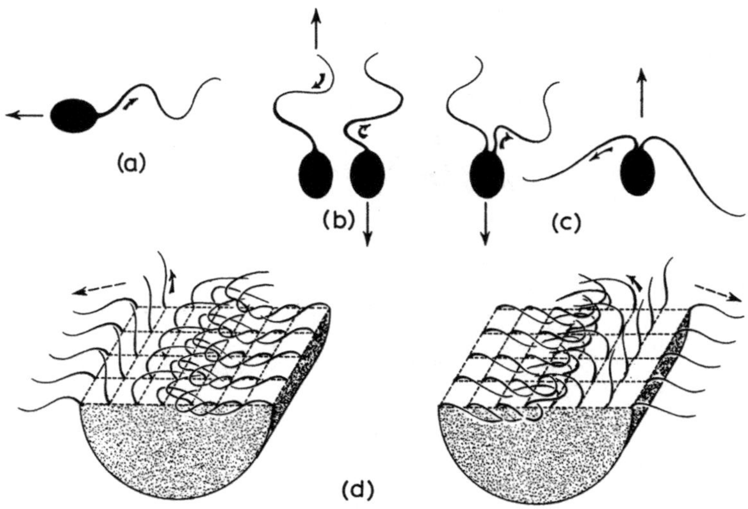

Figure 2. Ciliary activity of microorganisms. (a) Forward swimming (sperm cell). (b)-(d) Avoiding reactions. (b) Change in direction of bend propagation (Crithidia). (c) Change in timing of stroke phases (Chlamydomonas). (d) Ciliary reversal. Change in metachronal wave direction (Paramecium). Small arrows indicate direction of bend propagation. Large and broken arrows indicate direction of swimming.

is a symmetrical undulatory wave propagated along many long sperm tails, while the short cilia of Paramecium beat with an asymmetrical stroke with effective and recovery portions (Párducz, 1967). This has aroused some anxiety among electron microscopists since the axonemal morphology of say, sea urchin sperm and Paramecium is identical. However, more careful examination of stroke form reveals certain basic similarities, the most important of these for our purposes being that the bent regions of the axoneme are in all cases circular arcs that are separated by completely straight regions. The basic mechanism of bend initiation and propagation is probably reasonably similar in all simple 9 + 2 axonemes whose diameter is in the range of 0.2μ. This conclusion is supported by thermodynamic calculations which suggest a basic similarity of rate-limiting chemical reaction within differing cilia (Holwill, 1967). The varying lengths of the axoneme, the timing of stroke phase and other behavioral complexities account for variations in stroke form.

The morphological units corresponding to some of the main protein constituents of the ciliary axoneme are reasonably well-defined (cf. Gibbons, this symposium). In negative stain preparations 40A globular particles can be shown to comprise the microtubular walls. These particles belong to a class of proteins collectively called tubulin. A second protein – dynein – apparently comprises the arms or battlements attached to one side of the doublet microtubules and is the main ciliary ATPase. Divalent cations – Ca^{2+} or Mg^{2+} – are required co-factors for this enzyme. Other constituents, probably proteins, that are less well-studied form (1) a helical sheath around the central microtubules, (2) the links that join doublets, and (3) the spokes (radial links) that

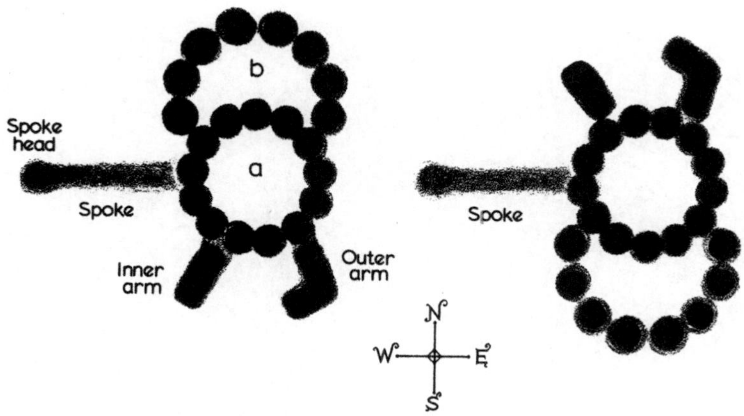

Figure 3. Asymmetry of attachments to subfiber a. Left: Viewed base to rip. Right: Viewed tip to base.

connect the central sheath and the doublets. This list must not be taken to be inclusive, however.

The concurrent examination of ciliary biochemistry and ciliary ultrastructure has led to the development of specific theories of the function of the constituents of cilia in motility. This paper concerns itself primarily with (1) structural considerations leading to the development of the sliding microtubule theory of motility and (2) the implications of the sliding microtubule theory for ciliary behavior.

Ciliary Structure

a) Microtubule Arrangement and Enantiomorphic Form

Ciliary microtubules are obviously flexible and apparently inextensible. They may be twisted in a complex three-dimensional curve during a beat, or they may run perfectly straight. In either event they are usually parallel to the longitudinal axis of the cilium, although they occasionally are helically wrapped instead (Phillips, 1969). The peripheral doublets are each composed of one complete microtubule – subfiber a – and one incomplete microtubule – subfiber b (Figure 3). Along most of the axoneme, subfiber a bears the two rows of dynein arms spaced at about 175Å intervals along the microtubule, projecting toward subfiber b of the adjacent doublet. It also bears centripetally-directed spoke protein. Subfiber a is backed by subfiber b lacking specific appendages. The common wall clearly belongs to subfiber a. This is seen in ordinary cilia at the tip where the subfiber b's terminate before the subfiber a's (Satir, 1965). In some cilia the subfibers splay apart before termination of subfiber b revealing the C-shape of this fiber (Phillips, 1966). At the tip the subfiber b's are capped over and terminate abruptly (Figure 4). The arms end about 0.2μ before the termination of subfiber b. A few images suggest that the spokes may persist for at least 0.1μ after the termination.

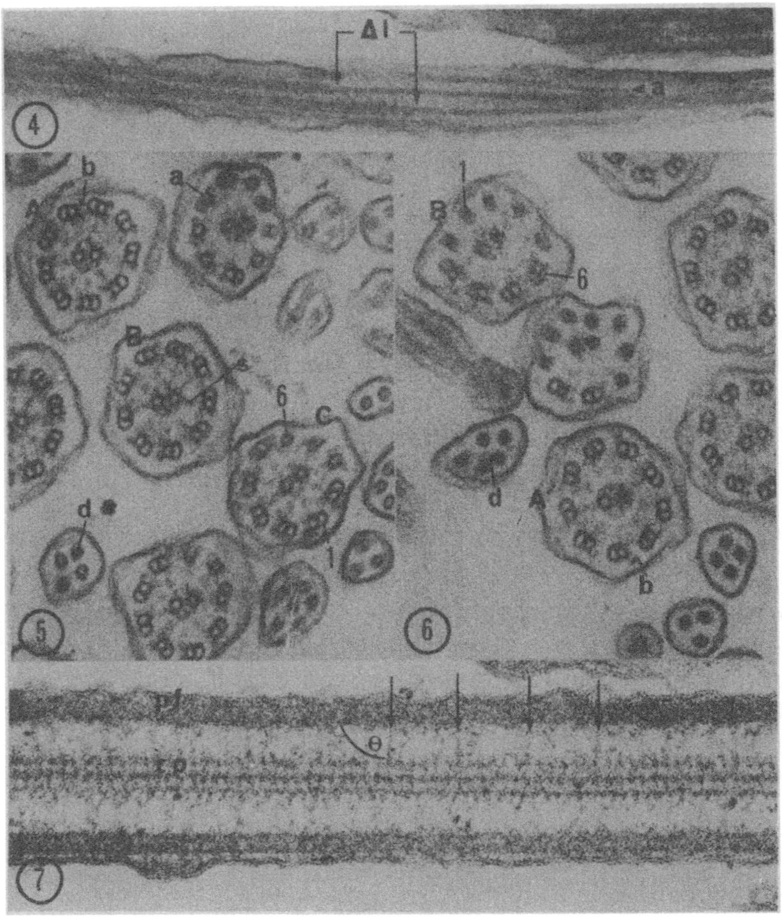

Figures 4-7. Mussel gill cilia.

Figure 4. Longitudinal section of tip. Arrows mark termination of subfiber b and give rise to a Δl of about $0.3\,\mu$. Note taper of subfiber a at (a). 55,000×.

Figure 5. R-pointing lateral cilia. Cilia A and B correspond to Figure 1 with bridge at (b). Cilium C shows critical tip-section corresponding to Figure 10. Note at (a) subfiber a continues as a complete microtubule, while subfiber b ends. Spokes are clearly seen at (s). A domino tip is shown at (d). Filaments No. 1 and 6 are labeled. 95,000×.

Figure 6. E-pointing lateral cilia. Cilium A shows axoneme viewed tip to base, and cilium B shows critical tip section corresponding to Figure 10. Labeled as in Figure 5. 95,000×.

Figure 7. Longitudinal section of straight region showing spoke periodicity. Arrows mark periodic spokes extending from subfiber a of peripheral element (pf) to the central sheath (cp). Note that θ is approximately 90°. 135,000× (Micrograph by N. B. Gilula)

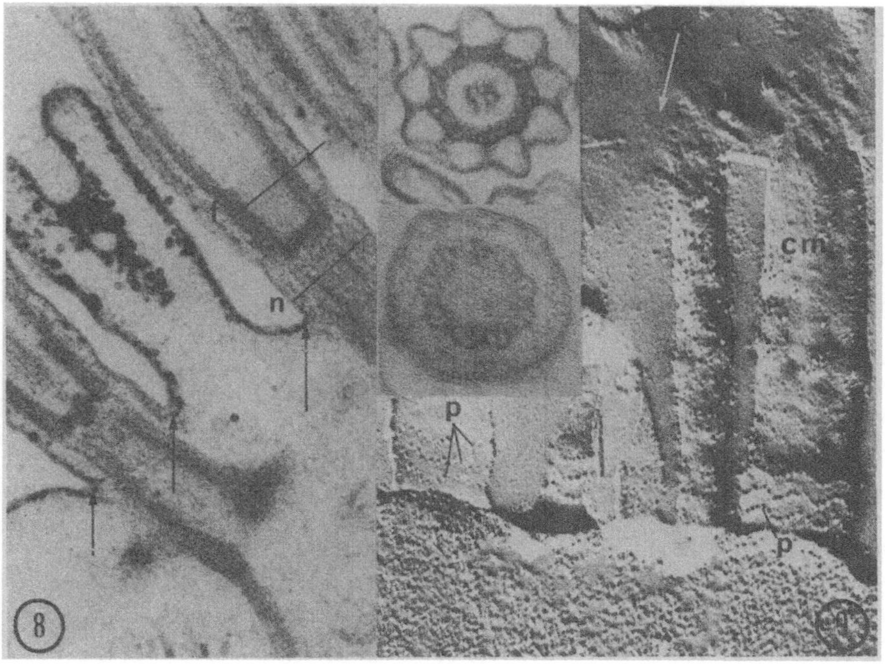

Figure 8-9. Mussel gill cilia.

Figure 8. Pyroantimonate localization. The black pyroantimonate precipitate along the cell and microvillar membrane ends abruptly at the juncture of ciliary and cell membrane (arrows) Regions corresponding to the "flower pattern" (f) and "necklace" (n) cross-sections shown in Figure 9 are indicated. 55,000×.

Figure 9. Freeze-etch preparation of ciliated cell surface. Arrow indicates direction of shadowing. The ciliary membrane (cm) is relatively smooth except in the "necklace zone" between the cell membrane and the basal plate, where three scalloped rows of particles (p) can be seen. 72,000× (Micrograph by N. B. Gilula). Inset. Upper. Cross-section through "flower pattern" region of axoneme showing fluting of the membrane and connection between membrane and ciliary microtubules. 84,000×. Lower. Cross-section through "necklace" region showing connections between microtubules and spheroids attached to the membrane. 108,000×.

The exact length of each subfiber is species specific. There seem at present to be two main classes of ciliary construction, one characteristic of certain vertebrate cilia and one characteristic of many invertebrates and microorganisms.

In the best studied case – that of mussel gill lateral cilia – all nine subfiber b's appear to be of the same length (differences of no more than $\pm 0.15\mu$ or 2-3 per cent of total length). On the other hand, subfiber a's taper as they terminate and are of quite different lengths (more than 1μ different) (Satir, 1968). These length differences between subfiber a's give rise to the characteristic domino-patterned tip sections seen in many cilia (Figures 5, 6) and to the taper of the tip.

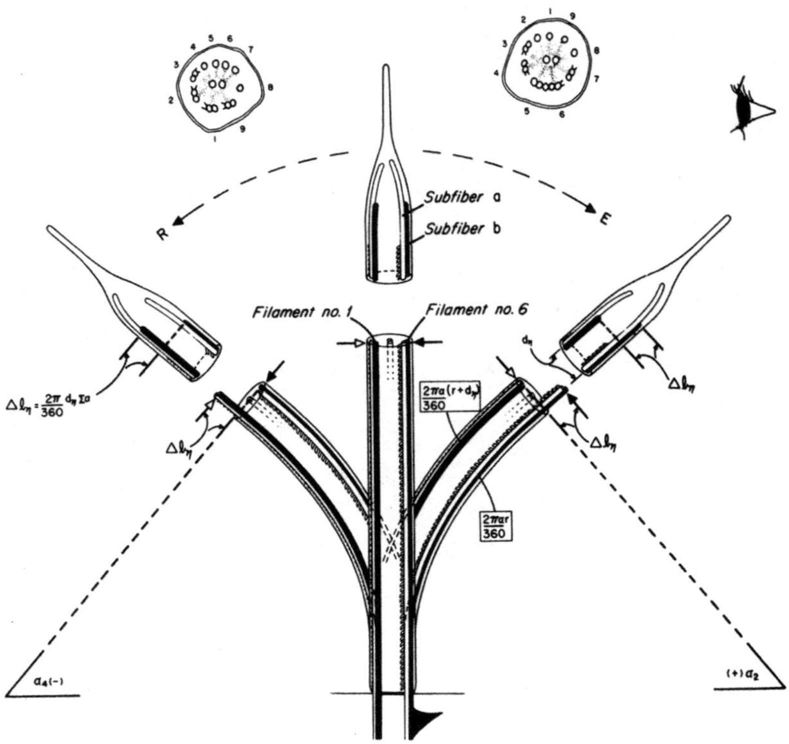

Figure 10. Sliding filament model. Behavior of two doublet peripheral filaments (No. 1 and 6) at the tip and base when a cilium is bent to either side of a straight position. Bending produces an apparent length difference (Δl_n) at the cilium tip, since the filaments are inextensible. Where filament No. 1 is apparently shorter, Δl_n (in this case, Δl_6) is positive (E-cilium), where filament No. 1 is apparently longer, Δl_n is negative (R-cilium). A cross-section through the tip at a level where some filaments are doublets and some singlets is shown for both R and E cilia at the top of the diagram. These compare to cilium C in Figure 5 and cilium B in Figure 6 respectively. (Reprinted by permission from J. Cell Biol.).

At the proximal end of the axoneme the doublets extend past the basal plate into the basal body (centriole) proper; usually a third subfiber, subfiber c, is joined to subfiber b in the more proximal part of the basal body. At this end the microtubules are embedded in dense amorphous material and their exact ends, which may be open, are difficult to discern. However, basal body microtubules in gill cilia apparently terminate within 0.1μ of one another.

It is likely that subfiber a is highly polarized since it must provide regular spatially-oriented sites for several appendages. When the site of spoke attachment is directed in a certain way (compass West, Figure 3) the dynein arms are North only when the microtubule is viewed from tip to base, South only when the microtubule is viewed from base to tip. It has been recognized for about a decade that all eukaryotic ciliary doublet microtubules have this single enantiomorphic form. As cilia develop, subfiber a apparently grows by subunit addition at the tip.

The peripheral microtubules are arranged around the central pair so that the axis of the cilium – which corresponds to the plane of beat in gill cilia and certain sperm, at least – passes between two doublets on one side (the effective stroke direction) of the axoneme and transects the doublet on the opposite side (the recovery stroke direction) (Figure 1). The transected doublet is conventionally labeled filament No. 1, and labeling proceeds so that filament No. 2 is that doublet microtubule whose subfiber b apposes the arms of filament No. 1. The doublets between which the axis passes are then filaments No. 5 and 6, and in certain cases these are further identifiable in axonemal cross-sections because they are specifically connected by a bridge. At the level of the basal body the amorphous material attached to these microtubules sometimes extends laterally to form a spur or basal foot.

The central microtubules are often the longest microtubules in the axoneme. They may extend to the very top of the cilium and sometimes they fuse at that point just before the cilium terminates. At the proximal end of the axoneme, they do not extend past the basal plate. Here, the ending is free, or the pair may be positioned in a socket of dense material. In some cases, one member of the pair extends further into the basal plate region than its counterpart.

A line connecting the centers of the central microtubules is always perpendicular to the axis of the cilium. The members of the central pair may be distinguished by the side of the cilium to which they are closest. A convenient notation is cp_3 – denoting the member closer to filament number 3 – and cp_8 – denoting the member closer to filament No. 8.

b) Matrix Organization and Central Sheath

Very recently, new information has become available from a number of laboratories on the organization of the ciliary matrix. A spoke periodicity is evident in both straight and bent portions of the ciliary axoneme. The major repeat along subfiber a is about 960Å (Figure 7). In some cases there is a secondary spoke dividing the period into about a 320Å, 640Å subperiod. This has been particularly well-studied for a dipteran sperm by Warner (1970), although here the period appears to be 880Å with a 320, 560 subperiod. The spokes end in a specialized knob, the spoke head. Warner interprets the exact arrangement of spoke heads as a two-start double helix of 1760Å repeat with a 40° pitch. Interestingly, a helical wrapping connecting the central pair and the peripheral doublets was deduced by Manton and Clarke in 1952 from micrographs of frayed cilia, but remained obscure in most sectioned material until now.

The spoke heads abut and perhaps attach to the central sheath. According to Warner, this sheath is an asymmetrically-wound single helix extending out 25Å from the central pair. It apparently has an inherent periodicity of about 160Å and an 8-10° pitch. The exact construction of the central sheath is somewhat more complex in mussel gill cilia, but the match of about 6 turns of sheath material to one major spoke period of about 960Å also holds here.

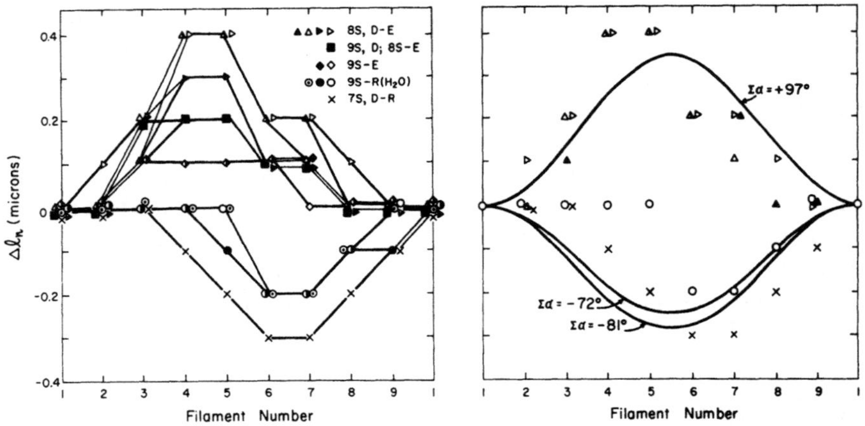

Figure 11. Δl_n vs. filament number. Left. Measured points from E vs. R cilia (complete tip notation given in Satir, 1968). Curves suggest that Δl_n for one cilium is a continuous function of distance from filament No. 1. The family of curves suggests that as tip type changes, Δl slowly increases or decreases. Right. Comparison of predicted values (curves) of Δl_n from equation (1) and measured points for $\Sigma\alpha = +97°$ (8 S, D−E cilia), $\Sigma\alpha = -72°$ (9 S −R(H_2O) cilia) and $\Sigma\alpha = -81°$ (7 S, D−R cilia) (Reprinted by permission from J. Cell Biol.).

c) The Ciliary Membrane and Basal Associations

The cilium is completely enclosed by what at first appears to be a simple continuation of the cell membrane (Figures 8, 9). The ciliary membrane has the typical unit membrane appearance in cross-section. Within limits, it appears to respond osmotically, swelling and shrinking with appropriate changes in external medium. The ciliary membrane seems reasonably independent of the axonemal microtubules, although occassional connections have been reported, However, as the membrane approaches the cell and the axoneme ends in the basal plate, a very precise series of associations between membrane and microtubules presents itself. This is species specific. For mussel gill cilia Gibbons (1961) has given a detailed description of these associations. About 0.2μ above the basal plate, a fibrous attachment extends toward the membrane from the midwall between subfibers a and b of each doublet. Then, the whole cross section takes on a "flower pattern". (Figure 9, upper inset). The membrane column is fluted in this region and narrow channels of membrane make intimate contact with each doublet. Abruptly, the entire membrane pinches in around the microtubules to form a collar. The collar zone begins at the basal (proximal) end of the basal plate and occupies about a 0.1μ length immediately distal to the plate. The collar may be asymmetric around the axoneme, approaching some microtubules more closely for longer distances than others. As the microtubules enter the flower zone, they approach each other and begin to assume their centriole-like placement. The axonemal diameter shortens by about 20 per cent through this region.

At the basal plate, the axonemal matrix is filled with an amorphous electron-opaque material. This material is about 48 mμ thick. Below this, the membrane collar widens and the flutes disappear. Within 50 mμ the axoneme is again filled with amorphous material. This is taken to be the beginning of the basal body proper. At this level, the midwall of each peripheral doublet is again connected to the membrane. The connection is very specific; short fibers extend from each midwall toward the membrane (Figure 9, lower inset). About halfway, they attach to structures that are oblately spheroidal in shape and whose edges are slightly osmiophilic. Longitudinal sections show that there are three rows of these spheroids. They are approximately 28 mμ in length, perhaps 40 mμ in width, and their osmiophilic edges are between 60-80Å thick. About 50 mμ proximal to these structures the ciliary membrane joins the cell membrane. Here again, short fibers extend from the micro-tubules to the membrane and demarcate the juncture.

The fine structure of the transition zone reflects a sharp transition between ciliary and cell membrane. In the mussel gill, the ciliary membrane differs from the adjacent cell membrane in its ability to precipitate pyroantimonate (Satir and Gilula, 1970). An electron-opaque precipitate forms along the cytoplasmic surface of the cell membrane when potassium pyroantimonate is added to osmium fixatives. The distribution of precipitate is not uniform, however, and the precipitate stops abruptly when the cilium extends outward from the cell surface (Figure 8). For the most part, pyroantimonate precipitate apparently localizes bound sodium ion and it is likely that the difference between ciliary and cell membranes reflects fundamentally different cation binding properties of the membranes.

Another sign of the sharp transition from ciliary to cell membrane is seen in freeze-etch preparations. Fracture faces of the ciliary membrane contain few particles except in the transition region. Here, the ciliary membrane contains three well-defined rows of particles that completely encircle the ciliary shaft, like a necklace (Figure 9). The necklace is scalloped and the scallops apparently correspond to the peripheral microtubules and to the spheroids at the distal edge of the basal body seen in thin section (Gilula and Satir, 1970).

Sliding Microtubules

Some cilia from microorganisms and from lamellibranch gill have been fixed in the metachronal wave positions, that is, in different stroke stages. The hypothesis that the peripheral microtubules do not change length during their stroke, but instead slide relative to one another as bending begins, predicts that, in different stroke stages, (1) morphological relationships of the microtubules will change qualitatively and (2) the geometry of the cilium will determine the amount of sliding quantitatively. For a cilium composed of straight regions and circular arcs, the total sliding of any filament relative to filament No. 1 will be:

$$\Delta l_n = d_n \Sigma\alpha \qquad (1)$$

where Δl_n = sliding of filament No. n in μ;

$\Sigma\alpha$ = the sum of angles subtended by the arcs in radians and

d_n = the distance in μ between filament No. n and No. 1 measured on the axis of the cilium (Satir, 1968).

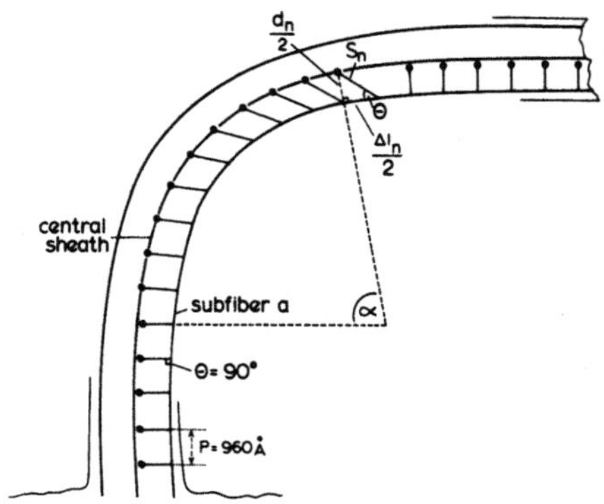

Figure 12. Schematic model of spoke attachment in a cilium with a single bend. In straight regions, spokes are perpendicular ($\theta = 90°$) to central pair and to subfiber a; they are not permanently attached to the central sheath, because they do not stretch as sliding occurs. If spokes were permanently attached to the central sheath (curved region) they would stretch as in Eq.(2) and θ would vary as in Eq.(3). Major spoke period (p) is indicated.

In gill cilia this difference may be seen in longitudinal sections (Figure 4) but it is easier to quantitate at present from serial reconstructions of cross-sectioned cilia. Also, in cross-sections the qualitative differences are most clear since in E-pointing cilia, Δl_n is positive while in R-pointing cilia, Δl_n is negative. Subfiber b of filament No. 6 will thus appear longer than subfiber b of filament No. 1 in E-pointing cilia; shorter in R-pointing cilia (Figures 5, 6, 10). Actually, the quantitative correspondence between predicted and experimentally – determined values for Δl_n is quite good (Figure 11).

Implications of the Sliding Model for Ciliary Behavior

a) General Features

The sliding microtubule hypothesis has certain interesting features. The first is that bend initiation and bend propagation are separable phenomena under this mechanism, that is sliding occurs all along the filament (from the base to the tip) when bending occurs, but no sliding necessarily accompanies propagation if the bend angle is unchanged. Manifestations of sliding by relative microtubule displacement usually occur at the tip but, at least in theory, also could occur in the basal body. A second feature is that the model accounts for the well-known constancy of axonemal diameter in 9 + 2 cilia. It strongly supports a constant basic mechanism of motility for all cilia and it predicts certain relationships between shape and tip configuration in cilia that have not as yet been examined critically. A third feature is that the model predicts that permanent connections between microtubules must be highly extensible. This feature is discussed in more detail below. Fourthly, the model has certain physiological implications. In the absence of sliding, the model predicts that a constant angle will be manintained between two ends of a cilium as waves traverse it. This appears to be the case in thiourea-treated spermatozoa examined by Brokaw (1968) and in most of the sperm tails swimming after laser microsurgery examined by Goldstein (1969).

b) Energy Transduction

Another feature of the model as presently conceived, is adirectionality: both bend initiation and propagation could proceed in either direction along the ciliary shaft. An important implication of this adirectionality might be that the cilium could operate in reverse, if sliding at the tip caused bending at the base of the organelle. This might be used in energy transduction in centriolar-based cilia-like 9 + 0 sensory systems.

In some systems where precise particle arrangements have been found within the cell membrane with the freeze-etch technique, these particles have been postulated to be sites of differential permeability to ions. This description is highly suggestive of an energy transduction role of the ciliary membrane at the basal body level, where differential ion permeability could result in differential activity of the microtubules. If the attachments between membrane and microtubules were permanent, as appears to be the case in the basal body region of gill cilia, sliding of the microtubules would necessarily produce distortions (strains) of these structures, perhaps affecting the alignment of the membrane particles. It is relatively easy to see how feedback control could operate to establish the ciliary stroke if this were the case.

c) Spoke Attachment

If the spokes were permanently attached to the central sheath (cf. Sleigh, 1969) as well as to subfiber a of each peripheral doublet, then as sliding proceeded the spokes distal to a developing bend would be stretched. Consider an idealized cilum projected in the plane of the axis. Suppose that in the straight region proximal to a bend of angle α, spokes were perpendicular to the microtubules (Figure 12), then distal to the bend they would be of length s_n and make angle θ with the microtubule, where

$$s_n^2 = (d_n/2)^2 + (\Delta l_n/2)^2 \qquad (2)$$

and

$$\cot\theta = \alpha \ (\alpha \text{ in radians}) \qquad (3)$$

For filaments No. 5-6, $d_n/2$ is half the axonemal diameter or 0.1μ and when $\Delta l_6/2 = 0.1\mu$ ($\alpha \sim 60°$) then $\theta = 45°$ and $s_6 = 0.14$. Bends of over 90° are not uncommon on cilia and flagella, and it seems probable that we would be able to detect regions where spokes were continuously attached during sliding if these occur. This situation is presently being analyzed in mussel gill lateral cilia. From preliminary evidence it appears that in the straight regions both proximal and distal to a single bend on a cilium, the periodic spokes are perpendicular to the microtubules (Figure 7). Therefore, as sliding proceeds in straight regions, the spokes are not continuously attached to the central sheath.

In bent regions, there is some evidence to suggest that some spokes may remain continuously attached as sliding proceeds. In bent regions along the axoneme the spokes are also periodic and the periodicity is the same as in the straight regions whether measured along the central sheath or along subfiber a. If the microtubule lengths between any two spokes in a single bend are measured, no difference is discernible between the length measured on subfiber a and on the central microtubule. In a few cases where the angle θ of several spokes in succession can be measured in the bent region, it decreases progressively.

Figure 12 shows a model of spoke attachment as it is presently conceived. We may suppose that the spokes play a major role in bend propagation. Note however that occasional 9 + 0 motile sperm do not appear to possess this elaborate matrix machinery (Afzelius, 1969; Manton and von Stosch, 1966).

d) Microtubule Activation

According to our present model, bending regions are initiated concomitantly with microtubule sliding. The growth of the bending region is not linear (Satir, 1967). In many but not all cilia, bend initiation is confined to the basal part of the organelle and isolated fragments of axonemes do not move. (cf. Goldstein, 1969).

Activation of the microtubules is probably sequential. An important observation on sperm is that bends in one direction are invariably followed by bends in the opposite direction. Two adjacent bends in the same direction are never observed. This is easy to explain if the wave is sinusoidal, but is more puzzling with a circular arc, straight region wave form. The observation can be extended to most, but probably not all, cilia. In a few cases, Sleigh (1968) apparently has observed monophasic strokes. However, this may represent a specialized evolutionary adaptation and should not be taken as the primitive situation.

The ciliary wave form could be produced either by (1) microtubules on differing sides of the cilium actively sliding in the same direction or (2) microtubules on one side actively sliding in different directions at different stages of beat.

It seems likely, however, that the gross polarization (enantiomorphism) of subfiber a is reflected mechanistically and that active sliding occurs only in one direction. Effective vs. recovery stroke could then be determined by (a) which microtubules are actively sliding and (b) the duration of the sliding phase. In this situation, activation of microtubules for sliding arising at any one point on the cilium (say at the bridge between 5-6) might spread symmetrically around the axoneme. Such spreading activation would produce bending in opposite directions. For example, in the sequence 5-6, 4-7, 3-8, 2-9, 1, the force produced by doublet microtubules 3 and 8 sliding in the same direction would cancel out and a straight region would intervene between two bends. The second straight region would occur during the refractory period between successive activations.

e) Ciliary Reversal

The relationship between metachronal wave direction and membrane potential in protozoa is well documented (cf. Kinosita and Murakami, 1967). In Paramecium, Naitoh and Eckert (1969) have shown that reversal is caused by a transient increase in Ca^{2+} permeability of the cell membrane, and a corresponding decrease in K^{+} permeability. Generally, the fact that the direction of the metachronal wave is a function of ciliary stroke form has been neglected, however. Alterations in metachronal wave direction are the result of alterations in the direction of the effective stroke of the cilium. There are two possible explanations for the latter alteration: (1) either the same microtubules slide to generate the effective stroke while the entire cilium swings or twists to a new position, or (2) different microtubules slide to generate the effective stroke in different directions. It seems unlikely that the cilia of protozoa could twist from the basal bodies since the orientation of kineties is so precise and the connections seem permanent. A series of fixations of Paramecium, for example, for electron microscopy after membrane potential has been set has not yet been attempted and the point cannot entirely be settled as yet. Twists in the axoneme above the transition zone are known to occur during ordinary beat but alterations in such twisting require mechanisms more complex than those under discussion. It is interesting in this regard that Naitoh (1969) has been able to reset the direction of non-beating glycerinated Paramecium cilia with ATP, Ca^{2+} and Zn^{2+}.

From the results of Kinosita (1954), (cf. Sleigh, 1966) it can be calculated that a change of 4 mV of membrane potential changes the effective stroke direction by 40°. If possibility (2) discussed above were correct, prolonged filament sliding would shift by one doublet microtubule for a 4 mV change in membrane potential. For example, instead of 5-6 sliding for the longest time as in the normal case, 6-7 or 4-5 now slide first. This perhaps need only be a switch in the origin of the sliding activation without any concomitant change in stroke timing or it could be both a timing and an activation change. Only in those cases of ciliary reversal where beating actually reversed by 180°, could the timing of the beat alone be altered. In this case, the sliding activation of filaments 1 and 2-9 might simply be longer than that of filaments 5-6.

f) Ciliary Co-ordination

In some cases, membrane depolarization precedes ciliary beat. However, the depolarizations measured thus far in ciliated systems are isotropic throughout one cell and probably throughout a tissue. Thus, these depolarizations can only act as pacemakers. It is not surprising then that they are related to the frequency of beat. There may, however, be membrane depolarizations accompanying sliding that are small and local such as those that accompany movement of the microtubular-based tentacle in dinoflagellates (Eckert and Sibaoka, 1967). These could affect relative beat phase and be a source of neuroidal transmission where such occurs.

ACKNOWLEDGEMENTS

This work was supported in part by grants from USPHS (HL 13849) and the AMA Educational and Research Foundation, and the committee on Research (UC Berkeley). A portion of this work was done in collaboration with Norton B. Gilula. I thank Norton G. Gilula, Stuart Goldstein and George Ojakian for helpful discussion and Clarence Clark for technical assistance. The assistance of the Scientific Photography and Electron Microscope Laboratories of the University of California is acknowledged.

REFERENCES

Afzelius, B. (1969). In Handbook of Molecular Cytol. (Lima-de-Faria, A., ed.) 1220.
Brokaw, C. J. (1968). Symp. Soc. Exp. Biol. 22, 101.
Eckert, R. and Sibaoka, T. (1967). J. Exp. Biol. 47, 433.
Gibbons, I. R. (1961). J. Cell Biol. 11, 179.
Goldstein, S. (1969). J. Exp. Biol. 51, 431.
Goldstein, S., Holwill, M. E. J. and Sylvester, N. R. (1970). J. Exp. Biol. 53, 401.
Holwill, M. (1967). Current Topics Bioenerg. 2, 287.
Kinosita, H. (1954). J. Fac. Sci. Tokyo Univ. (Zool.) 7, 1.
Kinosita, H. and Murakami, A. (1967). Physiol. Rev. 47, 53.
Manton, I. and Clarke, B. (1952). J. Exp. Bot. 3, 265.
Manton, I. and von Stosch, H. A. (1966). J. Roy. Micro. Soc. 85, 119.
Naitoh, Y. (1969). J. Gen. Physiol. 53, 517.
Naitoh, Y. and Eckert, R. (1969). Science 164, 963.
Párducz, B. (1967). Int. Rev. Cytol. 21, 91.
Phillips D. M. (1966). J. Cell Biol. 31, 635.
Phillips, D. M. (1969). J. Cell Biol. 40, 28.
Randall, J. R. (1969). Proc. Roy. Soc. London B 173, 31.
Satir, P. (1965). J. Cell Biol. 26, 805.
Satir, P. (1967). J. Gen. Physiol. 50 (6, pt. 2), 241.
Satir, P. (1968). J. Cell Biol. 39, 77.
Satir, P. and Gilula, N. B. (1970). J. Cell Biol. 47, 468.
Sleigh, M. A. (1966). Symp. Soc. Exp. Biol. 20, 11.
Sleigh, M. A. (1968). Ibid. 22, 131.
Sleigh, M. A. (1969). In Handbook of Molecular Cytol. (Lima-de-Faria, A., ed.) 1244.
Wade, J. and Satir, P. (1968). Exp. Cell Res. 50, 81.
Warner, F. (1970). J. Cell Biol. 47, 159.

Further information regarding the sliding microtubule model has been provided by two important papers:

Summers, K. E. and Gibbons, I. R. (1971). Pro. Nat. Acad. Sci. USA. 68, 3092.
Brokaw, C. J. (1971). J. Exp. Biol. 55, 289.

HABITUATION AND OTHER BEHAVIOUR MODIFICATION

HABITUATION IN THE PROTOZOAN SPIROSTOMUM AND PROBLEMS OF LEARNING

P.B. Applewhite

Yale University,
Biology Department,
New Haven,
Connecticut 06520, U.S.A.

The first thing to establish in studies on the molecular basis of memory is that the organisms chosen do, in fact, exhibit learning. This presents an immediate problem because a definition accepted by all is not available (Thorpe, 1963; Quarton et al., 1967; Hinde, 1970). More specifically, since we do not know what learning is from a chemical or physiological viewpoint we have difficulties in defining it precisely. For example, habituation is defined as a "waning of a response as a result of repeated stimulation" (Thorpe, 1963). If an addictive narcotic is given in a large enough dose to a person, he shows a behavioral response (euphoria) and repeated stimulation in the form of more doses eventually produces a waning of the behavioral response, i.e. his system has adapted to it. This certainly meets the definition of habituation but no one considers it a possible model system for learning. There is also the immunological response whereupon the second presentation of an antigen produces not only a larger titer of antibodies but also at a faster rate. This has been called immunological memory (Kabat, 1968) and certainly meets many definitions of memory but it too is not studied as a learning phenomenon. Why? The reason lies in the fact that "leaning and memory" are not precise enough terms to determine whether further study of phenomena agreeing with these definitions can be of any use in elucidating the molecular basis of learning and memory as psychologists and ethologists generally define it.

We are studying habituation to a mechanical stimulus in the protozoan Spirostomum. These protozoa contract to initial presentations of the stimulus, but eventually "learn" not to respond to it. All experiments (both behavioral and biochemical) reported on have been done in deionized water to eliminate any difficulties arising from bacteria being present in the culture medium. The site of the behavioral change is non-local in that a habituated protozoan is cut in two and both pieces still show habituation (Applewhite, 1968 a). Naive protozoa cut in two do not show habituation so the cutting itself does not produce a failure to contract to repeated stimulus presentations. If Spirostomum is first habiuated at one end, the other end also shows habituation indicating there is no sensory fatigue (depletion of a chemical substance) since the second end to be stimulated habituates with fewer stimuli, even though these sensory receptors were not previously habituated. An indicatation that the contractile mechanism is not fatigued is given by the fact that an electrical stimulus will produce contraction if given immediately after the tactile habituation. Protozoa habituated to a mechanical stimulus will also respond and habituate to an electrical stimulus showing the behavior is stimulus specific (Applewhite, Gardner, and Lapan, 1969). Protozoa given gradually increasing-in-intensity mechanical stimuli which eventually reach a maximum level will be as well habituated as controls receiving maximal level stimuli for the same number of stimuli (Applewhite, Gardner, and Lapan, 1969). Those receiving the gradual stimuli undergo 60 percent fewer contractions than the controls, indicating that the act of contraction per se is not fatiguing them and producing the habituation. Similar results are found in rats in habituation of a startle response to sound (Davis and Wagner, 1969) indicating their habituation is not caused by fatigue either. Furthermore, these same kind of experiments to eliminate fatigue as an explanation of habituation in Spirostomum have been done by us on the small flatworm Stenostomum and the results agree with those from Spirostomum. We must conclude, then, that habituation behavior is virtually identical in a protozoan and a metazoan and such behavior is not an isolated event in the animal kingdom. While we have eliminated fatigue, shown the behavior to be stimulus specific, and shown there is a time course of several minutes for the retention (memory) of the response, can we say habituation is a simple form of learning? Many would now say yes (Altman, 1966; Bullock, 1967; Carthy, 1965; Hoar, 1966; McConnell, 1966; Ochs, 1965; Pinsker, et al., 1970; Ramsay, 1968; Richter, 1966; Schone, 1961; Thorpe, 1963).

We habituated groups of protozoa by presenting them with a series of constant intensity mechanical shocks every 4 seconds so that eventually only a small percentage of them would be contracting. Photographic recording was done during this procedure so that we could count at each stimulus the number of protozoa that contracted to it. Using radioactive uridine and leucine we measured the change in RNA (Applewhite and Gardner, 1968) and protein (Applewhite, Gardner, and Lapan, 1969) synthesis during habituation and compared this to controls receiving no stimulation. We found an increase in both in the habituated groups and showed it was not due to permeability increases but rather due to increases at the transcriptional and translational levels. Many others have found such increase in other organisms during other forms of learning (Hyden and Eghyhazi, 1962; Hyden and Lange, 1970; Shashoua, 1970; Bogoch, 1968; Corning and Freed, 1968; Kahan et al., 1970; Machlus and Gaito, 1969; Beach et al., 1969; Bowman and Strobel, 1969). However, when protein synthesis is inhibited by 95 percent there is no effect upon habituation behavior and RNA synthesis inhibition by 89 percent only slightly interferes with habituation (Gardner and Applewhite, 1970 a), suggesting synthesis of protein (at least in large amounts) is not necessary for this behavior. Further confirmation of this comes from other studies. In comparing protein synthesis changes in protozoa given gradually increasing-in-intensity stimuli with those given constant intensity stimuli, we find no difference (Applewhite, 1970). Using Spirostomum devoid of nuclei and about 40 percent of their cytoplasm (Applewhite and Gardner, 1970), we have shown that such protozoa are unaffected in their habituation. If we compare habituated protozoa prepared this way with quiet controls also prepared this way, no protein increase can be found in the habituated group, substantiating the inhibition and gradual intensity experiments, but, an RNA increase is still obtained. We can only conclude that RNA synthesis, if it is relevant at all, during habituation is needed in larger amounts then protein is. However, arguments against RNA and protein synthesis changes being directly involved in memory coding have been made by us (Applewhite, 1967) and others (Glassman, 1969; Horridge, 1968), but much further work needs to be done until firm conclusions can be made.

Further support that no de novo macromolecular synthesis seems necessary for habituation to occur comes from temperature experiments with Spirostomum. Protozoa were habituated at temperatures ranging from 5°C to 32°C and it was found that the rate of acquistion of habituation is temperature independent (Gardner and Applewhite, 1970 b). This suggests, because of the Q_{10} values, that no synthesis is taking place, or more generally, no energy requiring process is occurring. However, during the recovery phase, that period of time during which the organisms are returning to their pre-stimulus sensitivity levels, their behavior is temperature dependent. This suggests synthesis, or some other energy consuming process, may be taking place during this period. On the basis of our radioactive labeling experiments, however, we can only detect an RNA increase. Any protein increase may be just too small to detect in the whole organism.

Since synthesis seems unnecessary for habituation, ion flow seems an attractive alternative to explain this phenomenon. We can detect no ion changes of Na, K, Mg, or Ca (using atomic absorption spectrophotometry) across the pellicle of Spirostomum during habituation, nor do we find any exchange of material with the solution Spirostomum is in during habituation, so we must deal with an internal system. We suggest that during habituation, ions diffuse out of a compartment adjacent to the contractile fibrillar system (Yagiu and Shigenaka, 1963) until some critical concentration is left. At this point the organism becomes habituated as no contraction can occur. Since the response to repeated stimuli is all-or-none, the actual process of diffusion would be expected to have no effect on contraction or the response to stimuli would become graded. If we propose that contraction in Spirostomum is similar to muscle contraction (Huxley, 1969) we would say that ions activate an ATPase, which hydrolyses ATP and causes contraction. Thus, if the ions activating the ATPase diffuse away, contraction will not occur to further stimuli and the organism becomes habituated. We have extracted an actomyosin-like substance from Spirostomum and are in the process of determining the chemistry of its function. During the recovery phase, the ions are actively transported (to agree with the temperature dependence found) back to their compartment until a critical concentration is again reached, and the organism is "reset" to contract to stimuli again. One can explain with this theory why placing Spirostomum in the cold after habituation produces less recovery than controls kept at room temperature (Applewhite, 1968 b). It is that at 5° the ions cannot be actively transported, because of energy deficiencies, back to their original compartment.

We cannot yet say which ions are crucial to this process but Ca and Mg would seem to qualify as they have an effect upon habituation (Applewhite and Davis, 1969). Since Ca (which can cause contraction) inhibits the effect of Mg (which can prevent habituation), both ions are probably needed to exert a fine control over the habituation process. The fact we have ruled out fatigue as an explanation suggests the flow of ions is not merely exhausted, but rather is turned off at some critical stage before depletion. The nature of this control is, of course, an area for detailed examination. Does habituation involve, then, information storage? At its simplest, it involves a binary process (that is either off or on as a result of the organism's previous experience) and such would represent the simplest kind of information storage (Shannon and Weaver, 1963).

REFERENCES

Altman, J. (1966). Organic Foundations of Animal Behavior. Holt, Rinehart and Winston, New York.
Applewhite, P. B. (1968 a). Nature 217, 287.
Applewhite, P. B. (1970). Communications in Behavioral Biology. 5, 67.
Applewhite, P. B. (1967). Yale J. Biol. Medicine 40, 205.
Applewhite, P. B. (1968 b). Nature 219, 1265.
Applewhite and Davis, S. (1969). Comp. Biochem. Physiol. 29, 487.
Applewhite, P. B., Gardner, F., and Lapan, E. (1969). Trans. N. Y. Acad. Sci. 31, 842.
Applewhite, P. B. and Gardner, F. (1968). Nature 220, 1136.
Applewhite, P. B. and Gardner, F. (1970). Physiol. and Behavior 5, 377.
Beach, G., et al. (1969). Proc. Nat. Acad. Sci. 62, 692.
Bogoch, S. (1968). Biochemistry of Memory. Oxford University Press, New York.
Bowman, R. and Strobel, D. (1969). J. Comp. Physiol. Psychol. 67, 448.
Bullock, T. H. (1967). In Neurosciences Research Symposium Summaries, ed. by F. O. Schmitt, et al., M. I. T. Press, Cambridge. Volume 2.
Carthy, J. D. (1965). Behavior of Arthropods. Freeman, San Francisco.
Corning, W. C. and Freed, S. (1968). Nature 219, 1227.
Davis, M. and Wagner, A. (1969). J. Comp. Physiol. Psychol. 67, 486.
Gardner, F. and Applewhite, P. B. (1970 a). Psychopharmacologia 16, 430.
Gardner, F. and Applewhite, P. B. (1970 b). Physiol. and Behavior 5, 713.
Glassman, E. (1969). Ann. Rev. Biochem. 38, 605.
Hinde, R. A. (1970). Animal Behavior. McGraw-Hill, New York.
Hoar, W. (1966). Comparative Physiology. Prentice-Hall, Englewood Cliffs, New Jersey.
Horridge, G. A. (1968). Interneurons. Freeman, San Francisco.
Huxley, H. E. (1969). Science 164, 1356.
Hyden, H. and Eghyhazi, E. (1962). Proc. Nat. Acad. Sci. 48, 1366.
Hyden, H. and Lange, P. W. (1970). Proc. Nat. Acad. Sci. 65, 898.
Kabat, E. (1968). Structural Concepts in Immunology and Immunochemistry. Holt, Rinehart and Winston, New York.
Kahan, B. E. et al. (1970). Proc. Nat. Acad. Sci. 65, 300.
Machlus, B. and Gaito, J. (1969). Nature 222, 573.
McConnell, J. (1966). Ann. Rev. Physiol. 28, 107.
Ochs, S. (1965). Elements of Neurophysiology Wiley, New York.
Pinsker, H. et al. (1970). Science 167, 1740.

Quarton, G. C. et al. Eds. (1967). The Neurosciences. Rockefeller University Press, New York.
Ramsay, J. A. (1968). Physiological Approach to the Lower Animals. Cambridge U. P., London.
Richter, D. Ed. (1966). Aspects of Learning and Memory. Basic Books, New York.
Schone, H. (1961). In Physiology of Crustacea, Volume 2, ed. by T. H. Waterman, Academic Press, New York.
Shannon, C. and Weaver, W. (1963). The Mathematical Theory of Communication. University of Illinois Press, Illinois.
Shashoua, V. (1970). Proc. Nat. Acad. Sci. 65, 160.
Thorpe, W. H. (1963). Learning and Instinct in Animals. Methuen, London.
Yagiu, R. and Shigenaka, Y. (1963). J. Protozoology 10, 364.

PHYSIOLOGICAL CORRELATES OF HABITUATION IN STENTOR COERELIUS

D.C. Wood
University of Pittsburgh,
Department of Psychology,
Pittsburgh,
Pennsylvania 15213, U.S.A.

Habituation in contractile protozoa, and Stentor in particular, is a behavioral modification which has been known since the end of the nineteenth century. In his well-known book, The Behavior of the Lower Organisms, H.S. Jennings summarized in 1906 the results of his earlier studies on Stentor and included a description of a phenomenon he called "acclimitization". Jennings noted that individual Stentor generally contracted in response to the first of a series of mechanical stimuli delivered by a hand-held glass needle, but that subsequent stimuli presented with rather short interstimulus intervals became progressively less effective in eliciting contractions. It is this progressive decrement in response probability during the course of iterated stimuli of constant amplitude the Jennings called "acclimitization" and I refer to as habituation.

Habituation as defined by psychologists has generally referred to a decrement of response probability or amplitude during repetitive stimulation if this decrement can be shown to be independent of sensory adaptation or effector fatigue (Harris, 1943; Thorpe, 1956). The latter two processes have been excluded from consideration in order to limit the process of habituation to events which occur within the central nervous system of vertebrates or at central synapses in invertebrates. This form of definition appears to have been adopted because habituation may be viewed as the most elementary form of behavior modification which can be considered as learning, and learning phenomena have been assumed to be the unique property of animals with complex nervous systems. Since it is evident that protozoa do not possess complex nervous systems, it has rather arbitrarily been held that simple learning phenomena, such as habituation, could not be observed in them (Harris, 1943; Thorpe, 1956).

At the same time reviewers of data on habituation have consistently noted the similarity between metazoan habituation and the response probability

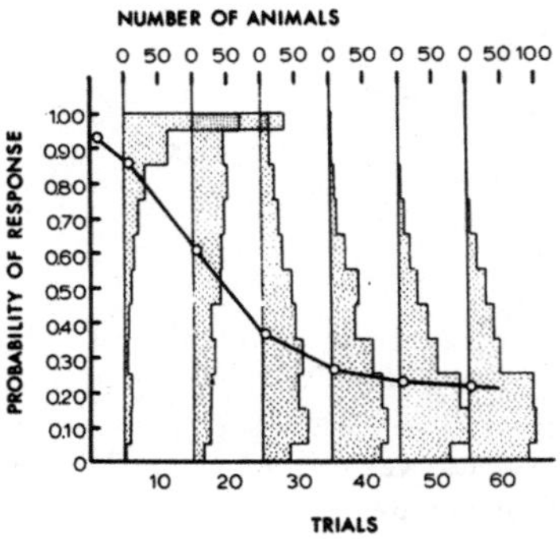

Figure 1

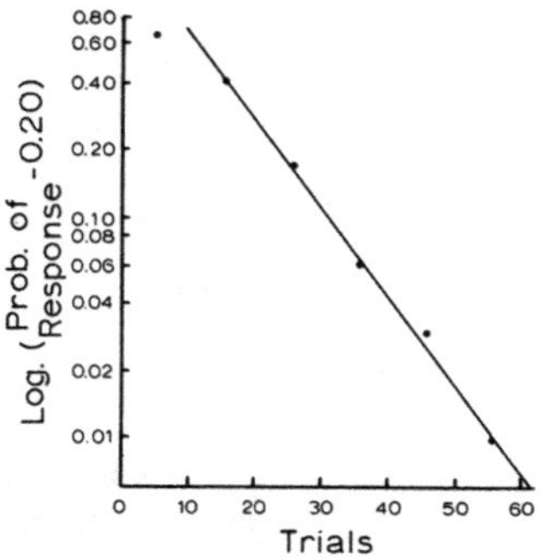

Figure 2

Figure 1. Average probability of response and variability of response to 60 mechanical stimuli of a 0.10 in. amplitude and delivered at a frequency of 1 /min. In this and subsequent graphs the first point represents the probability of response to the first stimulus and subsequent points represent the average probability of response to 10 stimuli (from Wood, 1970 a).

Figure 2. Logarithmic plot of the probability of response less the asymptotic probability of response showing that the observed response decrement curve is approximated by a negative exponential function of the number of trails (from Wood, 1970 a).

decrements noted in protozoa. Of course, if there exists a strong behavioral similarity between the response decrements seen in metazoa and protozoa then it becomes logically tenable to suppose that the electrophysiological and biochemical bases of these two processes might also be similar. In this event contractile protozoa may come to serve as model systems for the elucidation of simple learning phenomena much as the squid axon has served the neuro-physiologist and bacteria, phage, and drosophila have served the geneticists.

However, it is a priori rather difficult to imagine that behavioral modification in protoza and animals containing a complex nervous system should proceed via similar mechanisms. Therefore, the behavioral similarity between these two phenomena must be marked before one would feel justified in making inferences from the protozoan to the metazoan even if the inference is only to be used to formulate a testable hypothesis. For most behaviors a rigorous test or series of tests on which to base such a decision of similarity or difference is missing owing to considerable inexactitude in the characterization of the behavioral process. Fortunately metazoan habituation has been extensively characterized (Spencer, Thompson and Neilson, 1966) and this characterization can serve as an operational definition of it for the purpose of comparison.

Parametric characterization of the response probability decrement of Stentor has been achieved with very simple apparatus. Animals are tested in a 5 ml. beaker fixed to the end of a solenoid plunger whose excursion provides a reproducible and adjustable stimulus. The solenoid is actuated at regular intervals and the number of the animals which contract to each stimulus is recorded.

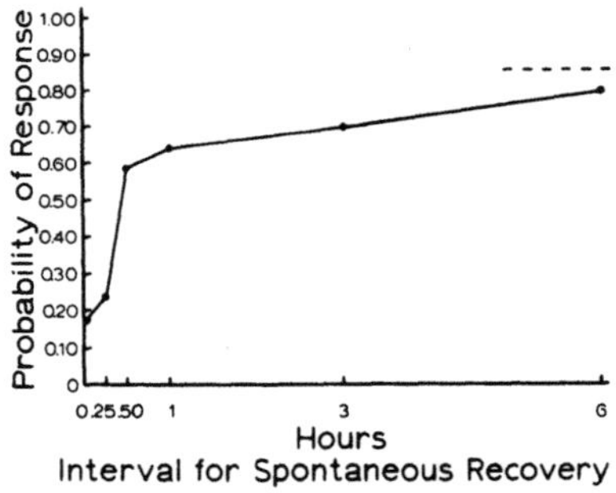

Figure 3. Probability of response on the first 10 retest trails as a function of the interval for spontaneous recovery. Dashed line indicates the average probability of response on trials 1-10 of the initial stimulation series (from Wood, 1970 a).

Figure 1 shows that the probability of an animal's contracting in response to a stimulus decreases as a function of trials over a period of 30 to 40 minutes when stimuli are presented at a rate of one per minute. A nonzero asymptotic level of responding is then attained. Metazoan habituation is characterized by a similar response decrement which is approximated by a negative exponential function of the number of trials. Figure 2 shows that such a negative exponential function also describes the behavioral data presented in Figure 1 rather well if one ignores the initial 10 trials.

Habituated metazoans recover their responsiveness to the previously iterated stimulus during a rest period following the stimulation. The probability or amplitude of response after the rest period is a negatively accelerated monotonic function of the rest period duration. In Figure 3 the spontaneous recovery of Stentor's responsiveness, after 1 hr. of 1/min. stimulation, is plotted as a function of the rest interval. Each point represents the response of a separate group of animals to 10 1/min. test stimuli presented at the end of the rest interval. Throughout most of its course the curve follows the expected form for spontaneous recovery. A significant level of response probability decrement is retained by the animals for as long as 3 hr. after the cessation of the original stimulation series.

If stimulation by the habituating stimulus is continued beyond the number of stimuli required to produce a zero level of response probability, then these additional stimuli can be shown still to be effective even though they cannot of course depress the response probability farther. Their effect is to depress the degree of spontaneous recovery observed after a given rest period. In the case of Stentor and many metazoan behaviors this phenomenon cannot be directly observed since a zero level of responding is never attained. Analogously, however, stimulation beyond that required approximate to closely the asymptotic level of responding has the same depressing effect on spontaneous recovery. Figure 4 shows that less spontaneous recovery is observed in Stentor after 2 hrs. of stimulation and 3/4 hr. of rest than is characteristic after 1 hr. of stimulation and 3/4 hr. of rest.

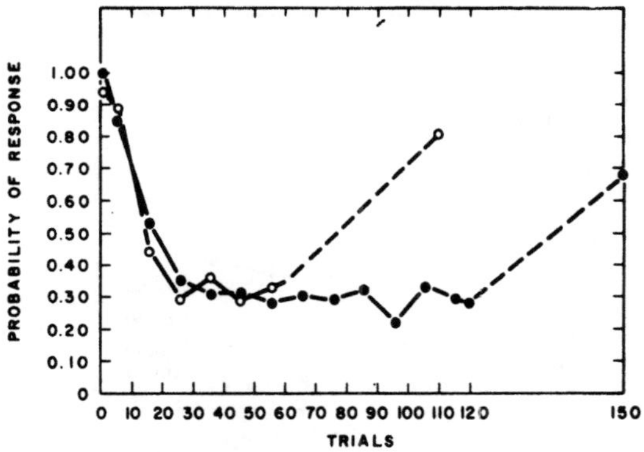

Figure 4. Probability of response to 10 1/min stimuli after 1 hr of 1/min stimulation and 3/4 hr of rest and after 2 hr of 1/min stimulation and 3/4 hr of rest. The probability of response after 2 hr of stimulation and 3/4 hr of rest (0.81) was significantly less ($p < 0.025$; t test for matched samples) than after 1 hr of stimulation and 3/4 hr of rest (0.68). Data were obtained from 19 pairs of animals matched for their total number of responses to the first 60 stimuli.

In similar fashion parametric characterizations have been made of the response probability decrement in Stentor while varying the interstimulus interval and the stimulus amplitude. Studies of the rate of response probability decrement after a period allowed for spontaneous recovery have also been performed. Since the flavor of this type of data must now be clear, it seems sufficient merely to indicate that Stentor's behavior was in fact in accord with the behavior change called habituation with regard to these parametric variations.

Another defining characteristic of habituation is the generalization of the response decrement from the site on the body surface initially exposed to the iterated stimulus to other areas on the body surface. For example an earthworm habituated by tactile stimuli applied to one body segment will show fewer avoidance responses than normal when it is stimulated on adjacent segments for the first time (Kuenzer, 1958). This type of generalization has also been observed in the protozoan Spirostomum by Applewhite (1968) though the mechanisms involved in these two examples of response decrement generalization may well be different. To test for generalization in Stentor, one delimited membrane surface adjacent to its frontal field was stimulated by a small probe mounted on a piezoelectric crystal. Sixty stimuli were applied at a rate of 1/min. to this locus and a response decrement was produced; then the stimulus was applied to the animal's body surface on the opposite side of the frontal field. The response probability decrement was observed at this new locus of stimulation also (Figure 5). Stimulus presentation was counterbalanced across loci on the animal's surface to control for any differences in initial sensitivity of the membrane areas to mechanical stimuli. The expected generalization of the response decrement has therefore been observed in

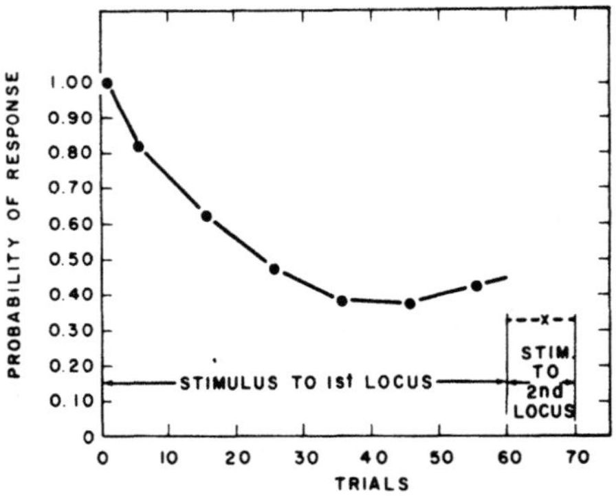

Figure 5. Probability of response versus trials for 60 1/min stimuli presented to one locus on the membranellar band and followed immediately by 10 1/min stimuli presented to a diametrically opposed locus on the membranellar band (N = 6).

Stentor also. Further discussion of this phenomenon will be presented later.

Dishabituation has also been specified as characteristic of response systems which undergo habituation. Dishabituation is observed when a novel stimulus presented after a train of habituating stimuli increases the animal's response to the habituating stimulus when it is presented again. Electric shocks and large amplitude mechanical stimuli have failed to produce dishabituation in Stentor (Wood, 1970 a). While there are of course an inexhaustible number of potential dishabituating stimuli that could be tried, nevertheless it presently seems unlikely that dishabituation will be noted in Stentor. Behavioral and electrophysiological analyses in metazoa have shown that dishabituation is attributable to an excitatory process which is independent of the processes which product habituation. It would appear that Stentor is devoid of this excitatory mechanism and is capable of exhibiting only the habituation phenomenon.

The behavioral analysis presented above demonstrates that the response probability decrement noted in Stentor is in every way analogous to the phenomenon of habituation noted in metazoa except for the failure to observe dishabituation. Since present evidence suggests that dishabituation in metazoa involves mechanisms separable from those producing habituation, the failure to demonstrate dishabituation of protozoan response probability decrements is not viewed as being crucial to the characterization of these behavior changes as examples of habituation. Consequently the term habituation will be used to describe these protozoan behavior changes and it is to be understood that the use of a common term to describe the behavior of protozoa and metazoa implies that I feel some commonalities will also be found in the physiological and biochemical changes which underlie these phenomena.

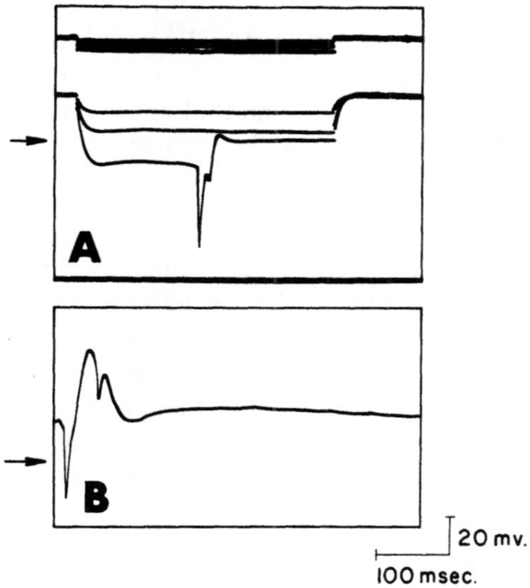

Figure 6. A) Intracellulary recorded transient responses to 2, 4, and 7×10^{-8} amp cathodal current pulses. Spike response had an amplitude of −42 mV. B) Record produced by mechanical stimulation immediately after the record shown in A. Response had an amplitude of −41 mV. The black arrows to the left indicate the 0 mV level with positive polarity being up (from Wood, 1970 b).

While this analysis has been concerned only with Stentor it is important to note that many similar studies have been undertaken on Spirostomum with similar qualitative results (Kinastowski, 1963 a, b; Applewhite, 1968). However, Spirostomum contracts more quickly (Jones et. al, 1970), reextends more rapidly, habituates only to a faster rate of stimulation and shows faster spontaneous recovery. But aside from the more rapid functioning of the relevant processes in Spirostomum the two animals appear to be similar.

If we now return to Stentor and consider it as a simple behavioral system I believe some conclusions as to the physiological basis of habituation in Stentor can be made on behavioral evidence alone. In order to make such an analysis a simple model must be proposed for the events which occur in an individual Stentor between the time of the stimulus and the response. Mindful of Occam's principle it seems sufficient to suggest that there are but two relevant processes occurring in the animal – a receptor process and an effector or contractile process. Mechanical stimuli appear to activate the receptor process which in turn may or may not trigger the contractile process.

Stentor have a reproducible threshold for contraction to electrical stimuli. If habituation produces a decrement in the ability of the animal to contract then one would expect that the threshold for contraction to electrical stimuli would be raised. During experiments in which Stentor's contraction threshold to electric stimuli was measured before and after habituation by mechanical stimulation, no alteration in the electrical threshold was observed. This result implies that the contractile mechanism of the animals was unaltered during the habituation process and that conversely the receptor mechanism was altered. This conclusion can be supported by other behavioral evidence but electrophysiological evidence is more convincing and is available.

The work of Chang, (1960), Eckert (1965 a, b), Eckert and Sibaoka, (1968) and others has shown that Noctiluca is capable of producing propagated action potentials which are coupled to the animal's bioluminescent flashes. Given this one example of a protozoan acting as an excitable tissue, it seems likely that other protozoa may also be capable of producing action potentials. Since Stentor's contractions are all-or-none and have an electrical threshold, they too fit into the pattern of behaviors mediated by action potentials. On the basis of this evidence microelectrode investigations of Stentor have been initiated.

Penetration of the animal's membrane resulted in the recording of an irregular, but generally positive, intracellular "resting" potential. Since the electrodes were rapidly encapsultated by the animal, little opportunity was given to characterize these anomalous "resting" potentials. Spontaneous contractions or contractions produced by electrical or mechanical stimulation were correlated with 10 to 50 mV. negative-going action potentials (Wood, 1970 b). Figure 6 shows that passage of current through a second intracellular electrode and mechanical stimulation from a small probe elicites action potentials of similar amplitude and wave form. Further a graded potential preceding the action potential is evident (though minimally evident in Figure 6) when mechanical, but not electrical stimuli are employed. This potential appears similar to a receptor potential.

After the penetrated animal had encapsulated the recording electrode, diphasic potentials were recorded in place of the previous negative-going potentials. Graded prepotentials were again recorded when mechanical stimuli were used, but not when electrical stimuli were used. The onset of these diphasic potentials were also shown to precede the onset of the animal's contraction by approximately 1.8 msec.

In summary, the electrophysiological evidence suggests a simple model is adequate to describe the sequence of events which underlies Stentor's contractile behavior. When mechanical stimuli are employed, this sequence sould appear to be as follows:

mechanical stimulus → prepotential → action potential → contraction.

Having digressed into a brief description of the electrophysiological behavior of Stentor we may now return to a consideration of the problem of habituation. As as result of habituation a mechanical stimulus which consistently produced contractions at the beginning of a stimulation series fails to do so later in that same series. The mechanical stimulus remains constant but the final element in the preceding sequential model does not always occur. Which process or coupling between processes is altered to result in this behavioral change?

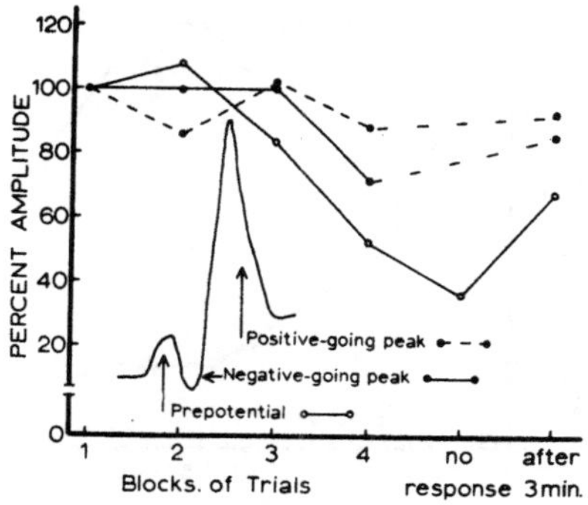

Figure 7. Percent potential amplitudes as a function of blocks of trials during the course of repetitive mechanical stimulation. After the no response trial a 3 min rest period was given before another stimulus was applied (from Wood, 1970c).

To answer this question Stentor were penetrated with microelectrodes and allowed to encapsulate them before stimulation and recording was begun. Then mechanical stimuli were applied once per minute until the animal demonstrated some degree of habituation by failing to respond to a stimulus. Subsequent to this non-response trial a 3 minute rest period was given before an additional mechanical stimulus was applied. It was expected that animals would recover some sensitivity to the mechanical stimulus during this 3 minute rest period and that the recorded potentials produced by the post–rest mechanical stimulus would partially or wholly return to the levels seem during the first stimuli. In Figure 7 the normalized amplitudes of the several phases of the electrical response are plotted as a function of blocks of trials. It can be seen that as stimulation proceeds the prepotential decreases progressively in amplitude and is minimal during the non-response trial. The prepotential decreases in amplitude significantly relative to the other two phases of the response which themselves show considerable, but not significant, changes. Since all potentials return to near their initial values after the 3 minute rest it can be concluded that the changes are reversible and not a function of damage done to the animal or alteration of the recording site. While the amplitude of the prepotential was decreasing with trials, the latency of the diphasic spike after the stimulus was increasing. Both of these observations support the conclusion derived from behavioral data that receptor function becomes depressed during repetitive stimulation and that this is the basis of the habituation phenomenon in Stentor.

As in the case of the electrophysiological studies, behavioral evidence is indicative of the type of chemical alteration we may expect to see correlated with habituation. In this regard one of the previously mentioned studies appears particularly indicative. It was previously noted that Stentor habituated by a punctile stimulus applied to one delimited body surface became simultaneously habituated to this same amplitude of stimulus when it was applied to a

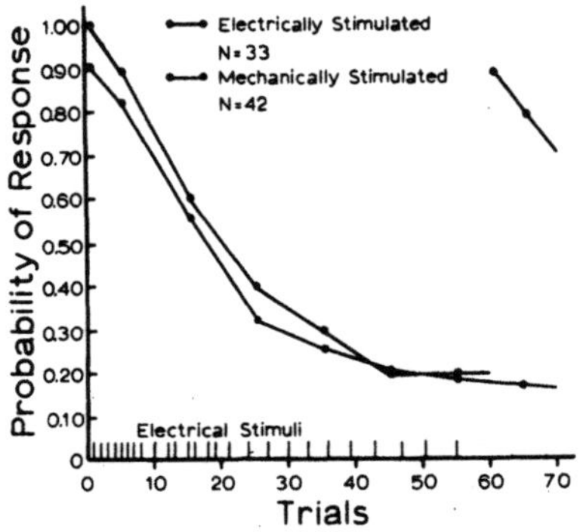

Figure 8. Comparison of response patterns of animals stimulated with the sequence of electrical stimuli shown along the abscissa and those stimulated with 0.10 in mechanical stimuli. During trials 61-70 both groups were stimulated mechanically (0.10 in 1/min stimuli).

different surface of the animal. Several interpreations of this generalization phenomenon are possible. For instant it can be argued that the second body surface was habituated by the mechanical stimulation provided by the contractions which occurred during the habituation procedure. These contractions are very rapid (occur in less than 10 msec.) and involve marked distortions of the animal's form (the animals shorten to less than 50 percent of their precontraction body length). Therefore it is reasonable to suppose that the contractions may serve as mechanical stimuli for all body surfaces and hence may produce habituation of all body surfaces. This possibility was checked by forcing the animals to contract to electrical stimuli and then testing their sensitivity to the mechanical stimulus. The electrical stimuli were presented in such a way that the temporal sequence of contractions produced by the electrically stimulated animals reproduced that observed in animals habituated by repetitive mechanical stimuli. As can be seen in Figure 8 electrically produced contractions do not result in marked habituation to the mechanical stimulus. Therefore the disturbance of the membrane surface produc d by the contractions does not appear to be causal in producing the generalization phenomenon.

Alternately, it might be argued that there is but one small area on the animal's body surface which is sensitive to mechanical stimuli and that this small area, acting as a unit, is habituated by the repeated mechanical stimuli. Generalization of habituation is then an inevitable result of the fact that only one sensitive surface can be habituated regardless of the site of stimulation. This explanation is counterindicated by the fact that diphasic potentials recorded from two different electrodes penetrating the same animal are often asynchronous and that the electrode nearest the site of the mechanical stimulation is always earliest in recording the response. This asynchrony in diphasic potentials is most easily understood if it is assumed that the diphasic potentials are propagated as the contraction which is correlated with them appears to be propagated (Jones et al., 1970). The fact that the earliest potential is recorded from an electrode site nearest the site of stimulation, independent of where the stimulus is applied, suggests that there must be more than one site on the animals body surface capable of being stimulated to produce spikes.

Applewhite (1968) has shown that generalization of habituation between two sites of stimulation occurs in Spirostomum even when the animals are transected after the habituating stimuli but before the test stimuli are applied at the second site. Since both pieces of a transected but unstimulated animal are sensitive to mechanical stimuli, each piece must contain a receptor surface. Therefore it is difficult to explain the phenomenon of generalization of habituation on the basis of a single desensitized receptor surface – at least in the case of Spirostomum and by analogy in Stentor also.

The hypothetical explanations of the generalization phenomenon previously entertained seem inadequate to account for some of the known relevant facts. An obvious alternative hypothesis, that the generalization is dependent on some diffusible substance, must therefore also be considered. Interestingly several studies have suggested that habituation in metazoa can be transferred from a habituated to a non-habituated animal-apparently via a diffusible stance (Ungar and Oceguera-Navarro, 1965; Westerman, 1963). Therefore the suggestion that a diffusible substance is important in the production of habituation is not without precedent. However, unless this diffusible substance can be identified and its functional relation to habituation shown, the hypothesis of its existence must be entertained with skepticism.

Our previous results and the hypotheses which seem best able to explain them suggest that a diffusible intracellular substance which is instrumental in the generation of the receptor potential is involved in the process of habituation. The most obvious class of substances fitting this description are the intracellular ions. Presumably one or more of the intracellular ions concentrations is instrumental in generating the receptor potential, though the responsible ion or ions have not yet been identified in Stentor as they have in Paramecium (Naitoh and Ecker, 1969). Further it is quire reasonable to assume that intracellular ion concentrations might change as a result of the habituation procedure and the contractions produced by it, since these contractions involve sizeable changes in the volume of the animal (Randall and Jackson, 1958). This is to say that contractions produce transmembrane fluxes of water which may well be associated with large transmembrane fluxes of ions. Therefore it seems reasonable to assume that there might be a loss of some intracellular ion normally maintained at a high concentration ratio relative to the dilute medium during the contractions produced by the habituation procedure.

To test this hypothesis the intracellular concentrations of Na^{+}, K^{+}, Ca^{2+}, Mg^{2+}, and Cl^{-} were measured using an ultramicroflame photometer especially designed for the purpose. Individual Stentor were washed in distilled water for a variable period of time and were then pipetted in 170 nl. of distilled water onto a quartz glass cover slip under a pool of liquid parafin (Keesey, 1968). The animals were then

TABLE 1. Intracellular Ion Concentrations in Habituated and Control <u>Stentor</u>

	K	Ca	Mg	Na	Cl
Habiuated group N = 30	12.45 ± 1.12*	49.08 ± 4.39	2.42 ± 0.31	0.10 ± 0.09	9.18 ± 0.96
Control group N = 27	12.53 ± 1.17	52.97 ± 6.97	2.31 ± 0.28	0.13 ± 0.06	9.40 ± 0.61

*Mean value ± standard deviation of the mean.

wet ashed by the addition of 51 nl. of 2N HNO_3. 20 nl. samples of this mixture were extracted for analysis of their Na^+ content. Mg^{2+}, Ca^{2+}, and K^+ concentrations were similarly determined after addition of phosphate and appropriate dilution of the mixture to minimize interference effects. Cl^- concentration was calculated from the concentration of Ag^+ not precipitated when 20 nl. of a $AgNO_3$ solution was added to a sample of 51 nl. of the test mixture. Since the animals were cultured in a medium containing only Na^+, K^+, Ca^{2+}, Mg^{2+}, and Cl^- as added inorganic ions, it was presumed that the concentration of all the major inorganic ions was measured.

Experimental animals were habituated by 60 1/min. stimuli, washed and analyzed. Control animals were taken simultaneously and handled in the same way as experimental animals but were not stimulated. Distilled water washes of 4, 8, 16, 32, 48, and 64 minutes were employed. The resultant plots of ion concentration vs. time in distilled water were fitted by computer with an exponential function to give the value of the ion concentration at the start of the wash period. Other information such as the slope of the logarithmic function and the asymptotic concentration of ion at infinite wash time are potentially obtainable from these data. However, the permeability of the ions out through the membtane was so slow that the asymptotic concentration was not approached in most cases even after 64 minutes of distilled water wash. Therefore estimates of this parameter and the slope of the logarithmic function were highly variable. Longer wash times could not be used because the animals did not survive for longer periods in distilled water.

In Table 1 the ionic concentrations of habituated and unstimulated control animals as extrapolated to 0 min. wash time are compared. It is evident from these data that no significant differences are to be found. It is more evident that there are no 2 or 3-fold changes in ion concentrations such as would be expected to account for the 2 to 3-fold reduction of the receptor potential amplitude. On the other hand these data are compatible with the previous finding that the amplitudes of the diphasic potential do not significantly change during the course of repetitive stimulation, since these potentials are presumably also dependent on intracellular ion concentrations.

Ionic concentrations might, however, be changing via mechanisms not directly measured here. For instance the exponential analysis indicated that much of the Ca^{2+} measured was in bound form within the cell. It appears possible that the concentration of bound Ca^{2+} might be increased rather markedly. The data suggested a similar change might be occurring with respect to K^+ and Mg^{2+}. Unfortunately the method of analysis proved inadequate to do any more than suggest this possiblity. Other tests of this proposition are currently being made.

Most of the previously cited data was generated to test the proposal that habituation in Stentor is analogous to metazoan habituation. On a behavioral level this analogy appears complete with the somewhat irrelevant exception of the dishabituation phenomenon. This similarity is at first glance somewhat surprising in view of the obvious differences between the two classes of animals in terms of complexity. However, the fact that habituation can be observed at the neuronal level in metazoa indicates that most or all of its characteristics are to be explained in terms of the functioning of single cells. The electrophysiological studies undertaken revealed that Stentor is capable of supporting receptor potentials and action potentials. Further habituation appears to be correlated with a decrement in the amplitude of the receptor potential. In metazoan nervous systems habituation has been attributed to a decrement in the amplitude of excitatory post synaptic potentials (Spencer et al., 1966; Castellucci et al., 1970). Therefore, in both protozoa and metazoa a decrement in the graded potential which precedes the action potential appears to be causal in the production of habituation. However this apparent similarity can be indicative of a further physiological similarity only if the metazoan EPSP decrement is attributable to post-synaptic membrane desensitization rather than a decrease in transmitter substance release by the pre-synaptic terminal. At present the mechanism producing the EPSP decrement in metazoa is not known. Nevertheless, the similarities between metazoan and protozoan habituation appear sufficiently strong at the present time to merit extensive biochemical analysis of the protozoan behavior change in the hope that it may serve as a model biochemical system. This biochemical analysis is presently being undertaken.

REFERENCES

Applewhite, P.B. (1968). Nature 217, 287-288.

Castellucci, V., Pinsker, H., Kupfermann, L., and Kandel, E.R. (1970). Science 167, 1743-1745.

Change, J.J. (1960). J. Cell. Comp. Physiol. 56, 33-42.

Eckert, R. (1965a). Science 147, 1140-1142.

Eckert, R. (1956). Science 147, 1142-1145.

Eckert, R. and Sibaoka, T. (1968). J. Gen. Physiol. 52, 258-282.

Haljamäe, H. and Wood, D. C. (1971). Anal. Biochem. 42, 155-170.

Harris, J. D. (1943). Psych. Bull. 40, 385-422. (1968).

Jennings, H. S. (1906). Behavior of the Lower Organisms. Columbia University Press, New York.

Jones, A.R., Jahn, T.L., and Fonesca, J.R. (1970). J. Cell. Physiol. 75, 1-8.

Keesey, J. C. (1968). J. Neurochem. 15, 547-562.

Kinastowski, W. (1963 a). Acta Protozool. 1, 201-222.

Kinastowski, W. (1963 b). Acta Protozool. 1, 223-236.

Kuenzer, P. (1958). Z. Tierpsych. 15, 29-49.

Naitoh, Y. and Eckert, R. (1969). Science 164, 963-965.

Randall, J. T. and Jackson, S. F. (1958). J. Cell. Biol. 4, 807-830.

Spencer, W. A., Thompson, R. F., and Neilson, D. R., Jr. (1966). J. Neurophysiol. 29, 253-274.

Thompson, R. F. and Spencer, W. A. (1966). Psychol. Rev. 73, 16-43.

Thorpe, W. A. (1956). Learning and instinct in animals. Methuen, London.

Ungar, G. and Oceguera-Navarro, C. (1965). Nature. 207, 301-302.

Westerman, R. A. (1963). Science 140, 676-677.

Wood, D. C. (1970 a). J. Neurobiol. 1, 345-360.

Wood, D. C. (1970 b). J. Neurobiol. 1, 363-377.

Wood, D. C. (1970c). J. Neurobiol. 2, 1-11.

Wood, D. C. and Haljamae, H. Analysis of nanogram quantities of Ca, Mg, Na, K, and Cl in biological samples by ultramicroflame photometry. (in preparation).

BEHAVIOR MODIFICATION IN PROTOZOA

E.M. Eisenstein, D. Osborn and H.J. Blair
Michigan State University,
Department of Biophysics,
East Lansing,
Michigan 48823, U.S.A.

ABSTRACT

A review is presented of several past studies which have shown behavioral modification in protozoa. At least two methodological problems inherent in these studies make it difficult to conclude unequivocally that learning has been shown: (1) often the behavioral changes seen over time could have been due to changes in the animal's environment rather than in the animal itself; and (2) it has not been clearly demonstrated that the temporal order of the stimulus and response events was the relevant variable responsible for the behavioral change rather than the total amount of stimulation *per se*.

Recent work on decrement in the probability of the contractile response to intermittent mechanical stimulation and the effect of electrical stimulation on *Spriostomum* is discussed.

1. INTRODUCTION

A major problem in studying the molecular bases of behavior modification is to find simpler experimental preparations in which one can locate and isolate the relevant changes. Many nervous systems are too complex. Neural elements involved in a particular behavioral act are not easily identified, and it is often difficult, if not impossible, to assess the contributions of intra-neuronal vs.inter-neuronal (i.e., connectivity) factors to such behavior. Protozoa (in particular, the ciliates) appear promising for such studies, since intercellular interactions can be eliminated from consideration. They show a variety of behavioral modifications including response decrement to an intermittently presented mechanical stimulus (habituation) (Kinastowski, 1963a, b; Wood, 1970a, b, c) and avoidance of an area where they have received electric shock (Bergstrom, 1968 a, b). In addition, the ciliates respond to a variety of stimuli such as light, chemical changes (particularly pH changes in the medium) and temperature. Some of them grow to be as large as several millimeters in length, enabling the investigator to observe single cells easily. The protozoan offers an opportunity to correlate molecular and behavioral changes in cells that are discrete, genetically similar, and simple in comparison even to the lowest phylum showing a distinct nervious system, i.e., the coelenterates. Protozoan research may offer promise in understanding intracellular events determining behavioral change (Eisenstein, 1967).

Past Behavioral Studies. A large body of the work on behavior modification in protozoans has been done on the paramecium. Early work by Day and Bentley (1911) showed that if a paramecium was drawn into a glass capillary tube the inside diameter of which was less than the animal's length, the paramecium, after swimming to the end, would make repeated attempts to turn around. After one to two hours, it would take progressively less time to complete a turn, and in addition, make fewer abortive turning attempts. Furthermore, if the paramecium was removed from the tube after such training, placed in an open dish of culture water, and replaced in the capillary tube after a ten to twenty-minute interval, it showed a "savings", that is, it took less time to complete a turn that it did the first time it was placed in the tube. Is this change in behavior evidence of learning? It certainly demonstrates at least two characteristics seen in most kinds of learning: (1) there is a progressive change in response to a given stimulus situation over time, and (2) there is evidence of retention of the response change (at least over a twenty-minute interval).

A criticism of this work as evidence of learning was made by Buytendijk (1919), who argued that paramecia, when subjected to mechanical stimulation, lost "tonus" and became more flexible, suggesting that only physical effects were involved. However, such an explanation may be misleadingly simple. It would be of interest to know what molecular changes in the paramecium allow this behavioral change to occur, and to consider whether such molecular changes associated with "use" bear any relationship to changes associated with long-lasting behavioral alterations that may occur in neural systems.

One of the most systematic efforts to explore learning-related behavior in paramecia has been that of Gelber (1952, 1954, 1956 a, b, 1957, 1965). A small culture of paramecia were placed in a depression slide and a sterile platinum wire was lowered into the center of the culture. The number of paramecia attached to or within the immediate vicinity of the wire were observed over a several minute period. This gave (as a control) a pre-training measure of the attachment tendencies of the culture. She then began a training procedure during which the wire was baited with the bacterium Aerobacter aerogenus (food material for Paramecium aurelia), lowered into the culture for fifteen seconds and removed. Twenty-five seconds later, the wire was lowered again. Generally, forty such training trials were given; however, the wire was baited with bacteria only on every third trial. This procedure gave the following results: (1) a longer interval between training trials resulted in greater clinging than a shorter interval; (2) a decrease in the clinging behavior occurred if, following training, several trials of wire were given without food (analogous to an extinction procedure); (3) if the culture was tested two hours after such an extinction procedure there was greater wire clinging than immediately after the extinction procedure (analogous to spontaneous recovery); and (4) the behavioral change lasted up to at least 10 hours after training and apparently survived fission within the culture.

Jensen (1957 a, b, 1965) has criticized the interpretation of these results as evidence of learning. His major thesis, based on his own work and on earlier studies by others, is that the procedures used to dmonstrate learning in paramecia have produced changes in the environment rather than in the paramecia. Jensen, and Jennings earlier (1899), demonstrated that paramecia show a clinging response to an object in their environment, and that this clinging, as well as aggregate behavior, is increased in an acidic environment. Jensen contends that the feeding procedure develops a zone rich in bacteria that produces CO_2 during metabolism. The paramecia are drawn into this area, and in the presence of CO_2 increase their clinging behavior, themselves producing CO_2 and thus further trapping themselves in an acidic zone. During a later test period they would be expected to cling more to a sterile wire, not as a result of learning, but because of changes in the acidity of the environment. As is often the case in such controversies the evidence for both positions is suggestive rather than conclusive. That CO_2-rich zones may have been a critical factor in Gelber's early work is supported because control cultures were not fed during the training period, and their environment was therefore less acidic. However, CO_2 gradients may not be the full explanation of Gelber's findings. The safest conclusion one can draw at this time regarding learning in paramecia is that it remains a possibility.

More recently, Bergstrom (1968 a, b) studied avoidance behavior in the ciliated protozoan, Tetrahymena, using a Pavlovian training procedure. He showed that when Tetrahymena were given an electric shock in the presence of light they later showed more light avoidance than controls given either shock alone or light alone. Furthermore, the degree of avoidance was a function of the number of light-shock pairings these animals received. On the surface this would appear as good evidence of an "association" or learning in this animal. Unfortunately, such an interpretation is confounded by the fact that the group receiving both light and shock received much more total stimulation and of different kinds than the group receiving either light alone or shock alone. Is a temporal association demonstrated between two stimuli (light and shock) or merely an effect due to more as well as different stimulation of one group relative to the others, i.e., senstivity to the light as a result of a greater amount of stimulation? The latter interpretation receives support from Bergstrom's results showing that groups given many shocks alone did begin to show some avoidance in the presence of light, even though shock was not given to this group in the presence of light (Bergstrom 1968b).

One control for assessing the possible contribution of temporal factors in behavioral changes of this kind would be to stimulate two experimental groups with the same total amount of light and shock but reversing the order of the two stimuli for the two groups. One would receive the light before the shock (forward conditioning) while the other would receive the light after the shock (backward conditioning). It is important that both groups receive the same amount of stimulation. If the first group avoids the light more than the second, then one can argue that temporal order is the fundamental variable accounting for this behavioral difference, and consider it in the same domain of behavioral plasticity as Pavlovian conditioning shown at other phyletic levels.

A commonly studied behavioral change in ciliates such as Spirostomum and Stentor is the decrement in the probability of contraction (habituation) to repeated and intermittent mechanical stimulation (Applewhite et al., 1969; Kinastowski 1963a, b; Wood 1970a, b, c). Kinastowski examined the effect of inter-stimulus interval on response decrement and its retention in Spirostomum. The stimulus consisted of a drop of culture fluid which fell into a small culture dish containing one of these animals; the resulting disturbance produced a contraction. He studied a large group of animals individually, noting the effect of varying the interval between stimuli on the decrement occurring over time. At interstimulus intervals of less than one per twelve seconds there was a marked decrement in the percentage of response over time. However, at one minute intervals there was no evidence of response decrement after 10 minutes (Figure 1). Recent unpublished work in the Laboratory of Eisenstein however has shown some habituation to stimuli at one minute intervals after 30 minutes.

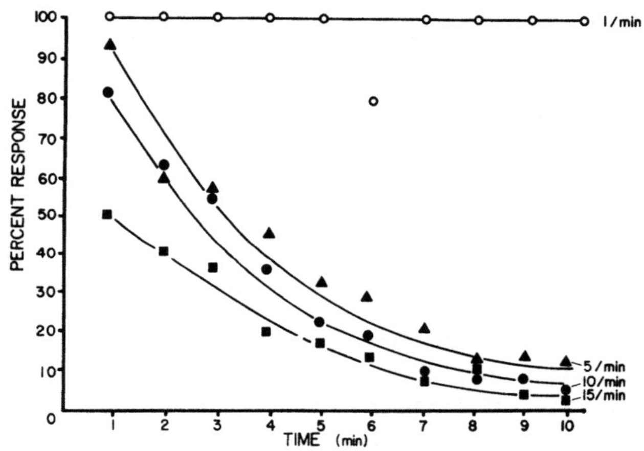

Figure 1. Effect of interstimulus interval on response decrement. A small drop of culture fluid was allowed to free fall into a slide well containing a single Spirostomum. The resulting disturbance of the culture produced a contraction. The percent contractions per minute for a large group of animals for each stimulus frequency are plotted. [Plotted from Kinastowski (22).]

Figure 2 indicates the effect of testing the animals at varying times after the initial habituation period. The first curve is from the previous Figure produced by stimulating at a rate of once per six seconds. These animals were habituated until the response level was very low, which took from eight to twelve minutes. Following initial stimulation, different groups were

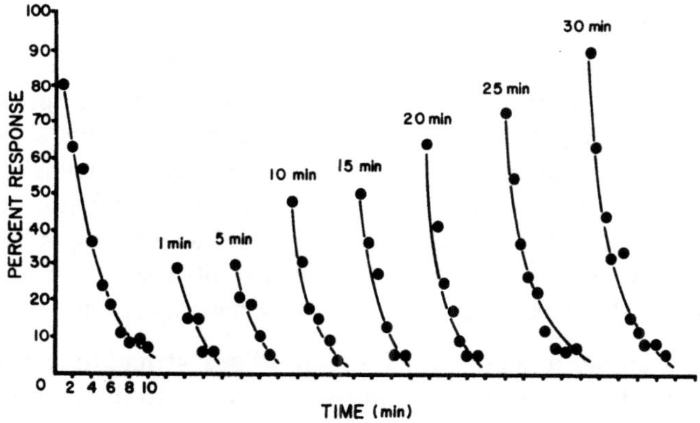

Figure 2. Effect of pauses of varying durations on response level in Spirostomum initially stimulated once per six seconds for ten minutes. This curve is seen in Figure 1 and reproduced here for comparison. At various times after this stimulation period different groups were stimulated again. The first five to seven minutes of each group are plotted. Note full recovery within thirty minutes [plotted from Kinastowski (23)].

stimulated for a second time at varying intervals after the original training period. The retraining times are marked above the curves. The data indicate that retention of this behavioral change is dissipated within 30 minutes. Kinastowski further demonstrated (Figure 3) that the effect of repeated habituation was cumulative. Following initial habituation, a ten minute rest was allowed followed by re-habituation. This was repeated several times. There was a reduction in the response level with each successive stimulation period.

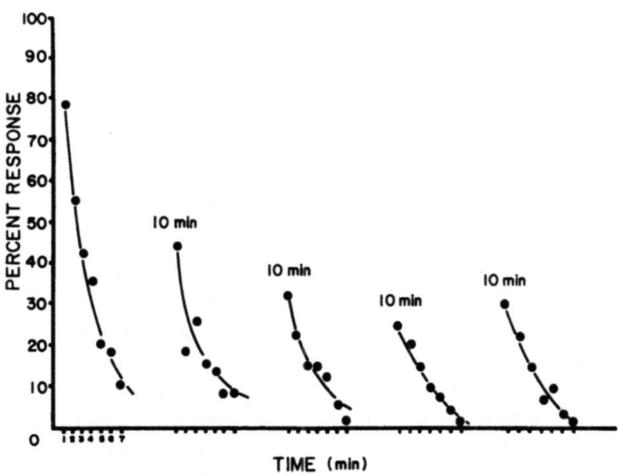

Figure 3. Effect of repeated stimulation of the same animals with ten-minute pauses interspersed. [Plotted from Kinastowski (23).]

2. Materials and Methods

In our laboratory we have been concerned with changes in the frequency of occurrence of the contractile response in the protozoan, Spirostomum ambiguum, to mechanical and electrical stimulation. Animals were obtained from Connecticut Valley Biological Supply, Southampton, Massachusetts. A single animal was used to start a clone. The culture medium, described by Carter (1956), contained heat-killed wheat seeds which supported a bacterial population upon which Spirostomum feeds. The pH was adjusted to 6.3 by adding a KH_2PO_4-KOH buffer. Cultures were maintained at room temperature.

Figure 4 shows a schematic diagram of our stimulating apparatus. Animals were placed in the well of a microscope slide 10 minutes before the stimulation period and their behavior observed through a binocular dissecting microscope. A brief mechanical stimulus was delivered to the edge of the slide by turning off a solenoid, spring driving a central metal core to the edge of the slide and then electromagnetically drawing it back. The resulting vibration of the slide well containing culture medium stimulated the animal to contract. Usually between one and four animals were studied simultaneously. Electric shock also can be delivered intermittently by placement of platinum electrodes along the well wall.

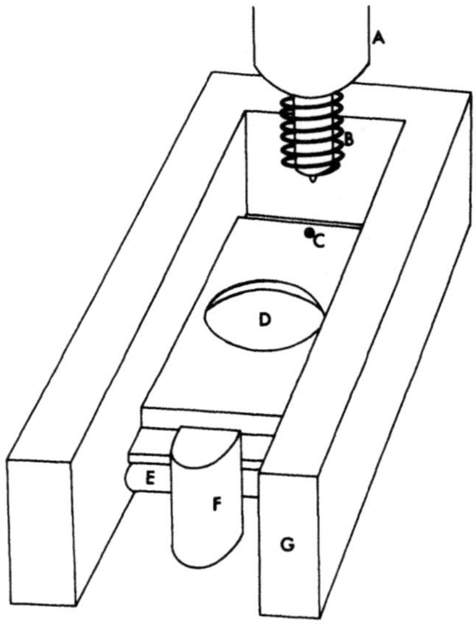

Figure 4. Apparatus used for delivering a mechanical stimulus to Spirostomum. One to four animals are placed in the well of a plastic slide (D) which is nineteen millimeters in diameter and three millimeters deep; 0.9 milliliters of fluid is placed in the well. The slide is placed over two rubber mounds (E), one at each end, and held loosely in place by plastic walls (F and G). A spring loaded central core (B) of a solenoid (A) is then driven against the edge of the slide (C). The resulting disturbance of the medium and response of the animal is observed through a binocular dissecting microscope placed over the well.

3. Results

Figure 5 is a trail by trial plot of the percent response of Spirostomum to a mechanical stimulus delivered at the rate of one per ten seconds for five minutes. Following this, one minute of retraining is given after a two-minute rest period. There is a decrease in response level during the first five minutes with a return to the starting level within two minutes. However, the rate of re-habituation is considerably more rapid than during the first stimulation period, corroborating Kinastowski's observation of a residual effect due to prior stimulation. In addition, the mean response level for the minute of retention is greater (less retention) after a five minute stimulation period than after a ten minute stimulation period.

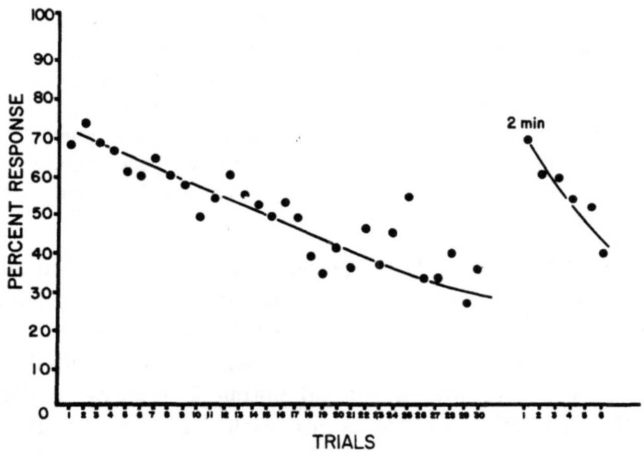

Figure 5. Trial by trial plot of the percent response to a mechanical stimulus delivered at one per ten seconds for five minutes. Following a two-minute pause an additional minute of stimulation was delivered. Note the rapid return of the response level on the first stimulus after the pause and the more rapid rate of decrement after the pause. (N = 57) (H. Joseph Blair, unpublished).

In order to determine whether repeated initiation of contraction itself leads to response decrement, electric shock was selected as a stimulus since it produces contraction and it has been suggested by work in our laboratory and by others that it produces little decrement, if any (Figure 6). A two millisecond biphasic pulse delivered at a frequency of one per ten seconds at three different current levels failed to produce evidence of response decrement over the same period of time during which the percent response decreased to mechanical stimulation (cf. Figures 5 and 6) (Jahn, 1966; Kinosita 1938a, b; Jennings, 1899; Naito and Eckert, 1969; Wood, 1970a). To examine whether the electric shock or electrolysis by-products prevented response decrementfrom occurring, animals electrically shocked for three minutes were than mechanically stimulated for five minutes and compared to mechanically stimulated but unshocked controls. Both groups showed response decrement to mechanical stimulation. In addition, habituation to mechanical stimulation also occurred in bacteria-free distilled water.

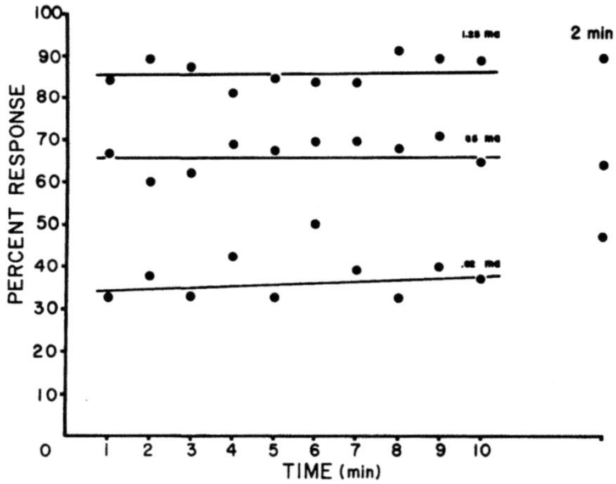

Figure 6. Percent response per minute to three different levels of current delivered at the rate of one stimulus per ten seconds for ten minutes. Following a two-minute pause an additional minute of stimulation was given. The stimulus consisted of a two millisecond biphasic square pulse delivered by a Grass S-8 stimulator. (N = 81) (H. Joseph Blair, unpublished.)

From these data a tentative hypothesis suggests that the response decrement due to mechanical stimulation represents a change in the animal prior to the initiation of the contractile response itself; one possible site of change is in the membrane processes associated with a graded receptor potential Wood (1970, c) showed a graded potential occurs in Stentor to a mechanical stimulus but does not occur with electric shock) which decreases with repetitive stimulation. Although graded potential changes to mechanical stimulation in Spirostomum have not been studied, Ettiene (1970) reports that he finds no measurable depolarization in Spirostomum when electric shock is used to produce contraction.

4. Discussion

One question to consider is whether the response decrement to repetitive mechanical stimulation "really" is learning. This is not a question to be answered by an arbitrary assertion or definition. It is an empirical question. It requires knowing the molecular substrate of the decrement and how this substrate is similar or dissimilar to that underlying such generally accepted forms of learning as Pavlovian conditioning and instrumental learning. This response decrement certainly shows several characteristics associated with learning: 1) it is a change over time to the same stimulus; 2) it may show retention up to several hours; and 3) it is reversible.

Behavioral characteristics not yet demonstrated and which most workers would like to see before they would agree that the above phenomenon is related to learning seen in organisms with a nervous system are: 1) stimulus discrimination, i.e., is the response decrement specific to the stimulus used to produce it, and not a general decrement to all stimuli to which the animal is capable of responding? 2) Can dishabituation be shown? If a more intense stimulus is presented out of the temporal order used for habituation, is there some erasure of the decrement (dishabituation is seen in a great many systems where habituation occurs)? Wood has not seen dishabituation in Stentor and we are not prepared at this time to say whether it does or does not occur in Spirostomum. 3) If Pavlovian conditioning is attempted using a contractile response (or some other behavior), will it make a difference in the response change to the conditioned stimulus whether the conditioned stimulus occurs before or after the unconditioned stimulus? Temporal order is a fundamental variable in learning, and as previously noted if it can be shown to be relevent in this system, it is reasonable to consider such behavior in the same domain of behavioral plasticity as Pavlovian conditioning shown at other phyletic levels. (Eisenstein 1967).

Our intent is to explore in this system the relevance for behavioral modification of stimulus parameters known to be important in learning in neural systems and characterize the associated molecular changes. Eventually, it may be possible to establish the causal sequence of molecular events between the stimulus and response accounting for this response decrement as well as to determine the relevant sequence of molecular events underlying other types of behavior modification.

ACKNOWLEDGMENTS

We wish to thank J. Thompson, and N. Novelly for their extensive contributions to the work reported from our own laboratory; to N. St. Pierre who provided valuable technical assistance in the design and maintenance of the equipment used as well as critical comments on the manuscript, and J. Berry and Charlene Sawallich who provided the drawings of the figures. In addition, we would like to thank Dr. David Wood, Dr. Philip Applewhite and Dr. D. Davenport for their helpful and critical comments on this manuscript.

Our work has been supported by NIH grant MH 18570-01 and NSF grant GB 23371 to E. Eisenstein and by General Research Support Grant FR-05656-02 from the General Research Support Branch, Division of Research Facilities and Resources, National Institutes of Health. Mr. Dustan Osborn was supported by PHS Training Grant No. GM-01422-06 from the National Institutes of Health.

REFERENCES

Applewhite, P. B., Lapan, E. A., Gardner, F. T. (1969). Nature 222, 49.

Bergstrom, S. R. (1968 a). Scand. J. Psychol. 9, 215.

Bergstrom, S. R. (1968 b). Scand. J. Psychol. 9, 220.

Buytendijk, F. J. J. (1919). Arch. Neerl. Physiol. 3, 455.

Carter, L. (1956). Exp. Biol. 34, 71.

Day, L. M. and Bentley, M. (1911). J. Animal Behav., 1, 67.

Eisenstein, E. M. (1967). The Rockefeller Univ. Press, N. Y., 653.

Ettiene, Earl M. (1970). J. Gen. Physiol., 56, 168.

Gelber, B. (1952). J. Comp. Physiol. Psychol. 45, 58.

Gelber, B. (1954). Am. Psychol. 9, 374.

Gelber, B. (1956 a). J. Genet. Psychol. 88, 31.

Gelber, B. (1956 b). J. Comp. Physiol. Psychol. 49, 590.

Gelber, B. (1957). Science 126, 1340.

Gelber, B. (1965). Animal Behav. 13, 21.
Jahn, T. L. (1966). J. Cell. Physiol. 68, 135.
Jennings, H. S. (1899). Am. J. Psychol. 10, 503.
Jensen, D. D. (1957 a). Science 126, 1341.
Jensen, D. D. (1957 b). Science 125, 191.
Jensen, D. D. (1965). Animal Behav. 13, 9.
Kinastowski, W. (1963 a). Acta Protozool. 1, 201.
Kinastowski, W. (1963 b). Acta Protozool. 1, 223.
Kinosita, H. (1938 a). J. Facultv Sci., Tokyo Imperial Univ., 5, 71.
Kinosita, H. (1938 b). J. Faculty Sci., Tokyo Imperial Univ., 5, 93.
Naito, Y. and Eckert, R. (1969). Sci. 164, 963.
Wood, D. C. (1970 a). J. Neurobiol. 1, No. 3, 345.
Wood, D. C. (1970 b). J. Neurobiol. 1, No. 4, 363.
Wood, D. C. (1970 c). J. Neurobiol. 2, No. 1, 1.

THE ROLE OF THE CLOCK IN CONTROLLING PHOTOTACTIC RHYTHMS

V.G. Bruce
Princeton University,
Department of Biology,
Princeton,
New Jersey 08540, U.S.A.

SUMMARY

A short review of the general properties and ideas concerning the possible mechanism of biological clocks in unicellular microorganisms is given. Phototactic rhythms are reviewed briefly, and a preliminary report describing mutant phototactic behavioral mutants in Chlamydomonas reinhardi is included.

1. INTRODUCTION

Many microorganisms possess biological clocks which regulate a variety of functions, including some which are behavioral. These clocks, or circadian rhythms, have approximately a 24 hr periodicity which can be synchronized by environmental alternations of light and dark. The rhythms generally persist in constant conditions and possess the important adaptive characteristic that the period length is changed very little at different temperatures within the physiological range. Often the adaptive function of the clock is not obvious, especially in microorganisms, but the diversity of organisms in which rhythms are found with common features, suggests that they are adaptive. The importance of biological clocks in the regulation of behavior is obvious and it is no surprise that the clock can be coupled to the phototactic behavior of microorganisms.

Circadian rhythms have been observed in fungi, algae, flagellates, ciliates, and other eukaryotic microorganisms. Rhythms satisfying the essential prerequisites of clocks, such as temperature compensation, have not been demonstrated in prokaryotic organisms, although a few reports suggest that such rhythms might occur in bacteria. Circadian clocks control such diverse functions as spore formation and growth patterns in fungi, photosynthesis, bioluminescence, motility and phototaxis in algae and flagellates,

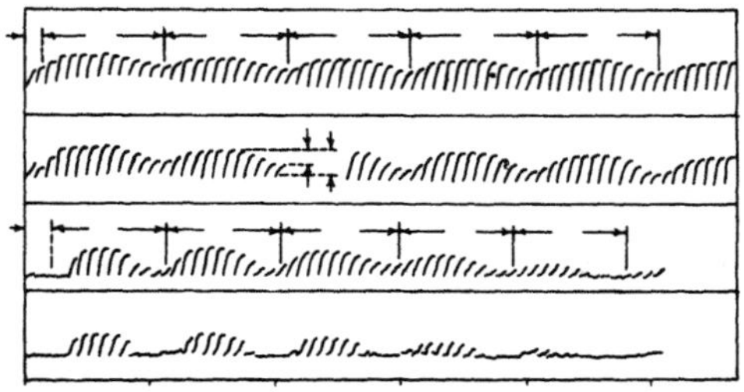

Figure 1. The circadian rhythm of phototactic responses of *C. reinhardi*, w - strain, at 22°C. Tracings of the chart records are shown for two cultures grown in continuous light and transferred to continuous darkness (test lights only) at hour zero. The period τ of the rhythm is measured between minima and the phase ϕ is the time from the initiating light – dark transition to the first minimum (extrapolated if necessary). The maximum and minimum responses in a cycle are used to determine r_1 and r_2 and the amplitude $A = r_1/r_2$ of the rhythm. Records 1 and 2 are for aliquots of one culture whereas 3 and 4 are records from separately grown cultures of a spontaneous mutant $w - c_1$ of this strain which has a slightly shortened period.

growth and mating reactivity in ciliates, and many others. Several physiological or behavioral activities may be clock-controlled in a single organism and these clocks undoubtedly serve an important role in the temporal organization of the organism.

a) General Properties of Clocks

Circadian clocks possess certain characteristic common adaptive features, such as approximation of the period length to 24 hr, temperature compensation, and entrainability to 24 hr light – dark cycles. These rhythms are endogenous, innate, and persist with remarkable precision in non-entraining conditions such as continuous darkness or light. Temperature changes generally can phase-shift the rhythm, and temperature cycles can entrain it, but the period length depends very little on temperature. The temperature coefficients and the response to temperature changes differ from one organism to another and also may depend on physiological conditions. The period length generally does not differ more than 10 per cent from 24 hr within the physiological temperature range and, although it is generally slightly lengthened with lowered temperature, the opposite effect is sometimes noted. There is also a compensation for the period length of the rhythm for variations in growth rate, since factors such as light intensity and media composition can markedly alter growth rates without greatly changing the period. The stability and precision of the clock is revealed by the long continued persistence of many of these rhythms with little loss of synchrony. Light – dark cycles in nature serve an important role in synchronizing clocks. The marked phase-shifting effect of light or dark signals is in sharp contrast to the general insensitivity of the phase of the rhythm to most disturbances. The phase-shift resulting from a light signal varies with the time of the cycle and it is reproducible and stable. A rhythm can often be induced by a single transition in light conditions (such as light to dark) with a characteristic phase relative to the transition.

Many factors can affect the expression of a rhythm. The loss of a rhythm can result from an inhibition of clock-controlled activity or uncoupling of the clock from the controlled function, as well as from a direct inhibition of the clock. For example, a phototactic rhythm may be lost as a result of a direct inhibition of phototaxis, or it may be lost with no inhibition of the phototactic response. Loss of rhythms is often noted in fungi where the growth medium may determine whether a zonation or banding growth pattern occurs. Sometimes certain conditions of continuous light may inhibit a rhythm whereas a lower intensity or different spectral range may not. If more than one function in a single cell is clock-controlled, it is sometimes possible to inhibit one rhythm without inhibiting another. In some organisms, for example Paramecium, where mating type rhythms are observed and can be scored only in starved cells, there is evidence that the clock runs while the cells are growing but it is not detectable by the assay methods used (Karakashian, 1965; Barnett, 1966). The variation in the expression of the rhythm also includes changes in the amplitude of the rhythmic component, but it does not include period changes, which reflect a basic clock parameter. Changes in phase relationships may result from altered coupling between the clock and the controlled function, or between the clock and the light–dark cycle. These are not common but they are of interest since they reflect changes in the way the clock can be coupled in the cell. No cases of dissociation of rhythms (running with different period lengths) have been reported in single cells although such phenomena are observed in multicellular circadian rhythms. I have discussed the factors which influence the expression of the rhythm at some length because of their importance for interpreting the results of experiments designed to elucidate the mechanism of the clock.

b) What is Known About the Mechanism?

Attempts to learn something about the mechanism of the cellular clock have been directed at two questions. What can be said about the localization and physical nature (organization) of the clock? What types of biochemical processes are involved in the clock? Experiments relevant to the first question were done by Sweeney and Haxo (1961) working with the single celled alga Acetabularia. These experiments indicated that a rhythm of photosynthesis in enucleated cells will persist for 30 to 40 days and that the phase of the rhythm can be shifted by light. On the other hand Schweiger and Schweiger (1965) transplanted nuclei between plants on different clock phases and showed that the nucleus also is rhythmic and when present it controls the phase of the rhythm. Barnett's (1966) experiments with Paramecium also indicated a controlling role of the nucleus in determining the phase of the rhythm. The genetic constitution of the nucleus has been shown to affect the expression of the rhythm in fungi (Stadler, 1959; Huong, 1967), as well as in other microorganisms. The physical organization of the clock must allow for the replication of the clock to be independent of the rate at which it operates, since clock

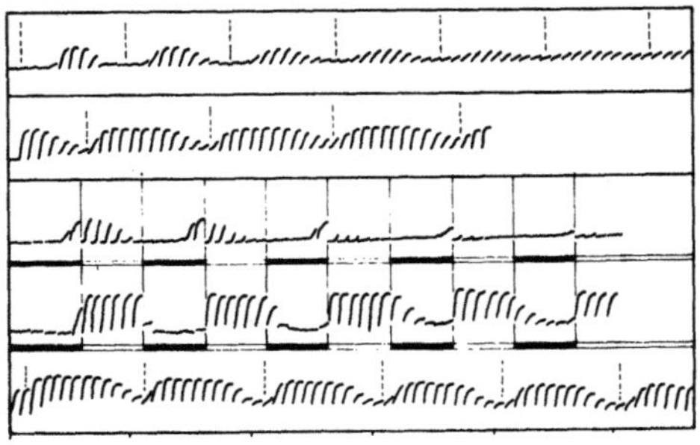

Figure 2. Record 1 is for a short period mutant w-27 (τ = 21 hr) and record 2 is for an altered phase mutant (ϕ = 15 hr) obtained by mutagenesis. Both cultures were tested in continuous dark after growth in continuous light. Record 3 illustrates the altered sensitivity to light of w − c_1. Record 4 is a control w- for comparison. Both were tested in a light − dark cycle after growth in continuous light. Record 5 is a continuous dark Lo-control for comparison with record 2. Dashed vertical lines are placed at the estimated minima.

rate is essentially independent of growth rate. A model for the clock, (Ehret and Trucco, 1967), which involves some structural organization within the cell considers these restrictions. In conditions of rapid growth when the cell replication time becomes less than the clock cycle length a rhythm is generally lost. There may be exceptions to this (Barnett, 1966), but it does seem plausible that under these conditions of rapid growth the organization of the clock may be broken down.

Inferences regarding the biochemical nature of the clock are based primarily on studies using inhibitors of macromolecular synthesis. Actinomycin was shown by Karakashian and Hastings (1962) to inhibit the bioluminescent rhythm in Gonyaulax within one cycle while the photosynthesis rhythm was inhibited more slowly. Actinomycin can also either advance or delay a rhythm in a single neuron of an isolated ganglion of the sea hare Aplysia studied by Strumwasser (1965). Technical difficulties precluded observing more than one cycle in a single ganglion but it was postulated that the drug affected the expression of the rhythm. In Acetabularia this drug knocks out the rhythm if the cells have a nucleus, whereas it has no effect if the cells are enucleated (Vanden Driessche, 1966). Actinomycin enhances the rhythm in Podospora (Huong, 1967). It is clear that actinomycin affects the expression of the rhythm in some organisms, but it is not clear to what extent it affects the clock. Cycloheximide inhibits protein synthesis in Euglena and, as shown by Feldman (1967), the period length of the rhythm is lengthened. There is a direct relationship between the period lengthening and degree of inhibition of synthesis. Other inhibitors, such as heavy water which can reversibly inhibit many cell processes, have been used to demonstrate that the clock can be phase-shifted or stopped. Partial deuteration has a slight period lengthening effect (Bruce and Pittendrigh, 1960). Although photosynthesis may be required for an appropriate expression of the rhythm in photosynthetic organisms, it does not seem

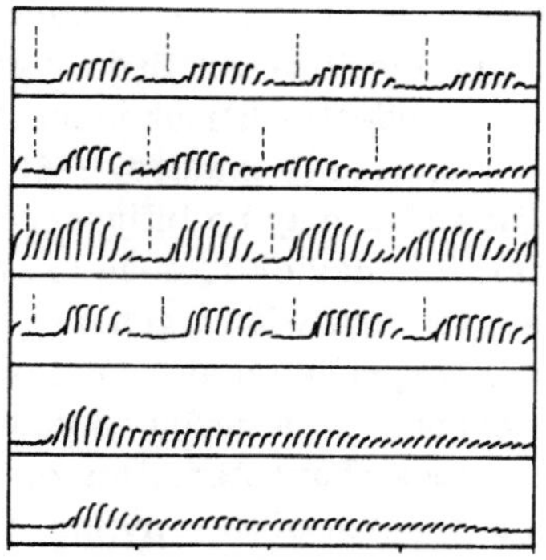

Figure 3. Records 1 and 2 show the rhythms in continous darkness after growth in continuous light of strains 89+ and 90-. Records 3 and 4 are mt+ progeny from a single zygote of a cross of 89+ × 90- and 5 and 6 are mt- progeny from this zygote. Dashed guide lines are placed at estimated minima.

to be required either to maintain or to phase-shift the clock. Using photosynthetic inhibitors Hastings (1960) showed that the clock control of bioluminescence in the dinoflagellate Gonyaulax was neither phase-shifted by pulses of inhibitors, nor insenstive to phase-shifting by light in the presence of the inhibitor. Edmunds (1970) has shown that a photosynthetically impaired mutant of Euglena has a clock which is entrained by light and Kirchstein (1969) has studied a motility rhythm in a permanently bleached Euglena and showed that this rhythm persists under conditions of anaerobic glycolosis. The expression of the rhythms in non-photosynthetic organisms may depend on the relative amount of respiration and glycolosis and there may be differences in the response to temperature changes of bleached Euglena under conditions of respiration and glycolosis (Kirchstein, 1969).

2. Phototactic Rhythms

There are a number of older reports describing phototactic rhythms in green algae of several types, in diatoms, and in flagellates, but I know of none describing them in bacteria or blue-green algae. These rhythms have been observed in a number of ways and they represent a rather complex behavioral pattern involving several factors operating simultaneously. An illustration is afforded by the observations of Palmer (1965) with Euglena obtusa. This euglena moves up and down on the mud flats of the river Avon in England in synchrony with the tidal flow in the river and can thus be exposed to the light at the times of low tide without being washed away. This behavior is mediated by means of a phototactic response which is clock-controlled and sensitive to light intensity. Positive migration to the surface occurs only during the day phase and only when the light intensity is not reduced by the shading effect of the muddy water at high tides. An interesting tidal behavior rhythm in a diatom was also described by Palmer and Round (1966).

In Euglena several of the factors which influence the overall phototactic behavior have been shown to be clock-controlled. Motility and phototactic sensitivity are controlled independently (Brinkmann, 1966), and growth and division can also be clock-controlled (Edmunds, 1969). Response can be towards or away from the light and it may be influenced by many factors in addition to the clock. The overall behavior is complex and may be influenced by the way in which it is assayed, but with a given testing arrangement a repeating pattern of phototactic responses may be obtained. This pattern can be thought of as the changing response to a repeated constant stimulus measured over several days. It is the clock characteristics of this pattern, such as the period length and phase relationships of the rhythm, that I am primarily interested in.

Most studies of phototactic and motility rhythms have utilized non-dividing or slowing-dividing cultures and in earlier work photoautotrophic cultures were employed. Continuous light inhibits the rhythm in Euglena and it was found by Pohl (1948) that a short, repeated light signal (20 to 30 min /2 hr) may provide enough energy for the cells and permit persistence of the rhythm. Motility, as well as phototactic sensitivity can be clock-controlled, and the results may be influenced by the physical nature of the testing set-up. Brinkmann (1966) used relatively deep (5 cm) cultures and showed that the turbidity at a given level could fluctuate with a circadian periodicity and that this was due to a fluctuation in the motility of the cells. The cells could be differentially phototactic and this was reflected by a change in the turbidity at the level of a horizontal light beam which resulted from phototactic accumulation of the cells after the light was turned on. In my studies I have used a system in which a vertical light beam is passed through a relatively shallow (4 mm) culture and the cells swim horizontally into the light beam.

Many studies, especially those by Brinkmann (1966) indicate that the period and phase of the rhythm in Euglena are uninfluenced by changes in the intensity of the assay-light. Omitting one or several light periods has little effect on the phase of the rhythm but supplemental light between the test signals can phase-shift the rhythm. Changes in the ratio of light to dark in the testing cycle may result in small period length changes (Betz and Brinkman, 1968) but the clock characteristics are relatively stable when the test light only is used and this is referred to as continuous dark testing conditions. In contrast to the relatively stable nature of the clock parameters the expression of the clock, (pattern of the phototactic responses) is more variable. This will become apparent in the description of the phototactic rhythm in Chlamydomonas.

3. Materials and Methods

a) Strains

The following strains of Chlamydomonas reinhardi were used in these experiments: strain w- obtained originally from Lutz Wiese (137F). $w-c_1$ (a spontaneous mutant), and strain Lo- obtained from Kwen-Sheng Chiang (137C).

Strains have been maintained by routine transfer on minimal medium agar slants kept in continuous light.

b) Media

Minimal medium described by Sueoka, Chiang, and Kates (1967) and referred to as 0.3 HSM was used for liquid cultures and 1.5 per cent agar added for slants. For mutagenesis a modified procedure of Gillham (1965) was followed using only autotrophic culture medium. Survival levels ranged between 1 per cent and 10 per cent. No selective method was used.

c) Technical Details of Phototactic Assay

Cultures were grown for phototactic testing in 20 ml of 0.3 HSM in 125 ml Erlenmeyer flasks with shaking in continuous light from cool-white fluorescents (1500 lux) at 21-25°C. Phototaxis was assayed using 10 ml samples placed in a plastic tissue culture flask (Falcon 30 ml size). The apparatus used for making the phototactic tests, more completely described elsewhere (Bruce, 1970), employed a vertical testing light beam. Cells are attracted to, and accumulate in, the light beam. This light thus serves to elicit the response, and the change in the transmitted light measured by a photocell serves as a measure of the response. The voltage changes are recorded on a strip-chart recorder and the chart drive is turned off between tests. Cells which accumulate phototactically during a test generally disperse completely before the next test signal. In addition to the test light a supplementary light which can illuminate the entire culture can be used to phase-shift or synchronize the rhythm. This light is always turned off during a phototactic test to avoid interfering with the phototactic response. Chart records are taped on cards and photographed for a permanent record. The amount of the phototactic response using this system reflects both the motility and the phototactic sensitivity.

4. Results

If autotrophic cultures of C. reinhardi grown in continuous light are then put into continuous dark testing conditions cell division stops very quickly but the cultures remain healthy and motile for days. As with many other organisms a circadian clock is initiated by the transition from light to dark and this may result in a rhythmic phototactic response pattern. There are characteristic features of this pattern which are illustrated in Figure 1. The magnitude "r" of the response depends on cell concentration and in most of my experiments this is high enough to give responses like those in record 1 if the cells are strongly phototactic. Three characteristics of the response pattern describe the rhythm. The period length τ (Figure 1) is best measured by the time between minima of the responses. The amplitude $A = r_1/r_2$ of the rhythm is a measure of the difference between the maximal and minimal responses in a cycle. The third characteristic of the rhythm is the phase ϕ. This can be defined in a number of arbitrarily different ways. Many of my experiments are done by transferring light grown cultures into continuous dark testing conditions and since the time of this transfer determines the time of subsequent minima I use this in determining the phase of the rhythm. It is frequently necessary to extrapolate from later minima to find the time of the first minimum when there is no pronounced minimum in the first cycle but several subsequent minima are observed. When the first minimum is observed there is no indication of a transient change in the period length. Two strains were tested in the experiment illustrated in Figure 1. Records 1 and 2 are for two aliquots of one culture of w- and records 3 and 4 are for two independently grown cultures of a short period variant w- c_1 of this strain. There may be differences in the pattern of responses between replicates which may get progressively more pronounced over a period of several days. These relatively gradual changes in the pattern are unavoidable since the physiological condition of individual aliquots can change during the several days during which they are tested. From records of the type shown in Figure 1 it is possible to estimate values of τ and ϕ for a given culture and by testing clones from a common parent stock grown under the same conditions to approximately the same cell density (rather than aliquots from a common culture) some estimate of the reproducibility of the clock parameters can be obtained. For example, in one experiment with 8 mt-cultures the values of τ ranged from 24 to 24.5 hr and the values of ϕ ranged from 4 to 5 hr. In another experiment with 16 independent mt+ cultures the values of τ ranged from 24.5 to 25 hr and ϕ ranged from 5 to 7 hr. This variability may be somewhat reduced if aliquots from one culture are tested simultaneously.

The amplitude of the rhythm can be rather markedly reduced if the culture is grown to too high a cell density before it is introduced into the testing conditions. Phototactic responses are good in such cultures but the rhythm deteriorates because the cells respond strongly all the time. Good rhythms (pronounced minima with amplitude ratio A close to one) may be initiated from exponential phase cultures grown in continuous light but as the cell density gets to the point where the growth begins to slow down the rhythm becomes less pronounced. The supplementary background light which can be used to provide environmental test conditions of a light–dark cycle or of continuous light may affect the expression of the rhythm. The entraining and phase-shifting effects previously described for _Euglena_ (Bruce and Pittendrigh, 1958) also pertain to _Chlamydomonas_ but the expression of the rhythm in the latter is more sensitive to two aspects of this environmental light. The environmental light conditions for the first 12 to 24 hr in the test conditions can markedly alter the way in which the phototactic rhythm is expressed in subsequent darkness. Secondly, continuous light inhibits phototactic response and the rhythm in _Euglena_ whereas in _Chlamydomonas_ different strains may respond in a variety of ways in these test conditions. Working with a given strain, a reliably reproducible rhythmic pattern of phototactic responses can be produced in _Chlamydomonas_ if cultures are grown to late exponential phase in continuous light and if rhythms are initiated by transfer to dark test conditions. However, strains may differ from one another due to selection occurring in routine maintenance of stocks.

Wild type strains of C. reinhardi obtained from different sources may differ in clock characteristics and in phototactic sensitivity. Most mt+ strains which I have tested have period lengths slightly longer than 24 hr (up to 25 hr). On the other hand mt- strains may have period lengths ranging from 21 to 24 hr. No consistant difference in phase between mt+ and mt- strains has been noted. Constant light test conditions inhibits the phototactic response of some strains, stimulates it in others, and in some a rhythmic response pattern may be expressed. Mutants with altered clock and response characteristics have been obtained using nitrosoguanadine as a mutagenizing agent. The short period mutant shown in Figure 1 was a spontaneous one but others with period lengths in the range of 21 to 22 hr have been obtained with the mutagenizing treatment. One of these, as well as a second type of clock mutant is illustrated in Figure 2. The second mutant has altered phase relationship to the initiating transition from constant light to dark. However, the expression of the mutant phase in this strain seems to be sensitive to culturing conditions. Figure 2 also illustrates the fact that some mutants have altered sensitivity to light. Normally, as in the case of Euglena the rhythm of the culture will show maximal response during the day phase of a light–dark cycle, with reduced response occurring during the night phase. In this mutant, light completely inhibits the response in constant light and gradually inhibits it in light–dark cycle although a good rhythm is observed in constant dark (Figure 1). Mutants with impaired motility also occur but they are not useful for the phototactic studies.

The reliability of the pattern of phototactic responses as a measure of the behavioral phenotype shows up in genetic crosses. For example, some of the progeny from a zygote of the cross 89+ × 90- were tested, (Figure 3). Records 1 and 2 are the parental types, one of which has a short period (21 hr). Records 3 and 4 are for two mt+ progeny, one with normal period and the other with shortened period (22 hr). Records 5 and 6 are for two mt- progeny which are almost arhythmic. Two other mt- cultures were very similar to those shown here and two other mt+ cultures resembled that in record 4. This experiment indicates that the short period of the parental mt- strain can be transferred to some of the mt+ progeny.

5. Discussion

The changed period or phase which may occur in mutants probably can result from several causes. They may be a consequence of some change in a compensation mechanism or they may be more basic and reflect a change in the primary rate-determining mechanism. Further understanding of the nature of the change might be found by determining whether it is expressed in different physiological conditions. The effects of different temperatures, and of inhibitors on the period length can also be studied. It is important to know whether the mutant characteristic is expressed in more than one rhythm. This can be determined in Chlamydomonas since there is a clock-controlled growth of cultures maintained in steady-state (Bruce, 1970), as well as a clock-controlled motility rhythm (unpublished observations).

This study is a preliminary one and mutants with more strikingly altered clock-characteristics as well as more genetic crosses are needed before much can be said about the genetic aspects of the system. No methods of selecting for clock mutants are available but I hope to be able to enrich a culture in mutants and to find some with more interesting properties.

ACKNOWLEDGEMENTS

The author gratefully acknowledge support from N.S.F. grant GB 7553. This study was also aided by the Whitehall and the John A. Hartford Foundations and the Eugena Higgens Trust Fund allocations to the Dept. Biol., Princeton University. The technical assistance of Mrs. E. Horn and Mrs. N. Bruce is very much appreciated.

REFERENCES

Barnett, A. (1966). J. Cell. Physiol. 67, 239.

Betz, A. and Brinkmann, K. (1968). Fifth Intl. Congr. on Photobiol. (Abstract), p. 42, Hanover, N. H.

Brinkmann, K. (1966). Planta (Berl.) 70, 344.

Bruce, V. G. (1970). J. Protozool. 17(2), 328.

Bruce, V. G. and Pittendrigh, C. S. (1958). Amer. Nat. 92, 295.

Bruce, V. G. and Pittendrigh, C. S. (1960). J. Cell. Comp. Physiol. 56, 25.

Edmunds, L. N. (1969). Science 165, 500.

Edmunds, L. N. (1970). Science 167, 1730.

Ehret, C. F. and Trucco. (1967). J. Theoret. Biol. 15, 240.

Feldman, J. F. (1967). Proc. Nat. Acad. Sci., Wash. 57, 1080.

Gillham, N. W. (1965). Genetics 52, 529.

Hastings, J. W. (1960). Cold Spr. Harb. Symp. Quant. Biol. 25, 131.

Huong, N. V. (1967). Ph. D. Thesis, Faculte des Sciences D'Orsay, U. de Paris.

Karakashian, M. W. (1965). In Circadian Clocks, ed. by J. Aschoff, p. 301, North Holland Publ. Co., Amsterdam.

Karakashian, M. W. and Hastings, J. W. (1962). Proc. Nat. Acad. Sci., Wash. 48, 2130.

Kirchstein, M. (1969). Planta (Berl.) 85, 126.

Palmer, J. D. (1965). Biol. Bull. (Abstracts) 129, 390.

Palmer, J. D. and Round, F. E. (1966). Biol. Bull. (Abstracts) 131, 400.

Pohl, R. (1948). Z. Naturforschg. 3b, 367.

Schweiger, H. G. and Schweiger, E. (1965). In Circadian Clocks, ed. by J. Aschoff, p. 195. North Holland Publ. Co., Amsterdam.

Stadler, D. R. (1959). Nature 184, 169.

Strumwasser, F. (1965). In Circadian Clocks, ed. by J. Aschoff, p. 442. North Holland Publ. Co., p. 442.

Sueoka, N., Chiang, K. S., and Kates, J. R. (1967). J. Mol. Biol. 25, 47.

Sweeney, B. M. and Haxo, F. T. (1961). Science 134, 1361.

Vanden Driessche, T. (1966). Biochim. Biophys. Acta 126, 456.

RHYTHMS IN DINOFLAGELLATES

J.W. Hastings
Harvard University,
Biological Laboratories,
Cambridge,
Massachusetts 02138, U.S.A.

Microorganisms, like other plants and animals, have evolved in a periodic environment, where night inexorably alternates with day. As a consequence, and with the same periodicity, the light intensity, temperature, humidity, and other physical factors also vary, and processes in the cell which are dependent on these factors are similarly affected.

Rhythmic phenomena in organisms which occur as a direct consequence of such environmental changes are called exogenous rhythms; in the absence of environmental periodicity there is no rhythm. An example of such a rhythm. An example of such a rhythm is shown in Figure 1. The pH of the culture medium containing the photosynthetic alga, Gonyaulax polyedra, varies as a result of carbon dioxide fixation in the light and its release by respiration in the darkness. The pH continues to vary rhythmically only so long as light and darkness alternate at regular intervals.

Endogenous rhythms are those which can be shown to be independent of environmental changes – at least independent to some extent. Such rhythmic phenomena have been postulated to involve an innate biological mechanism, one which serves to control and vary the capacities of various physiological and biochemical processes with respect to the time of day. The fact that this mechanism involves true temporal control – as distinct from sequence (e.g. as in transcription) has been clearly demonstated. The mechanism has thus been referred to as the biological clock, and the daily or diurnal rhythms as circadian (about one day) rhythms.

1. Circadian Rhythms in Gonyaulax

We have studied circadian rhythms in a relatively simple unicellular form, the marine dinoflagellate, Gonyaulax polyedra. This organisms is found ubiquitously and sometimes abundantly (e.g. in red tides) in the oceans. It

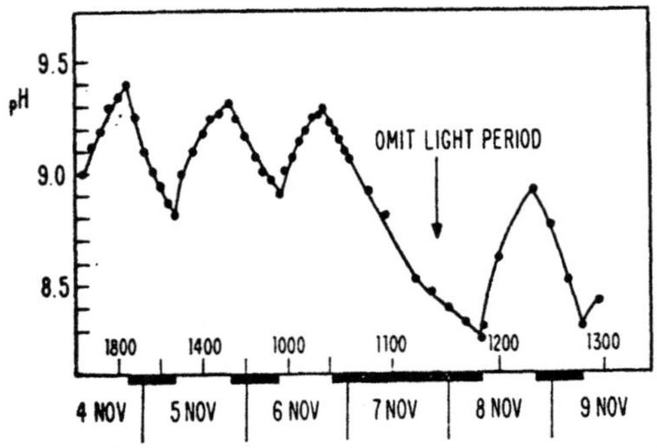

Figure 1. An exogenous rhythm: the change in pH of a culture of Gonyaulax polyedra exposed to alternating light and dark periods as indicated on the abscissa. The pH (recorded automatically) is directly dependent on the prevailing light conditions, increasing when the culture is illuminated and decreasing as long as the culture is in the dark. This point is illustrated in the experiment where, when one light period was omitted, the pH continued to fall.

grows photosynthetically and rather slowly, even under optimal conditions. Like many dinoflagellates, it possesses a thick external "armor", a polysaccharide (probably cellulose) test. It is motile, possessing two flagella.

The organism displays several circadian rhythms which we have studied, and it seems likely that there may be more that could be followed if needed. This multiplicity of overt rhythms is in itself of considerable usefulness in studying mechanism: one can study how the several rhythms relate to one another and to the controlling mechanism.

The Luminescent Flashing Rhythm

The organism is brilliantly bioluminescent, emitting flashes of light when stimulated at night. When stimulated in the daytime, however, relatively little light is emitted. This may be quantitatively measured by integrating the light output during a brief (1-2 min) stimulation. When cells are removed from the light–dark cycle and placed in an environment of constant light and temperature, this rhythm continues (Figure 2).

The Luminescent Glow Rhythm

In undisturbed cultures a relatively dim but measurable glow occurs towards the end of the dark period. This lasts for only a few hours each day, and may be accompanied by occasional spontaneous flashing which can be noted on a recording as a much brighter spike of light. In this case one measures the intensity of the light output in order to monitor the rhythm (Figure 3). In cultures kept in constant conditions (except for brief times in the dark to make the measurements) the rhythm persists without apparent abatement.

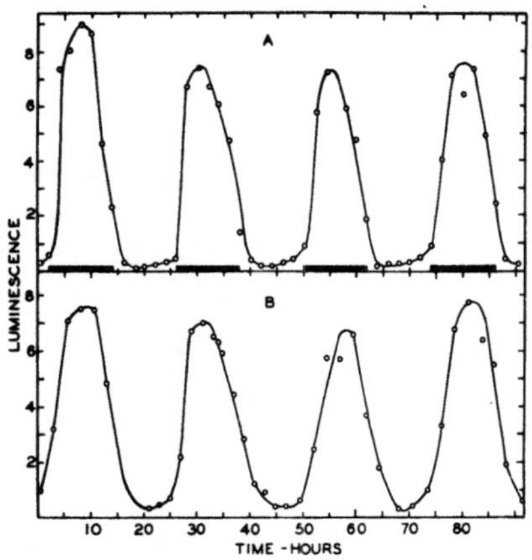

Figure 2. These curves illustrate the nature of the rhythm of flashing luminescence in Gonyaulax. The curve at the top shows the rhythmicity in cultures exposed to alternating light and dark periods of 12 hours each (LD 12:12). When such cells are transferred to conditions of constant light (120 foot-candles) and constant temperature (21°C) the rhythm persists with a period of about, but not exactly, 24 hours (curve B).

The Cell Division Rhythm

In both the laboratory and in the ocean in natural populations, mitoses in many species of dinoflagellates are restricted to a particular time of day; in Gonyaulax this falls towards the end of the dark period. This rhythm illustrates a significant and interesting feature of circadian control: physiological processes may be gated. Here not all cells divide each day since the growth rate may be relatively slow. Those which do divide during a given day do so at a certain restricted time – when the gate is open. The result is a rhythmic but not synchronous population, which thereby exhibits a staircase-shaped growth curve. This phenomenon also continues with cells kept under constant conditions (Figure 4).

The Photosynthetic Capacity Rhythm

Although cells in the dark are obviously unable to carry out photosynthesis, one can test their capacity to photosynthesize by putting them in the light and assaying them under optimal conditions. When this was done it was found that the cell's ability to photosynthesize varies considerably as a function of time of day. As might be expected, the capacity is greatest during the day. Under constant conditions the rhythmic changes in capacity persist for many days (Figure 5).

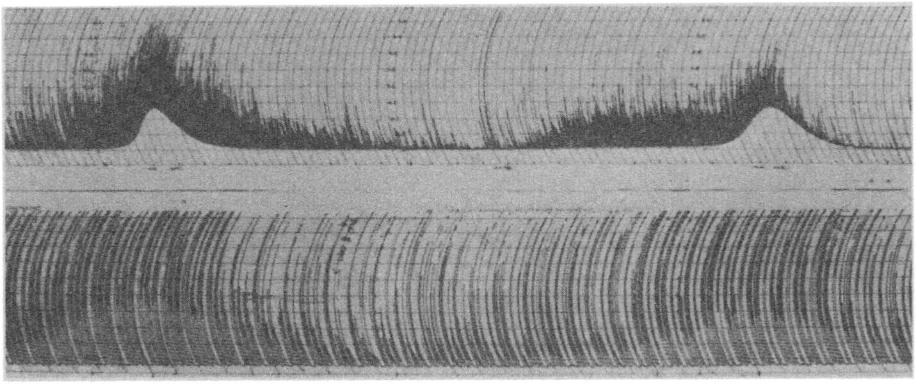

Figure 3. The luminescent glow rhythm, measured from one vial of cells kept in constant darkness (top); and (bottom) from 6 vials kept in constant dim light, except for brief periods every hour when the vial was placed in the dark in a phototube chamber to measure luminescence. The change in the baseline level is the steady glow; the vertical lines are from spontaneous flashing of individual cells. Temperature 23°C.

2. Properties of These Rhythms

As noted above these several rhythms all persist under constant conditions with a circadian period. The fact that their periods are circadian (e.g. about 1 day) and not exactly 24 hours is of critical interest and importance, for it indicates that the timing relies on an internal mechanism rather than on external physical periodicity (Figure 6). This circadian period is a function of environmental conditions, but the effects are relatively small. The effect of temperature, for example (Figure 7), is especially instructive. At temperatures 10° apart the clock mechanisms runs at frequencies which are not greatly different (26.5 hr at 27°; 22.8 hr at 17°). This phenomenon – referred to as temperature independence – is a hallmark of circadian rhythms, and is, of course, a rather crucially important property for a true timing device. Actually, as illustrated with Gonyaulax, the system is not temperature-independent. The period is relatively temperature-independent and in Gonyaulax, its period is actually somewhat longer at a higher temperature – just the opposite of what might be expected if temperature were increasing the rate of underlying metabolic reactions. This result prompted our suggestion that the biological clock mechanism involves temperature compensation reactions – and that it should not be simply viewed as temperature-independent.

It is evident that circadian systems are phase labile to light. The rhythm of an organism maintained on a 24 hour light–dark cycle always shows a 24 hour period rather than its circadian period (Figure 6). A displacement in longitude results in appropriate phase shift, and this may be simulated in the laboratory by scheduling artificial lights. But phase shifting does not actually require exposure to a new light–dark cycle. With an organism kept under constant conditions, single light flashes (simulating as it were, dawn or dusk) can reset a clock with full effectiveness, if administered at the correct

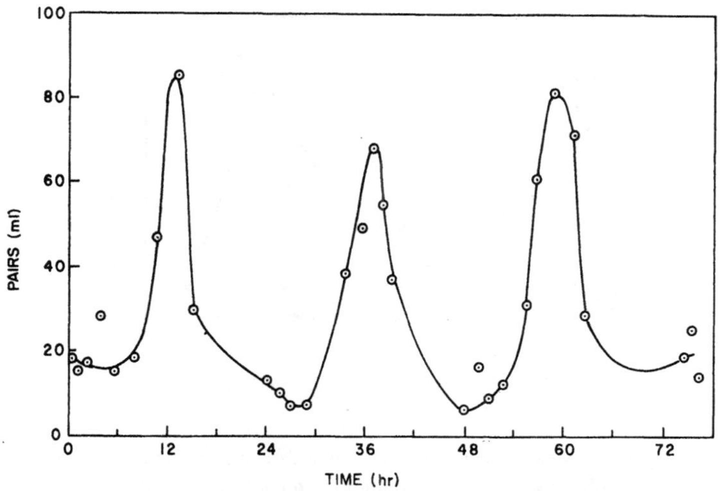

Figure 4. The number of paired cells present in a cell suspension of Gonyaulax polyedra on the twelfth, thirteenth, and fourteenth days of continuous dim light (100 ft-candles) at 19°C. G. polyedra was grown in a light–dark cycle with light from 1100 to 2300, and was transferred to continuous dim light at 1100 (at the end of a dark period). The measurements shown were started twelve days later. The average generation time between the tenth and fourteenth days was 3·8 days. Daughter cells remain attached for a while after division so that "pairs" constitute a good index of the mitotic activity.

time (Figure 8). Relatively little is known about the critical (biochemical) part of the receptor system. The action spectrum in Gonyaulax reflects the general pigment content of the cell.

3. Control of Several Rhythms

The relative phases of the several rhythms are illustrated in Figure 9 with cells grown on a light–dark cycle. The concept that there exists a clock mechanism carries with it the implication that several processes might be thereby controlled – or "plugged in". In fact, there is very little experimental evidence relating to this question.

In the experimental sense there is a distinction between the "mechanism" and the controlled process. It has been shown that there are rhythmic phenomena that can be blocked by using inhibitors without any substantial effect on the operation or phase of the clock. For example, photosynthesis in Gonyaulax can be blocked using the highly specific drug, dichorophenyl dimethyl urea (DCMU); yet the glow rhythm of bioluminescence continues all the while. Furthermore the rhythm of photosynthetic capacity will resume in phase following the removal of the inhibitor.

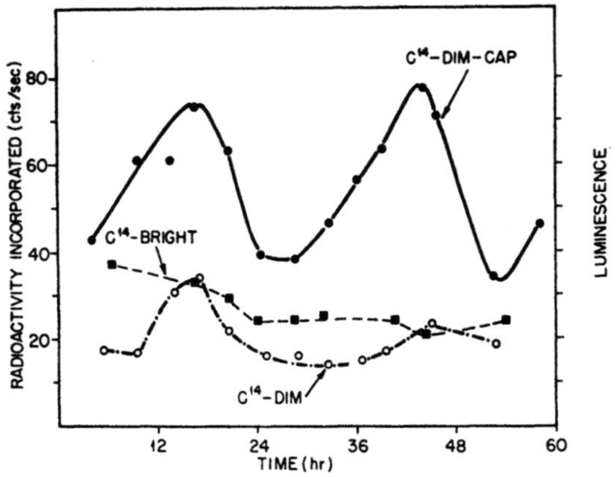

Figure 5. Measurements of photosynthesis and photosynthetic capacity of Gonyaulax cells maintained in continuous light. Cells were grown in LD 12:12 and transferred to constant light at the end of a dark period, 16 hours prior to zero hours on the graph. Dim light was 110 ft-candles and bright light was 960 ft-candles; temperature, 25 ± 0.3°C. ^{14}C-Dim-cap refers to the photosynthetic capacity of cells cultured in constant dim light, and records the relative amounts of $^{14}CO_2$ incorporation when aliquots were incubated with a tracer in saturating bright light for 15 minutes. ^{14}C-Dim refers to relative rates of photosynthetic activity in cells cultured in dim light, and records $^{14}CO_2$ incorporation when aliquots were incubated with tracer for 60 minutes in dim light. ^{14}C-Bright refers to relative rates of photosynthesis (or photosynthetic capacity) in cells cultured in bright light, and records the relative amounts of $^{14}CO_2$ incorporated when aliquots were incubated with tracer for 15 minutes in bright light.

4. Rhythms in Isolated Cells

The fact that microorganisms exhibit circadian rhythms in culture fails to deal with the question of the single cell. With Gonyaulax it has been possible to isolate and observe single cells, and to demonstrate that circadian properties pertain. For example, by isolating daughter cells in a capillary microdrop and making regular observations thereafter it was possible to determine the time interval until the subsequent divisions. As would have been predicted, division times cluster around 24, 48, 72, and 96 hours, e.g. n × 24, since the "gating" restricts divisions to a single time of day. Similarly, the rhythm of photosynthetic capacity has been demonstated in isolated single cells.

To demonstrate the persistence of circadian rhythms under constant conditions it is always necessary to use dim light or darkness, and with isolated cells the rhythms do in fact persist under these conditions. By contrast, rhythmic activity essentially disappears under conditions of constant bright light. To distinguish whether the loss of rhythmicity arises from the lack of rhythmicity in every cell or from a loss of synchrony between cells, isolated Gonyaulax cells were observed. It was possible to show that the first of these

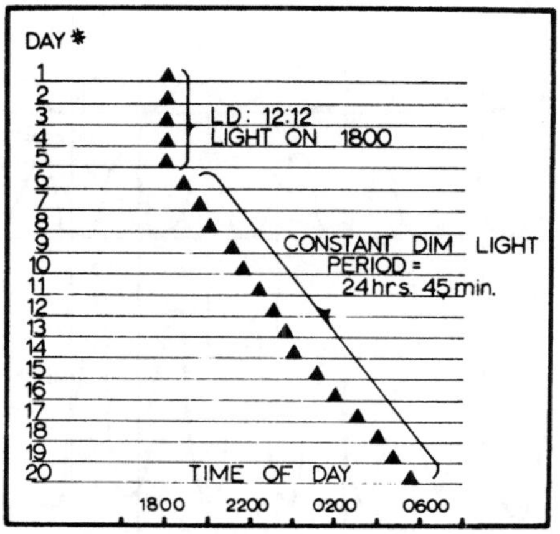

Figure 6. This shows the time of day at which the maximum in the luminescent glow occurred on each of 20 successive days. The values were obtained by measuring the luminescence from this vial approximately every two hours, similar to the fashion illustrated in Figure 3, bottom. For the first few days the culture was kept on a daily light – dark cycle, and the peak occurred at the same time each day. Subsequently the light remained on continuously and whereas the rhythm continued, its maximum occurred about 45 minutes later each day, indicating that the free-running period in this case was 24 hours, 45 minutes. Temperature 24°C.

possibilities holds, i.e., each cell loses rhythmicity. This has been demonstrated both with the rhythm of cell division and with the rhythm of photosynthetic capacity.

5. Biochemical Mechanisms

Although there are relatively few biochemical studies of these phenomena, an increasing number of laboratories are making contributions in this area. It is this aspect of the problem – namely the molecular mechanisms involved in circadian rhythms – with which my laboratory is now concerned. Let me divide the consideration into the two aspects alluded to above, namely the clock and its hands.

These two aspects are distinguished in the scheme set forth in Figure 10 where the clock mechanism is distinguished from clock-controlled processes. A premise of our study of biochemical changes is that there exists a cellular rhythmic mechanism whose key properties include the following:

1). It continues to operate rhythmically with a period of about but not exactly 24 hours in the absence of entraining agents or rhythmic cues in the environment; and is temperature compensated.

2). Its phase is established and is resettable by environmental light cues.

We are excluding exogenous rhythms from this consideration.

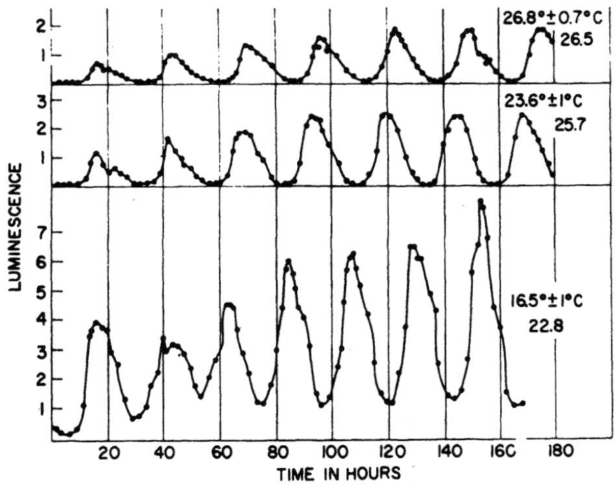

Figure 7. Characteristics of the persistent rhythm of luminescence in Gonyaulax at the three different temperatures noted. The cells were grown on conditions of light – dark 12:12 hours at 22°C and transferred at the end of a dark period to constant light (100 ft-candles) at zero time on the graph. The luminescence capacity was measured approximately every two hours. The average period in hours measured for each is noted on the graph below the temperature.

There are several general kinds of questions which one would like to consider. For example, if one takes the working hypothesis of Figure 10, then there may be many more physiological systems which exhibit rhythms; on the other hand, there may be many functions which are not tied into this mechanism. There are certainly some which may be included in this latter category, and it would be useful to learn which cell functions are circadian and which are not. One might thereby gain more insight concerning the role and importance of rhythms in the functioning of microbial forms.

Another question of interest, again with reference to Figure 10, relates to the coupling, or the clutch between the "clock" and its "hands". We should like to understand the physio-chemical nature of this coupling. Experimentally, one could approach this question by attempting to dissociate overt rhythms one from another, i.e. to alter their relative phases. Up to now this has not been achieved with microbial forms, although relative phase angles of two rhythms may differ under different conditions.

Another related question concerns the possible existence of a specific substance or substances involved in the control of rhythms. This might be a product of the clock mechanism and might intervene at the level of the output. If diffusible, and if it were to provide feedback to the mechanism itself, then it might be important in cell-to-cell communication.

Let us then focus on the two major questions posed by the representation of Figure 10, namely (1) the nature of the rhythmic mechanism and (2) the way in which the physiological processes are controlled.

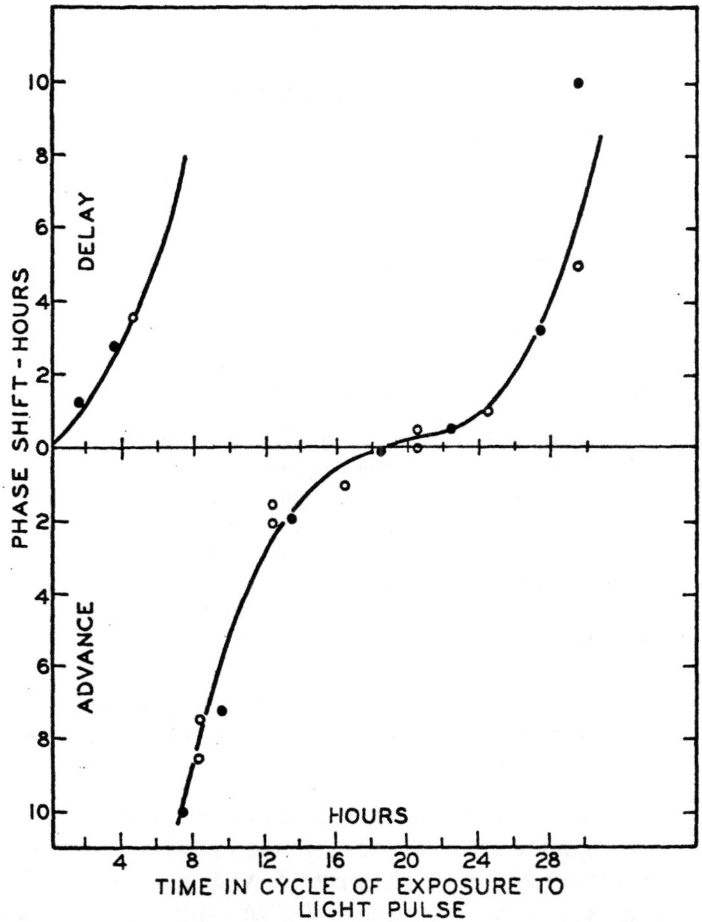

Figure 8. The relationship between time in the cycle when a light pulse is administered and the resulting phase change. Phase shift is plotted on the ordinate as either a dealy or an advance. The abscissa is measured in hours subsequent to the end of the last light period.

The mechanism itself has escaped explicit description at the molecular level. In fact, it has not yet been possible to define either the biochemical systems or the cellular components which are critically involved. Many studies were concerned with attempts to block rhythms in one way or another by the use of metabolic inhibitors. In general, these failed to reveal any specific chemical effects.

One of the earliest specific ideas concerning the chemical mechanism was based on the notion that RNA transcription might be programmed on a circadian basis, thereby resulting in time-of-day specific cellular syntheses. This hypothesis later received strong support from our observation that a rhythm in Gonyaulax was blocked both by Actinomycin D – a drug highly specific for blocking DNA-dependent RNA synthesis – and with a slight lag, puromycin, which inhibits protein synthesis (Figure 11). Although supporting observations were obtained by some workers, several others failed to support

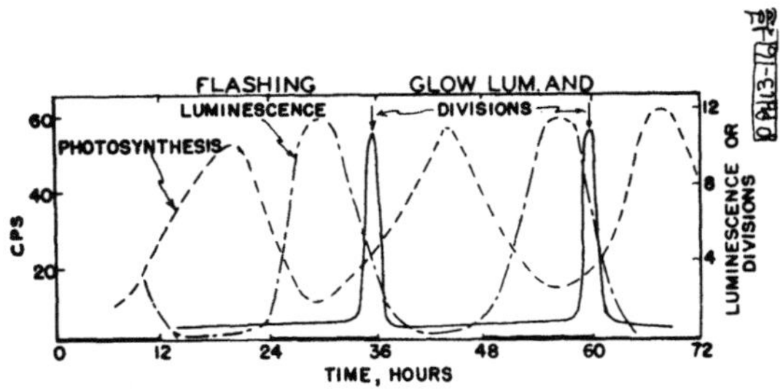

Figure 9. This figure schematically illustrates the several diurnal rhythms on Gonyaulax and their phase relationships to the daily light – dark cycle (LD 12:12). The rhythm of flashing luminescence (induced by mechanical agitation) has a broad maximum in the middle of the night. The rhythm of photosynthesis is maximum during the light period and the rhythms of cell division and steady luminescent glow have maxima at approximately the same time, at about the end of the dark period. Very little light emission actually occurs in the glow in contrast to the flashing emission, which is very bright. The scales are therefore not comparable.

the hypothesis. There remains, to be sure, considerably support for an hypothesis of this general nature, and experiments are continuing in several laboratories to test the theory.

All hypotheses envisaged have involved a loop of some sort, represented in Figure 10 by the circular set of arrows. In the hypothesis involving RNA synthesis, the subsequent step might be protein synthesis, followed by one or more steps leading back to the reinitiation of RNA synthesis in the subsequent cycle. Such a model suggests that an appropriate reversible blockage of one or another of the steps would delay the rhythm by a time related to the duration of the blockage. But, in fact, no response of this kind has ever been reported as the result of exposure to an inhibitor or other chemical agent. The action of Actinomycin D has never been reversed in a sensitive rhythmic system, while in analogous experiments with puromycin no phase shifting occurred in Gonyaulax.

Although this result does not lend support to the RNA hypothesis, the fact that inhibitors of protein synthesis are not 100 per cent effective (based on measurements with Gonyaulax) leaves open the possibility that the synthetic pathways involved in the clock mechanism may be immune or cloistered. Substantial but not large effects upon the period of rhythms have been reported both in Gonyaulax with chloramphenicol and colchicine, and in Euglena using actidione. But these do not really cause any appreciable phase shift, and are more reminiscent of the fact that the period may be altered by a number of chemical and physical factors, including temperature, and light intensity. One is also reminded of the spectacular effect upon the rhythm of Euglena of substituting D_2O for H_2O in the medium, reported by Bruce and Pittendrigh in 1960.

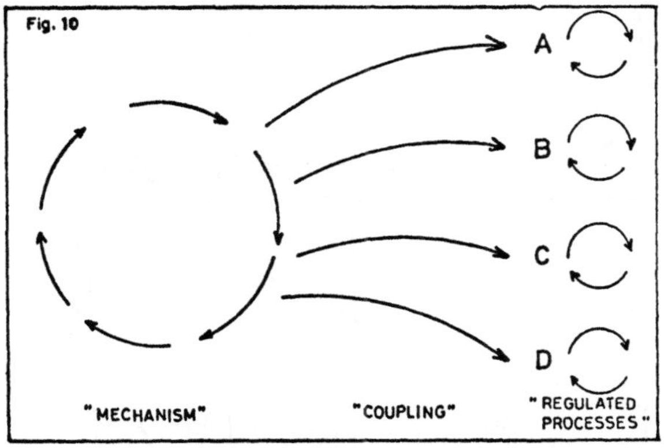

Figure 10. Schematic representation of a hypothetical model for the biochemical steps involved in circadian rhythms. It is intended to distinguish an autonomous rhythmic mechanism which is phase-sensitive to appropriate light or temperature treatments, from the cellular phenomena (A, B, C, ect.) which are controlled.

All of these more or less negative results are in contrast to the fact that the phase of the rhythm may be readily manipulated by either light or temperature. Phase-shifting by light is the more spectacular; clearly a product of a photochemical reaction can perturb the rhythm.

In clear contrast, permanent temperature-induced phase shifts require a rather long exposure to low temperature. This has not been studied very much but, from the few reports, it appears that low temperature stops either the operation of or the coupling to the mechanism. In Gonyaulax this requires that the temperature be below 14°C, and that this lower temperature be maintained for periods of at least about 24 hours. Thereafter, the phase of the rhythm is precisely determined by the time at which the temperature is raised.

In summary, the mechanism of the biological clock appears to be largely insensitive to a great variety of metabolic inhibitors. In a number of instances various inhibitors of macromolecular biosynthesis have been found to have effects, but experiments with different rhythmic systems give different results. The mechanism can, however, be very effectively perturbed by either light or temperature treatments, suggesting that some kind of experimental phase modification to the system might be possible with chemical agents, and that this might clues as to mechanism.

The second general question to which we have addressed ourselves concerns the nature of the biochemical changes during the rhythmic cycle. A priori one would imagine that this matter might be investigated with less indirection. But, in fact, it now seems clear that one cannot always conclude that the quantity or activity of a component in cell extracts accurately reflects the physiological situation in the living cell. This has been strikingly demonstrated in our studies of the biochemical basis for the rhythmic changes in bioluminescence in Gonyaulax.

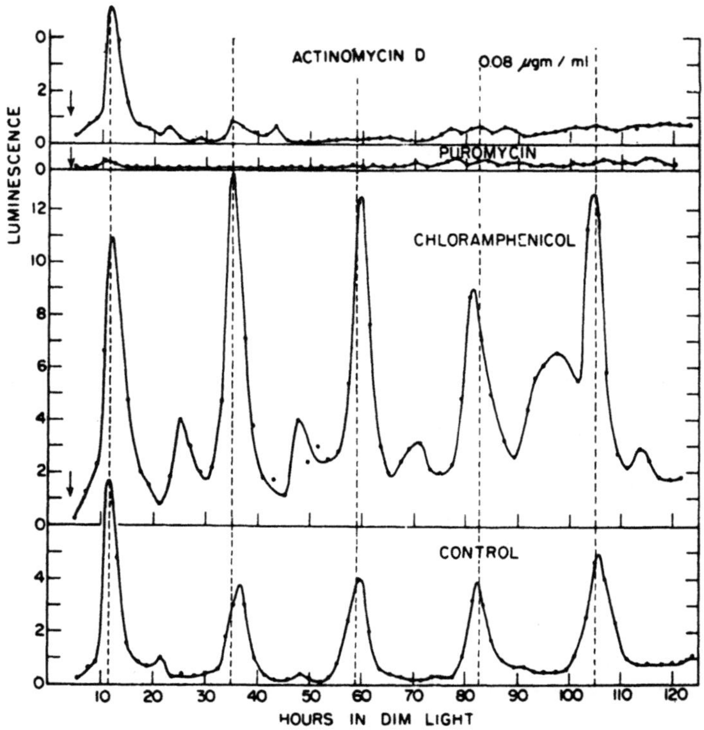

Figure 11. Effects of actinomycin D (0.08 μg ml^{-1}), puromycin (10^{-5} M) and chloramphenical (3×10^{-1} M) upon the persistent rhythm of bioluminescent glow. Cells were grown in light – dark 12:12 and placed in constant dim light and constant temperature (21° C) at the end of a light period (zero time on the graph). Inhibitors were added at the time indicated by the arrows. Luminescence is expressed in arbitrary units. The vertical grid lines are for guidance only.

In cell-free extracts of Gonyaulax it was found that a soluble enzyme and substrate could be isolated which, when appropriately recombined in vitro, would result in bioluminescence. In a rhythmic Gonyaulax system it was found that the extractable enzyme activity also varied with time of day, being substrate gave an unexpected result: the maximum in extractable substrate occurred during the day. This apparent paradox was resolved following the observation that the process of filtering the cells resulted in violent bioluminescence flashing during the night, but only a dull glow by day. It was therefore hypothesized that differential substrate utilization was occurring. This idea was supported by experiments in which flashing was inhibited prior to harvesting, whereupon greater quantities of substrate could be isolated from cells at night. These rhythmic changes in enzyme and substrate activity are illustrated in Figures 12 and 13.

The nature of the activity difference was not discovered, i.e. whether it was by virtue of amounts (i.e. synthesis and destruction), due to activity (i.e. activation and inhibition), or to a differential extraction efficiency (different quantities liberated during extraction at different times of day). Present results support the second (activation and inhibition) hypothesis. But this has become largely academic for the moment, for our presumptions concerning the

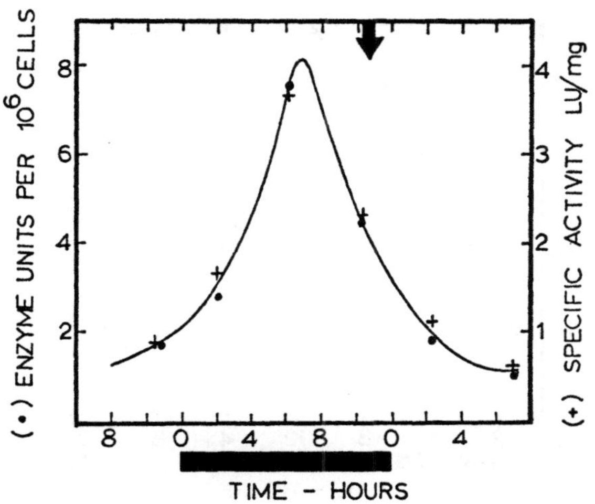

Figure 12. Measurements of the amount of extractable enzyme activity (ordinate, •) per 10^6 cells as related to time of day. The cultures were maintained on the light – dark cycle shown (12 hours of light, 12 hours of dark). Equal amounts of protein are extracted from the cells at different times of day, as indicated by the fact that specific activity (ordinate, +) closely parallels the activity. The bold arrow at the time indicates the time of day when the maximum in the glow of luminescence occurred in the cultures.

nature of the luminescent system in vivo were incorrect. Bioluminescence in Gonyaulax has now been shown to derive not only from a enzyme-substrate system, but also from a complex particle, apparently a cell organelle. This has been termed the scintillon, and the active particle has been successfully isolated from cells and purified. The matter of concern reduces – though the difficulty is not reduced – to the question of circadian control of the activity of this organelle. Such a situation implicates also physiological control mechanisms rather than simple enzyme synthesis and destruction. It thus underscores the view that biological control systems are in many instances concerned with a complicated target system whose control is subtle. Studies concerned with this aspect of the problem are continuing.

In summary, we have been able to find biochemical rhythms which occur in concert with and relate to a corresponding biological rhythm. But the origin and control of these biochemical rhythms is still uncertain. Of special concern is our understanding of the in vivo organization and control of the physiological systems which are under the control of the cellular circadian clock.

6. SUMMARY

The biochemical pathways involved in the generation and control of biological rhythms and cycles have not yet been described. Indeed, it is not even

K*

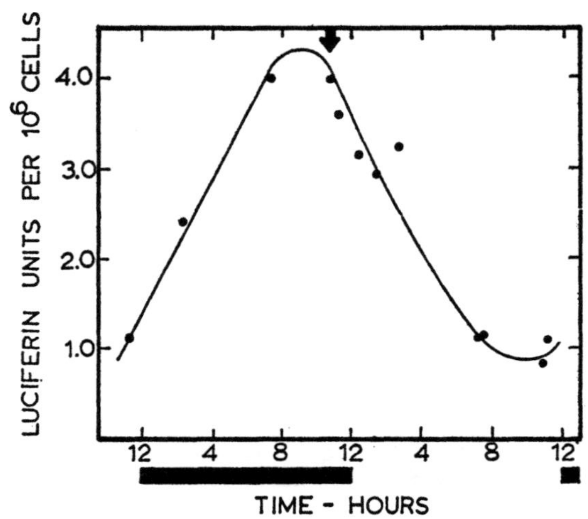

Figure 13. Measurements of the amount of extractable substrate (luciferin) from cultures maintained as described in the legend to Figure 9. The peak of substrate occurs somewhat later than the peak of enzyme.

possible to state with assurance what kinds of biochemical pathways are critically involved. The evidence available at the present time, derived largely from studies with specific inhibitors, implicates pathways in the biosynthesis of macromolecules. Although these results are mostly obtained from experiments with microorganisms, it is anticipated that the results may be equally applicable to higher forms.

The phenomenon at the cellular level may be viewed as a regulatory phenomenon, analogous in some ways to regulatory mechanisms which intervene in the great majority of biological processes. Rhythmic phenomena, however, are unique in the sense that they involve a time-dependent regulation, such that cells are able to vary the capacities of various physiological and biochemical processes with respect to time of day. The crucial point is indeed this: regulation is not simply with regard to the sequence of physiological processes, but is with respect to absolute time.

In considering the problems one should distinguish the rhythmic mechanism per se from the systems controlled by this mechanism. These have often been referred to as the clock and its hands, respectively. The mechanism itself must provide feedback regulation wherein time is the relevant parameter. Experiments with a variety of inhibitors have shown that this function is not disturbed by a large variety of metabolic inhibitors, including those which actually inhibit the target systems. Thus one may inhibit a rhythmic process without disturbing the rhythmic mechanism – the clock itself. The biosynthesis of both RNA and protein synthesis have been implicated as participants in the rhythmic mechanism in some systems. A recent proposal based on these observations holds that daily rhythms result from a sequential linear transcription of the genome, and that this recycles on a repetitive daily basis.

The second aspect of the problem relates to the way in which the hands of the clock are controlled. The possibilities may be considered in two broad classes: 1) a rhythmic de novo synthesis and breakdown of one or more of the components involved in the system; 2) a mechanism involving activation and repression. The theory involving a daily reading of the genome implies that de novo protein synthesis occurs with each rhythmic cycle. This has not been demonstrated, however, and a number of current investigations are concerned with the elucidation of the nature of the biochemical changes in systems which exhibit rhythmic fluctuations in activity – whether, for example, they undergo changes in quantity or in activity.

GENERAL REFERENCES

Aschoff, J. (1965). "Circadian Clocks". North Holland Publ., Amsterdam.
"Biological Clocks". (1960). Cold Spring Harbor Symp. Quant. Biol. 25.
Brown, F. A., Hastings, J. W. and Plamer, J. (1970). "The Bilogical Clock". Academic Press, N. Y.
Bunning, E. (1967). "The Physiological Clock". Springer Verlag.
Hastings, J. W. (1959). "Unicellular Clocks", Ann. Rev. Microbiol. 13, 297-312.
Sweeney, B. M. (1969). "Rhythmic Phenomena in Plants". Academic Press, N. Y.

CIRCADIAN RHYTHMS IN NEUROSPORA

D.O. Woodward and M.L. Sargent
University of Illinois,
Botany Department,
Urbana,
Illinois 61801, U.S.A.

1. Introduction

By comparison with some organisms, only a moderate amount of research on circadian rhythms has been carried out with the fungus *Neurospora*, although it is fast becoming one of the better characterized systems. The first report of a rhythm in Neurospora was in a strain called patch (Brandt, 1953) and, since that time, other strains have been described which exhibit rhythmicity, e.g. clock (Sussman, Lowry, and Durkee, 1964), and timex (Sargent and Woodward, 1965). In addition, this paper describes conditions under which most *Neurospora* strains manifest some degree of rhythmicity. Little has been done with any of these rhythmic strains in terms of studying the biochemistry of the rhythm or in attempting to elucidate the mechanism(s) involved in generating oscillations. The beginnings of such studies on *Neurospora* are discussed in this paper.

On the basis of what is known about the biochemistry of rhythms in organisms other than Neurospora, a number of clues are suggested which may eventually help to explain the mechanism by which oscillations are generated. For example, investigations with *Gonyaulax* and *Acetabularia* demonstrate the inhibition of expression of a rhythm by *Actinomycin D.* However, the loss of expression of a rhythm caused by inhibitors of transcription or translation in many organisms appears to involve an inhibition of some biochemical system coupled to an oscillator rather than affecting the oscillator itself. In *Acetabularia*, rhythms persist in anucleate cells; furthermore, the anucleate cells are not sensitive to *Actinomycin D* (Sweeney, 1967). Thus, a nuclear product may have an influence on the expression of the rhythm but is apparently not responsible for generating the oscillations (Vanden Driessche, 1966). However, the plant which donates the nucleus (transplantation) rather than the one that contributes the photosynthetic apparatus controls the phase of the photosynthetic rhythm. Does this mean that the phase of the oscillator can be

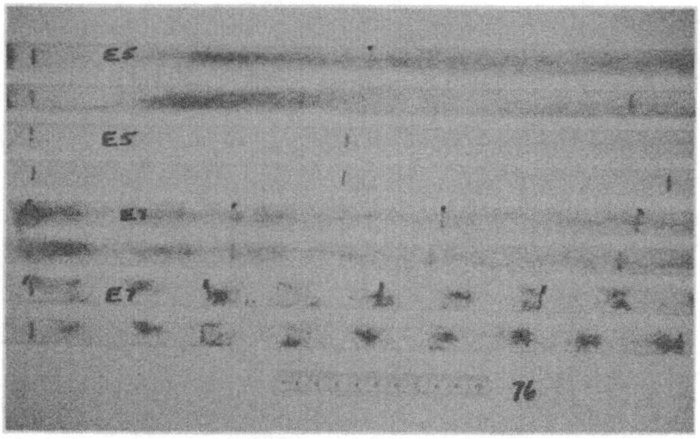

Figure 1. Growth-tube cultures of wild-type (E5a, pan$^-$) and rhythmic (E7a, bd) strains grown under standard conditions. The first and third pairs of tubes contained the Casamino-acids medium, while the second and fourth pairs contained the glucose - arginine medium. Pen marks on the tube delimit 48 hr growth intervals.

influenced by biochemical systems coupled to it, or are there two oscillators, either one of which can control cytoplasmic activities? The answers to these and other questions related to mechanism have not yet been answered with any resounding clarity, but at least certain hypotheses are either eliminated or rendered unlikely on the basis of such inhibitor studies.

2. Characterization of Neurospora Rhythms

Our own research with Neurospora has been based on the assumption that the mechanism(s) involved in free-running circadian oscillations are biochemical in nature and subject to standard biochemical analyses. Thus, faced with the same problem that all workers in this field have had of not knowing the kind of biochemistry to study, we were led to experiment with several different hypotheses, seeking clues concerning the basic process involved. Pittendrigh et al. (1959) pointed out some advantages of working with Neurospora in this regard.

Figures 1 and 2 illustrate two Neurospora stains whose rhythms can be monitored by morphology; the bd mutant by periodic conidiation and clock (Sussman, Lowry, and Durkee, 1964) by hyphal branching. In addition to these means of monitoring an oscillator, other monitoring systems have been identified in the bd mutant. Some of these may turn out to be more useful since they involve biochemical parameters rather than morphological characteristics. For example, in strain bd there is a periodic production of CO_2 (Figure 3), which is consistent with the same rules of circadian rhythmicity as is the production of conidia. Moreover, the rhythm can be monitored in standing liquid cultures which provide sufficient mycelium for extensive biochemical analyses. In addition, controls for regulating DNA content (Kaltenborn and Sargent, unpublished), and mitosis (Nambooderi and Lowry, 1967) can apparently be plugged into the basic oscillator(s).

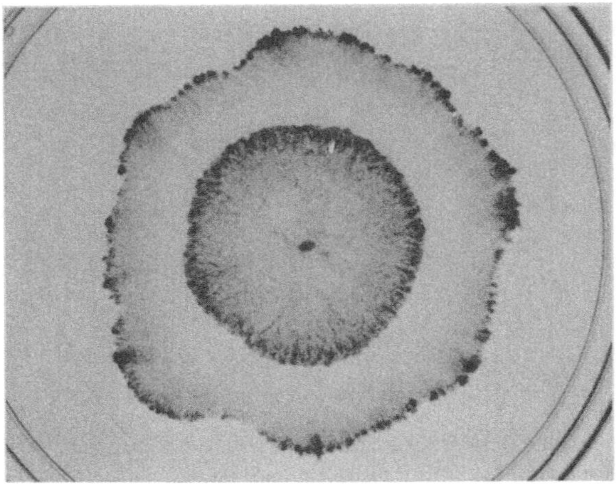

Figure 2. Appearance of clock strain when grown on complete medium at 25°C (courtesy of A. Sussman).

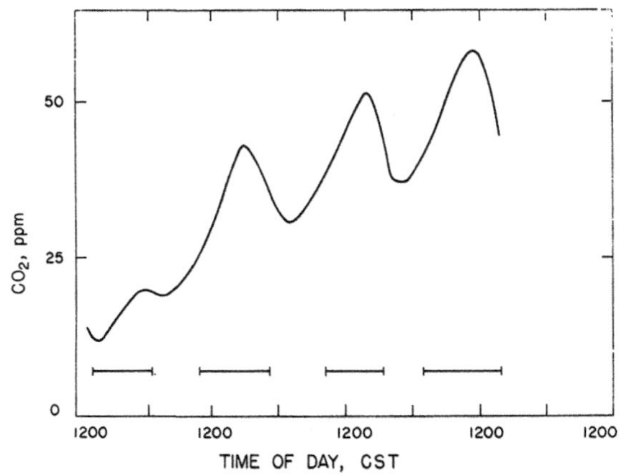

Figure 3. Rhythm of CO_2 production by the bd strain growing in a growth tube under standard conditions on glucose – arginine medium. A $N_2 \cdot O_2$ mixture (79 per cent N_2, 21 per cent O_2) passing through the growth-tube at 22-24 cc/min was continuously monitored for CO_2 in a Grubb Parsons Infra-Red Gas Analyzer. Bars (├──┤) represent times at which conidation was occurring.

Timex is a rhythmic strain of Neurospora that we previously characterized to some extent (Sargent, Briggs, and Woodward, 1966). This strain carries two genes that are known to influence the expression of rhythmicity by periodic production of conidia (bd and inv). The inv gene is the structural gene for the enzyme invertase (Sargent and Woodward, 1969b) and produces very little rhythmicity by itself, but enhances the expression of the bd gene when both are present. The bd (band) gene is characterized by a periodic production of conidial bands when growing on an agar surface, the biochemical basis of which is not understood. Time shows a temperature compensation typical of circadian rhythms (Figure 4). The period of the rhythm was relatively constant between 18°C and 35°C, which includes all temperatures under

Species	Source†	Rhythmicity on ‡	
		minimal sucrose	glucose-arginine
N. intermedia (NITa)...............	AMS	−	−
N. sitophila (Eng Sit 21a)............	AMS	−	−
N. tetrasperma....................	AS	−	−
N. crassa (STA 4)..................	FGSC	−	−
Strains of N. crassa:			
Abbot 12a....................	DDP	−	+ (> 8)
SY4f8a.......................	NHG	−	−
Lindegren 1A	RHD	−	+++ (> 7)
Em a.........................	DDP	−	−
Taiwan (Tai II 17a)	AMS	+ (4)	++ (4)
Puerto Rico 18A................	NHH	−	−
Liberia 4A	NHH	−	−
Singapore 2a...................	NHH	++ (> 5)	++ (> 7)
Philippine Islands (P. I. 42)..........	AMS	+ (3)	+ (> 6)
Costa Rica (C. R. 20502A)	AMS	−	−
inos 89601A	AS	+ (> 5)	+++ (> 6)
ad-4 F6A.....................		−	++ (> 7)
SF-26	HGG	−	+ (> 5)
L5D (lactose utilizer)		+ (> 6)	++ (> 6)
aur 17A......................	AS	−	+ (> 5)
arg-10 B317a..................	RHD	+ (3)	+ (> 8)
4-121 (altered trehalase)...........	AS	−	+ (> 5)
arg-8 P50a....................	RHD	−	+++ (> 7)
inos 37401a....................	FGSC	−	+ (> 6)
bd E7a.......................		++ (> 4)	++++ (> 14)
patch a	FGSC	+ (> 11)	+ (> 10)
inv 63 (partial mutant)		−	++ (> 8)
clock CL 11A	AS	++ (> 12)	+++ (> 20)
inv E1A......................		−	+ (> 4)
inv, bd E3A		+ (5)	++++ (> 14)

† Abbreviations are FGSC, Fungal Genetics Stock Center; RDG, R. H. Davis; HGG, H. G. Gratzner; NHG, N. H. Giles; NHH, N. H. Horowitz; DDP, D. D. Perkins; AS, A. Sussman; AMS A. M. Srb. All other strains were isolated in the authors' laboratories.

‡ The minimal sucrose medium contained Vogel's salts, 1.5 per cent sucrose, and 1.5 per cent agar. The glucose-arginine medium contained Vogel's salts, 0.3 per cent glucose, 0.5 per cent arginine, and 1.5 per cent agar. Appropriate supplements were added when required. Density of conidial bands ranged from no bands (-) to dense, well-defined bands (++++). The number of conidial bands observed is enclosed within the parentheses following the band density designations; > 12 means that 12 bands were produced before the growth front reached the end of the growth tube, thereby terminating the experiment.

which measurements can be made. Temperature affected the rate of growth (Q_{10} 2-3) but the Q_{10} for the period remained relatively constant (Q_{10} about 1). When dark-grown at 25°C, timex produces a band of conidia every 22.7 hr and can be easily entrained by light to give a 24-hr cycle. Growth rate is uniform from day to day under the conditions used and is also quite constant over a 24-hr period. Relative humidity had no effect on the rhythm.

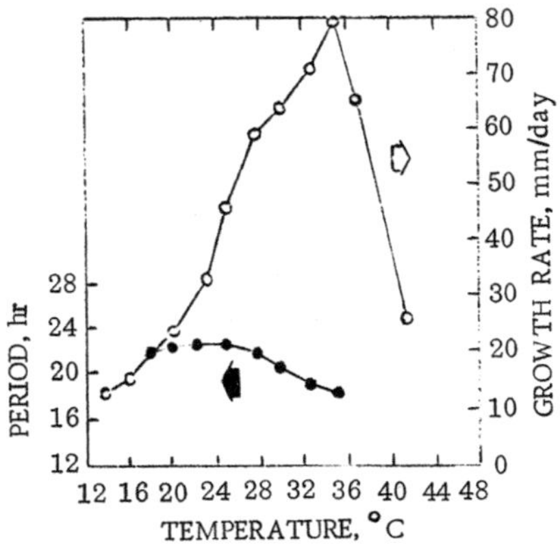

Figure 4. Temperature effect on growth rate (○) and period (●)of the rhythm. Timex was grown under standard conditions except for the temperature on the yeast-extract medium. Each point represents the average of data from six growth-tubes. The standard errors for growth rate ranged from 0.2 to 1.6 mm /day, and from 0.07 and 0.17 hr for the period measurements. (From Sargent, Briggs, and Woodward, 1966).

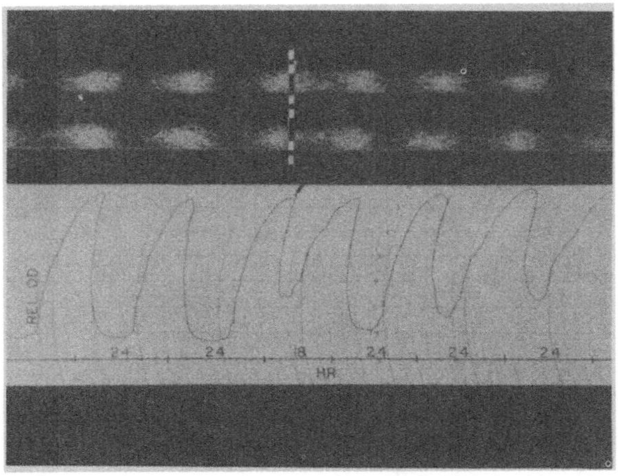

Figure 5. A 6.0 hr phase shift advance recorded by photography and a densitometer tracing. Timex was grown under standard conditions on casamino acid medium. The light exposure (fluorescent light 90 min, 450 ft-c) was given when the growth front was at the position indicated by the broken line across the tubes and the black mark at the top of the densitometer tracing. ×1/4 (from Sargent, Briggs, and Woodward, 1966).

Phase-shifting of timex by light is illustrated in Figure 5 and the phase shift response curve is shown in Figure 6. The complete inhibition of rhythmic expression by light of very low intensities is illustrated in Figure 7. The rhythmic expression of conidiation is eliminated with increasing light intensities. The threshold is approximately 0.72 ergs cm^{-2} sec^{-1}. The conidial

TABLE 2. Effect of Carbohydrates on bd Rhythmicity

Sugar	No. of bands	Band density	Period of rhythm, hr	Growth rate, mm/day
None	7-8	++	24.8	32.0
Acetate	>15	+++	21.5	29.4
Glycerol	2-3	+	Circadian	34.0
Ribose	7-8	+	23.2	28.5
Xylose	5-6	++++	21.8	38.5
Glucose	3-4	+++	Circadian	45.8
Fructose	3-4	++	"	45.0
Mannose	203	++	"	43.3
Galactose	6-7	++	23.6	29.5
Raffinose	4-5	+++	Circadian	35.7
Sucrose	3-4	+++	"	44.0
Maltose	3-4	+++	"	46.3
Lactose	4-5	++	"	31.9
Trehalose	4-5	+++	"	39.4

Growth-tube cultures of E7a, bd, were grown under standard conditions on Vogel's salts, 1.5 per cent agar and 0.3 per cent carbohydrate. Circadian: 20-24 hr.

band increases in size with increasing intensities until all the bands merge. What this means in terms of biochemical mechanisms is not clear, but these data on temperature compensation and phase shifting do clearly indicate that this Neurospora rhythm is typical of all other eucaryotic circadian rhythms. Our attempts to identify the photoreceptor have not yet been successful, although the action spectrum (Figure 8) for the photoreceptor involved looks very similar to the absorption spectrum of certain carotenoid pigments. The use of an albino Neurospora mutant which produces no detectable carotenoid (less than 5 per cent), however, revealed an equivalent light response to that of the fully pigmented strain. A carotenoid in very low concentrations or a flavin-containing compounds with a similar absorption spectrum are not eliminated as possible explanations.

3. Nutritional Studies

One of our attempts to find clues about the biochemistry of rhythmic Neurospora strains in general was directed toward a study of the effect of nutrition on rhythmic expression. A series of experiments with the bd strain led to the development of a glucose-arginine medium which produced a strong conidial banding pattern. This medium was used to test a large number of

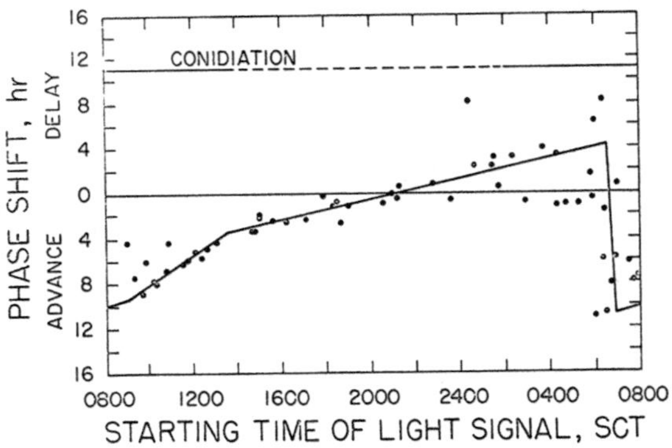

Figure 6. The phase shift response curve for timex. Light signals were 45 min in duration and 1430 ft-c in intensity. The solid black bar indicates the normal interval of conidiation within the daily cycle of timex. Each data point represents a single culture (from Sargent and Briggs, 1967).

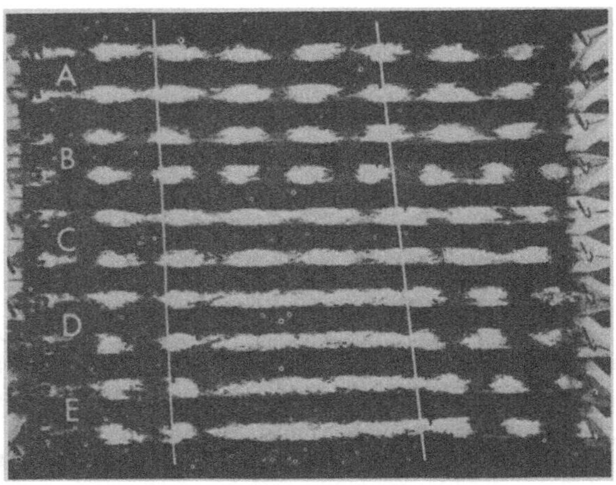

Figure 7. Inhibition of rhythm by light. The tubes were exposed to fluorescent light for the 72 hr growth interval between the lines. Intensities: A) 0; B) 4.20×10^{-2}; C) 4.12×10^{-1}; D) 4.24; and E) 5.45×10 ergs cm^{-2} sec^{-1}. ×1/4.

Neurospora strains, and many of these that did not express a rhythm on a minimal sucrose medium did exhibit a detectable rhythm on glucose–arginine (Table 1). In the process of developing this medium, the effects of several amino acids and sugars on rhythmic expression were observed. The response of bd to various sugars is shown in Table 2. Some of the sugars produced a stronger band density than did other sugars, but the period of the rhythm differed only slightly, depending on the sugar used. These effects of sugars on the period in strain bd are not significant by comparison with their effect on clock; sugars control both the expression (Berliner, 1966) and period (Berliner, 1965) of the clock strain. The period for clock was shown to vary over a wide range

TABLE 3. Effect of Amino Acids on bd Rhythmicity

Amino acid	No. of bands	Band density	Period of rhythm, hr	Growth rate, mm/day
A				
L-arginine...........	10+	++++	22.2	46.7
L-tryptophan.........	10+	+++	24.0	31.3
L-histidine..........	10+	+++	24.3	39.2
L-alanine...........	10+	++	20.0	48.5
(d, *l*)-hydroxylysine • HCl .	12+	++	22.4	26.8
B				
L-aspartic acid........	8-9; 4+	++++; ++	21.8	41.4
L-threonine..........	4-5; 5+	++; +	20.9	43.7
L-asparagine.........	5-6; 4+	+++; +	21.2	40.7
L-glutamine.........	4-5; 2-3	+++; +	21.2	37.5
L-ornithine • HCl.......	4-5; 5+	+++; +	21.8	41.8
L-citrulline..........	4-5; 6+	+++; +	23.2	35.6
C				
None..............	3-4	+++	Circadian	40.9
L-isoleucine.........	3-4	+++	"	43.3
L-phenylalanine.......	4-5	+++	"	41.9
L-proline...........	3-4	+++	"	42.4
L-glutamic acid.......	3-4	++++	"	44.6
L-valine............	3-4	+++	"	38.3
Urea..............	6-7	+++	21.5	38.7
D				
L-leucine...........	3-4	++	Circadian	43.3
L-tyrosine...........	2-3	++	"	41.6
L-serine............	4-5	++	"	39.2
L-methionine.........	2-3	++	"	47.2
L-glycine...........	2-3	+	"	38.4
L-hydroxyproline......	2-3	+	"	39.2
L-cystine...........	2	+	"	40.4
L-lysine • HCl.........	1	+	"	31.0
E				
L-cysteine • HCl.......	–	–	–	0

Growth-tube cultures of E7a, bd, were grown under standard conditions on Vogel's salts, 0.3 per cent glucose, 1.5 per cent agar, and 0.5 per cent amino acid. Heat-labile amino acids were filter-sterilized; media were titrated to pH 5.8 after addition of acidic or basic amino acids. Circadian = 20-24 hr.

on different carbon sources. It should also be noted that rhythmicity does not persist in bd when grown on sugars without amino acid supplementation.

Similar experiments were carried out with different amino acids (Table 3), some of which gave stronger banding patterns and more persistent rhythms

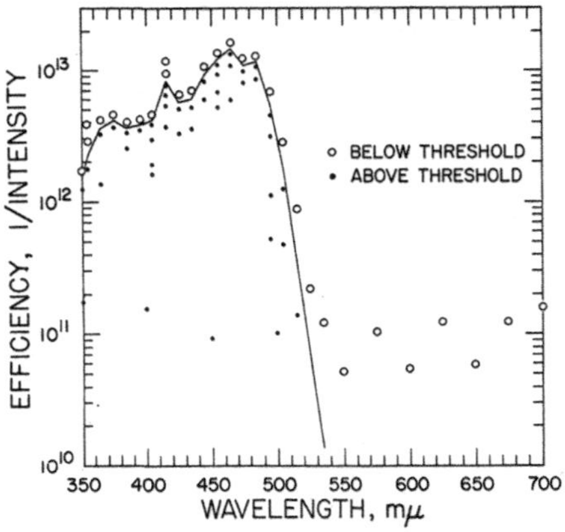

Figure 8. Action spectrum for inhibition by continuous light. The light intensity used is expressed as Einstein's cm^{-2} sec^{-1}. Each data point represents a single experiment in which three treated cultures were compared with three control cultures (from Sargent and Briggs, 1967).

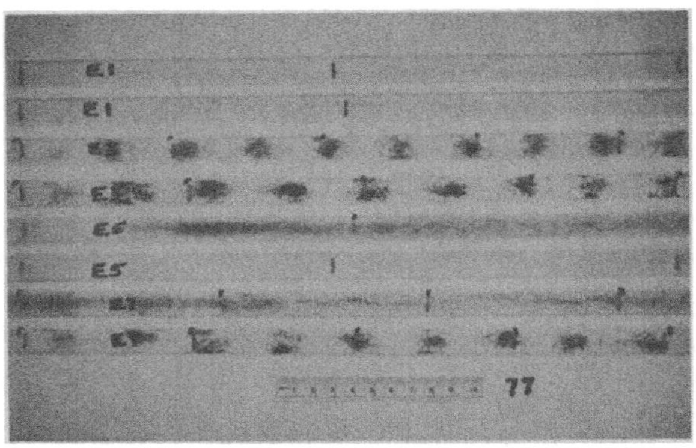

Figure 9. Growth-tube cultures of progeny from the tetrad in which the bd and invertase genes segregated. The strains E1 (inv, pan, A), E3 (inv. bd, A), E5 (pan, a) and E7 (bd, a) were grown under standard conditions on the casamino acids medium (top tube of each pair) and the glucose – arginine medium (bottom tube of each pair). Pen marks on the tubes delimit 48 hr growth intervals.

than others. The amino acids in group A strongly promote conidiation and persistency; those in group B weakly promote conidiation and persistency; those in group C are without effect; those in group D inhibit conidiation normally shown on glucose and L cysteine is toxic. It is not clear what the amino acids in group A have in common to strongly promote conidiation and persistency. As in the case of the different sugars, the period of the rhythm differed somewhat, depending on the amino acid used. Tryptophan and histidine, for example, gave a 24-hr rhythm while alanine showed a 20-hr rhythm. The

TABLE 4. Ascus E Isolates in Growth Tube Culture

Medium	Strain	No. of bands	Density of band	Period	Growth rate mm/day
Casamino acid	E_1(inv- bd+)	4-5	+	Circadian	83
	E_3(inv- bd-)	>12	++++	22.1	39
	E_5(inv+bd+)	0	−		80
	E_7(inv+bd-)	4-5	++++	Circadian	48
Glucose arginine	E_1(inv- bd+)	4-5	+	Circadian	88
	E_3(inv-nd-)	>12	++++	22.1	41
	E_5(inv+bd+)	0	−		82
	E_7(inv+bd-)	>12	++++	22.1	42

significance (if any) of these differences awaits a more critical testing of the reproducibility of such small effects.

The possible involvement of amino acids in some phase of rhythmic expression and/or generation is not be be taken too lightly, since this is not the only system in which effects by amino acids on rhythmic expression have been observed. Berliner (1965) observed an effect on control of the period in clock (from 18-110 hr) by amino acid mixtures. Similar observations have been made in organisms other than Neurospora (Jerebzoff, 1965) in which mixtures of amino acids influence persistency and period in both circadian and non-circadian rhythms.

Amino acid effects on conidiation in Neurospora have also been observed (Subramanian et al., 1968; Dicker et al., 1969) and the same amino acids that we observed to be effective in inducing rhythmic expression tend to be effective in inducing conidiation.

Again, it is interesting to observe a similar phenotypic nutritional response in the clock mutant. (Sternberg and Sussman unpublished private communication). This mutant strain normally exhibits a rhythm by sparse mycelial growth alternating with dense mycelium. The dense mycelium results from increased branching of the hyphal system. D-tyrosine causes severe growth inhibition which can be reversed by *l*-tyrosine. Mixtures of *d*- and *l*-tyrosine (with the *d* form in 2-fold excess) result in partial inhibition of clock with less dense mycelium than normal. Such a culture of clock is arhythmic; the branching hyphal system never fully develops. However, if the *l*-tyrosine is increased to the same concentration as *d*-tyrosine, full rhythmicity is restored. The *d*- forms of other amino acids and amino acid analogues were similarly tested and similarly inhibited, but the addition of *l*- forms relieved inhibition of growth, but rhythmicity was not restored; thus it is specific for tyrosine. In normally growing clock strains there is a derepression of tyrosinase. This, along with mutritional studies, suggests to Sternberg and Sussman (unpublished private communication) that the tyrosine –phenylalanine pool size may be involved in the causal mechanism.

Our previous studies (1969) showed a tendency for strains with modified carbon-source metabolism (invertase deficiencies) to show rhythmic conidiation. Colonial mutants (morphological mutants) in general have tendencies to

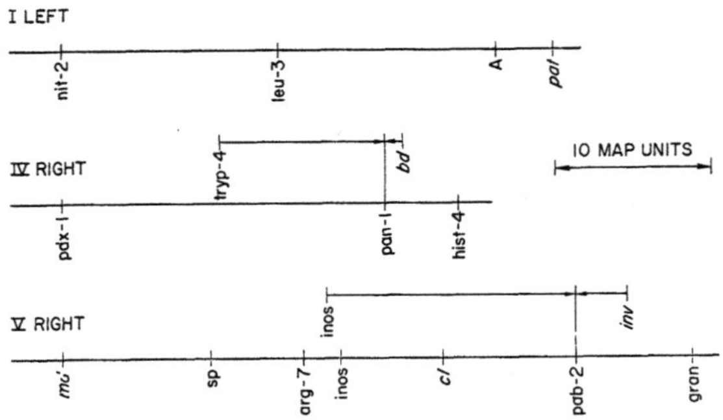

Figure 10. Location in the Neurospora linkage groups of inv, bd, and other loci responsible for rhythmic expression.

show rhythmic phenotypes. Brody (1966, 1967) has shown in the case of two morphological mutants that an alteration in carbon source metabolism is involved. The fact that inv and cot-2 map in the same region may therefore be significant. Esser (1969) made a similar observation in Podospora, i.e., that slow-growing morphological mutants tend to show rhythmic growth. If these observations reveal anything at all about rhythms, it must be that some of the outward manifestations of rhythms in fungi that can be brought about by modifying carbon source metabolism must be plugged into the oscillator directly or indirectly. Moreover certain types of disturbances can lead to the oscillation being manifest in the form of some morphological characteristic which is dependent on carbon source metabolism. Thus, from an optimistic point of view, this information may be useful in tracing back in the direction of the biochemistry of the oscillator, or at the very worst it can serve as another monitoring device.

4. Genetics of Timex

A cross of the timex strain was made with wild type and a tetrad was isolated in which the bd and inv genes segregated. Individual phenotypes of the four progeny of this tetrad were measured on two different media (Table 4, Figure 9). The bd gene alone showed no damping and dense banding on glucose–arginine medium, whereas an additional genetic block (inv) is required for persistency on casamino acid medium.

Additional genetic analyses were made in order to map the bd and inv genes. These linkage relationships are shown along with the locations of other Neurospora genes that produce a rhythmic phenotype (Figure 10). From this, it is obvious that there are several steps at which one can produce a hookup to an internal oscillator or, alternatively, there are several oscillators that different biochemical systems are capable of being coupled with.

5. Oxygen Effect on Rhythmicity

The bd gene may actually provide the best clues toward understanding the biochemistry of a Neurospora oscillator, since it shows a more pronounced

TABLE 5. Effects of Aeration on Neurospora Rhythmicity

Strain	No. of bands	Density of bands	Period of rhythm hr	Growth rate mm/day
Minimal sucrose				
Lindegren 1A - A	>7	+++	Circadian	57.0
C	0	–	–	71.5
N. tetrasperma - A	2	+	Circadian	85.0
C	0	–	–	68.0
N. intemedia (NITa) - A	0-4	+	–	46.5
C	0	–	–	47.5
N. sitophila (Eng. Sit. 21a) - A	0	–	–	86.0
C	0	–	–	81.0
N. crassa (STA4) - A	1-4	++	Circadian	87.5
C	0	–	–	85.0
Abbott 12a - A	2	++	Circadian	80.0
C	0	–	–	84.0
Sy4f 8a - A	0	–	–	85.0
C	0	–	–	73.5
Puerto Rico 18A - A	0	–	–	29.0
C	0	–	–	25.0
Liberia 4A - A	2	+	Circadian	89.0
C	0	–	–	97.5
Emerson a - A	>4	+++	Circadian	87.0
C	0	–	–	87.0
Minimal-glucose				
bd a (SHK 1-72) - A	>7	++++	21.8	48.2
C	2-3	+++	Circadian	46.8
Glucose-arginine				
N. crassa (STA4) - A	>5	+++	21.2	80.0
C	0	–	–	81.5

Growth-tube cultures were grown under standard conditions on the media indicated. Circadian, 20-24 hr. A - aerated; C - control.

rhythm than any of the other strains produced by single gene mutations. Moreover, bd is strictly circadian by all criteria. There is no guarantee, however, that what has been rather arbitrarily defined as circadian means anything more than possibly a closer coupling with the oscillator. Since we are presumably measuring different biochemical systems plugged into an oscillator in some way, a short circuit between the oscillator and the biochemical monitoring clue could simply result in what we call non-circadian. If this it true, many non-circadian rhythms might operate by the same basic mechanism as circadian rhythms, and thus would be potentially useful in a study of mechanisms except for the fact that they are usually more difficult to control and to quantitate. But even if bd only represents more sound circuitry between the oscillator and the biochemistry of the condition response, it may help to follow the circuit back to the oscillator. Unfortunately, not much is yet known about the biochemistry of the bd gene. The rhythm of CO_2 production, however, represents a starting place and prompted the question of whether O_2 in any way affects the expression of rhythmicity. When growth tubes were aerated, several wild-type strains which had not been observed to exhibit rhythmicity showed at least some evidence of circadian rhythmicity (Table 5). On the other hand, certain other strains under the most optimal conditions that we have found for expression still exhibit no rhythmicity. But if our past experience with Neurospora is any indication, then conditions can probably be found for which any strain will reveal the oscillation as judged by some biochemical or morphological criterion.

6. Discussion of Mechanisms

What the O_2 effect on expression actually means is not clear. Pittendrigh (1970, personal communication) has shown in recent unpublished studies, which extend his original observations (Pittendrigh, 1954), that oxygen is somehow involved in phase setting the oscillator. His experiments show that a Drosophila rhythm can be delayed by replacing O_2 with N_2, and the subsequent phase of the rhythm is delayed in proportion to the length of time left in N_2. The phase of the culture after returning to an O_2 atmosphere is in the same position on a 24-hr scale as it was when the N_2 was introduced to the culture. In other words, it appears as if the clock stops in the absence of O_2. Thus, some of the wild-type Neurospora strains that show a rhythm only when the external O_2 supply is high may in fact be defective in utilizing O_2 or in transporting it to a site available to the clock mechanisms. This may implicate mitochondria and ATP production as an essential part of the clock mechanism. Is, also, the differential sugar effect and amino acid effect related to O_2 consumption or utilization? We hope that experiments now in progress will help to answer that question.

There appears to be no easy way to distinguish a causative oscillation from the many rhythmic processes which the oscillator theoretically controls. The only unique property of the oscillator as distinct from other rhythmically varying biochemical processes are period and phase – both of which the oscillator imparts to the processes it controls. Therefore, a reaction sequence which belongs to the oscillator might be identified by the fact that changing it in a specific way alters either the phase or the period of the rhythms we observe. Abolishing rhythmicity by inhibitors, in most cases, may simply affect the process coupled to the clock. Thus the oscillator may be operating as usual in the presence of inhibitor, but is no longer measurable because of an inhibited monitoring system.

Most attempts to change the phase or period by nutrition or inhibitors, etc., have been unsuccessful. Slight changes in the period of Neurospora strain bd were observed under different nutritional environments, but we cannot be sure that these small differences are meaningful. Clock is different from these and other systems since light has no effect on the phase and nutrition drastically alters the period. If the differences are meaningful, it could mean one of two possible things: (1) It could mean that some aspect of carbon source metabolism is directly involved in the generation of oscillations and thus can influence the length of the period; or more likely, (2) it could mean that information transfer from oscillator to coupled system is not a one-way street (Sweeney, 1969, cites evidence that it is one-way), and information can be fed back to the oscillator through some of the systems coupled to it.

Some rhythms are affected by Actinomycin D, but there is no change in phase or period of bd up to a concentration that totally inhibits growth (Sargent, 1969). Inhibitors of protein synthesis have, in general, been observed to have no effect on rhythms, although Feldman (1967) reported cycloheximide to affect the period of a rhythm. Thus, the use of inhibitors has not led to a solution of the problem. We apparently have at our disposal only processes which show the presence of the oscillator but are probably not themselves a part of it. An exception to this may be the unusual effect of oxygen on rhythmicity and, if so, this may provide the closest link to the biochemistry of the oscillator.

Sweeney (1969) has suggested that an oscillator which is coupled to so many different functions in so many different types of cells must involve a basic and universal property of living systems. Since inhibition studies seem to exclude transcription and/or translation, at least in some systems, she has suggested membranes as another common denominator of cellular organization. There is certainly some reason to believe that most, if not all, cellular enzymes are membrane bound in vivo. Moreover, current studies on mutations which affect membrane structure or stability show that such mutations exert a pleiotropic effect on a variety of enzymes (Woodward, 1968; Puig et al., 1967; Schnaitman, 1969). Membranes also exhibit a property not well understood but which appears to involve conformational transitions transmitted along the surface of a membrane. This could constitute a kind of communication system or information transfer to a large number of biochemical systems. A striking example of the sensitivity of a membrane system is illustrated by the effect of colicin on bacterial membranes (Nagel de Zwaig and Luria, 1967; Nomura and Witten, 1967). A single molecule of colicin can kill a bacterial cell by attaching to a cell envelope receptor; the subsequent effect of this is to trigger a series of events that affect a specific biochemical target (e.g., protein synthesis or nucleic acid metabolism). The specific target that is affected depends on the type of colicin that attaches.

It remains to be seen whether membranes are involved either in generating oscillations or the more likely possibility of transmitting the oscillation to different biochemical systems from an oscillator. Membrane structure and function need to be much better understood before the answer to this question can be determined, but theoretically it stands as a contender for the role of being able to transmit information to many enzymes and hence many biochemical systems that are bound to membranes.

REFERENCES

Berliner, M. D. (1965). Canadian J. Micro. 12, 1068.
Berliner, M. D. and Neurath, P. W. (1965). J. Cell. Comp. Physiol. 65, 183.
Brandt, W. H. (1953). Mycologia 45, 194.
Brody, S. (1966). Proc. Nat. Acad. Sci. 56, 1290.
Brody, S. (1967). Proc. Nat. Acad. Sci. 58, 923.

Dicker, J. W., Oulevey, N., and Turian, G. (1969). Arch. Mikrobiol. 65, 241.
Durkee, T., Sussman, A. S., and Lowry, R. J. (1966). Genetics 53, 1167.
Esser, K. (1969). Mycologia 61, 1008.
Feldman, J. R. (1967). Proc. Nat. Acad. Sci. 57, 1080.
Jerebzoff, S. (1965). In: Circadian Clocks. J. Aschoff Ed. North Holland Publishing Co. p. 183.
Nagel de Zwaig, R. and Luria, S. E. (1967). J. Bact. 94, 1112.
Nambooderi, A. N. and Lowry, R. J. (1967). Am. J. Bot. 54, 735.
Neurath, P. W. and Berliner, M. D. (1964). Science 146, 646.
Nomura, M. and Witten, C. (1967). J. Bact. 94, 1093.
Pittendrigh, C. S. (1954). Proc. Nat. Acad. Sci. 10, 1018.
Pittendrigh, C. S., Bruce, V. G., Rosensweig, N. S., and Rubin, M. L. (1959). Nature 184, 169.
Puig, J., Azoubay, E., and Pichinoty, F. (1967). Compt. Rend. 264, 1507.
Sargent, M. L. (1969). Neurospora Newsletter 15, 17.
Sargent, M. L. and Briggs, W. R. (1967). Plant Physiol. 42, 1504.
Sargent, M. L., Briggs, W. R., and Woodward, D. O. (1966). Plant Physiol. 41, 1343.
Sargent, M. L. and Woodward, D. O. (1965). Genetics, 52, 472.
Sargent, M. L. and Woodward, D. O. (1969a). J. Bact. 97, 861.
Sargent, M. L. and Woodward, D. O. (1969b). J. Bact. 97, 867.
Schnaitman, C. A. (1969). Biochem. Biophys. Res. Comm. 37, 1.
Stadler, D. R. (1959). Nature 184, 170.
Subramanian, K. N., Padmanaban, G., and Sarma, P. S. (1968). Biochim. Biophys. Acta 151, 20.
Sussman, A. S., Durkee, T. L., and Lowry, R. J. (1965). Mycopath. Mycol. Appl. 25, 381.
Sussman, A. S., Lowry, R. J., and Durkee, T. (1964). Amer. J. Bot. 51, 243.
Sweeney, B. M. (1969). Rhythmic Phenomena in Plants. Academic Press, N. Y.
Sweeney, B. M. and Haxo, F. T. (1961). Science 134, 1361.
Sweeney, B. M., Tuffli, C. F., and Rubin, R. H. (1967). J. Gen. Physiol. 50, 647.
Vanden Driessche, T. (1966). Biochim. Biophys. Acta 126, 456.
Woodward, D. O. (1968). Fed. Proc. 27, 1167.

PROTEIN SYNTHESIS AND TEMPERATURE COMPENSATION IN CIRCADIAN RHYTHMICITY

J.F. Feldman and S.B. Stevens

State University of New York at Albany,
Department of Biological Sciences,
Albany,
New York 12203, U.S.A.

ABSTRACT

In Euglena gracilis and several mutants of Neurospora crassa a correlation exists between the Q_{10} of the circadian rhythm and the extent to which the period of the rhythm is lengthened by inhibitors of protein synthesis. A model is proposed in which the temperature-compensation mechanism of the circadian clock includes a device to compensate for changes in the rates of protein synthesis.

One of the most intriguing properties of a circadian clock system is its response to temperature. In contrast to most chemical and metabolic systems, the rate of operation of a circadian clock, as measured by its period length or frequency, is relatively constant over a wide range of physiological temperatures – i.e., the Q_{10} of the rhythm has a value close to 1. This constancy of period length has suggested to some investigators (Brown and Webb, 1948; Ehret and Trucco, 1967) that the circadian clock is temperature-independent – i.e., its rate is determined by some physical process whose rate is proportional to the absolute temperature.

On the other hand Q_{10} values close to 1 could also be obtained by a temperature-compensation system (Bruce and Pittendrigh, 1956; Hastings and Sweeney, 1957) in which the individual components are temperature-dependent chemical reactions with high Q_{10} values (about 2) but which interact in such a way that the rate of the final output of the system does not vary much with temperature. Such a mechanism could also be called temperature-adaptation.

Several observations seem to favor the temperature-compensation type of model: (1) Q_{10} values less than 1 have been reported in several systems (Hastings and Sweeney, 1957; Brinkmann, 1966). An "over-compensation" explanation (Hastings and Sweeney, 1957) seems the most plausible for

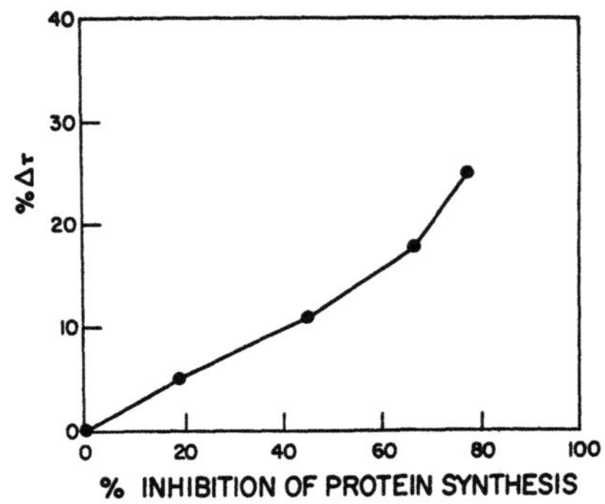

Figure 1. Relationship between percentage inhibition of protein sunthesis and percent lengthening of the period of the circadian clock in Euglena gracilis.

such an observation. (2) Circadian systems can be phase-shifted, or reset, by temperature steps or temperature pulses. The systems therefore can detect differences in temperature regimes and appear to adapt to the new conditions rather than to ignore them. In fact, Pavlidis et al. (1968) have proposed some additional details of a mathematical temperature-compensation model which account for a large part of the data on phase-shifting by temperature steps and pulses. (3) In certain microorganisms the Q_{10} value of the rhythm can be modified by growth on different media (Jerebzoff, 1965; Berliner and Neurath, 1965; Brinkmann, 1966). The involvement of chemical reactions in the temperature-responding system is strongly suggested by data of this type. (4) At extreme physiological temperatures the Q_{10} of the rhythm often rises significantly above 1. This suggests that a temperature-compensation mechanism may break down beyond certain temperature limits.

The circadian clock in Euglena gracilis controls a rhythm of phototactic response (Bruce and Pittendrigh, 1956). The Q_{10} of this rhythm in autotrophic cultures ranges from about 1.05 to 1.1. The period of the rhythm can be lengthened by various inhibitors of protein synthesis, the most striking results being obtained with cycloheximide (Feldman, 1967a, b; Brinkmann, 1971).

In the initial report of these observations (Feldman, 1967a) it was noted that a given concentration of inhibitor produced a much greater percentage inhibition of protein synthesis than percentage lengthening of the period (Figure 1). For example, at 50 per cent inhibition of protein synthesis there was only a 10 per cent lengthening of the period. It was suggested, with little additional evidence for support at that time, that this observation may result from the operation of the temperature-compensation mechanism of the clock – i.e., that protein synthesis is necessary for the operation of the clock but that the temperature compensation mechanism includes a device to compensate for changes in the rates of protein synthesis. Such a device would exert its effect whether changes in this rate were induced by temperature changes or by an inhibitor.

TABLE 1. Period Lengthening of Circadian Rhythm in *Euglena* by Cycloheximide

% Inhibition of Protein Synthesis	Equivalent Change In Temperature (°C)	Period Length (in hours)	Equivalent Q_{10}
0	0	24	–
50	–10	26	1.08
75	–20	28	1.08
		Q_{10} of rhythm	1.05-1.1

TABLE 2. Effect of Temperature and Medium on Period Lengths of Circadian Rhythm in Clock Strain of *Neurospora crassa*

Temperature	Period length (in hours)	
	Gray's Complete Medium	Vogel's Minimal Medium
20°C	31.1	47
25°C	24.0	35
30°C	20.1	26
Q_{10}	1.5	1.8

We now present additional information from clock systems in *Euglena gracilis* and *Neurospora crassa* which is consistent with this speculation.

1. The *Euglena* System

The properties and assay of the *Euglena* clock system have been described elsewhere (Bruce and Pittendrigh, 1956; Feldman, 1967a). We wish here to present no new data, but rather some new calculations from previously reported information (Feldman, 1967a). If one assumes that the Q_{10} of protein synthesis itself is 2, then, by definition, lowering the temperature by 10°C results in a 50 per cent reduction in the rate of protein synthesis and a second 10°C drop (total of 20°C drop) results in a rate reduced by 75 per cent from its original rate. Therefore, inhibition of protein synthesis 50 per cent by cycloheximide is equivalent to a 10°C drop in temperature, and 75 per cent inhibition of protein synthesis is equivalent to a 20°C drop in temperature. The data in Figure 1 show that the average period lengths at 50 per cent and 75 per cent inhibition are about 26 and 28 hours respectively. From these values one can compare the effect on period length of a 10° drop in temperature with the effect of 50 per cent inhibition of protein synthesis or similarly a 20°C drop in temperature with a 75 per cent inhibition of protein synthesis (Table 1). This can be done by calculating an "equivalent Q_{10}" – i.e., the ratio of the frequency of clock operation at 0 per cent inhibition to the frequency at 50 per cent inhibition, or the ratio of the frequency at 50 per cent to the frequency at 75 per cent inhibition. These equivalent Q_{10} values fall between 1.05 and 1.1,

TABLE 3. Period Lengthening of Circadian Rhythm of Clock Strain of Neurospora crassa by Cycloheximide

% Inhibition of Growth	% lengthening of Period (and period length in hr.)	
	Gray's Medium	Minimal Medium
0	0% (24 hours)	0% (25 hours)
40	14% (27 hours)	54% (54 hours)
50	36% (32 hours)	185% (100 hours)
65	69% (40 hours)	320% (148 hours)
75	84% (44 hours)	
80	116% (51 hours)	
90	292% (94 hours)	415% (181 hours)
Q_{10} of rhythm	1.5	1.8
Equivalent Q_{10}	1.3-1.5	1.7-2.8

very close to the real Q_{10} values obtained by measuring the change in period length at different temperatures. This correlation is consistent with the model described above – (a) that protein synthesis is rate-limiting for the clock, and (b) that any change in the rate of protein synthesis is compensated for by some clock device, whether that change is caused by temperature changes or by the addition of an inhibitor.

2. The Neurospora System

This model predicts that a correlation should exist between the temperature coefficient of a rhythm and the extent to which its period length can be affected by inhibitors of protein synthesis. If one could utilize a circadian system with a Q_{10} value different from that found in Euglena, one would predict that its response to cycloheximide should also be different. Better still would be the use of a system whose Q_{10} can be varied so that one could determine whether a correlation exists between Q_{10} and period lengthening by inhibitors.

The use of three mutants of Neurospora crassa, – band (bd), patch (pat), and clock (cl) – allow such an analysis. All strains exhibit a circadian rhythm of morphological change: band and patch have a rhythm of conidiation (Sargent et al., 1966; Pittendrigh et al., 1959) and clock a rhythm of hyphal branching (Sussman et al., 1964). Sargent et al. (1966) have shown that band has a Q_{10} between 0.95 and 1.21 and Feldman (unpublished data) has shown that patch has a Q_{10} of about 1.0-1.2. For both band (Sargent, personal communication) and patch (Feldman, unpublished observation) cycloheximide at concentrations up to 75 per cent inhibition of growth causes less than a 4-hour change in period length. The Q_{10} of clock, however, depends on the medium on which it is grown. Table 2 shows data for calculating the Q_{10} of the period lengths on two different media. On Gray's complete medium the Q_{10} is 1.5 and on Vogel's minimal medium it is 1.8. Table 3 shows the period lengths of clock at different levels of inhibition of protein synthesis on these two media. From these data two conclusions are apparent: (1) On both media where the clock strain has a significantly higher Q_{10} than either patch or band, cycloheximide has a much greater effect on the period length of clock than it does on the period length of patch or band. (2) Cycloheximide has a greater effect on clock on Vogel's medium (with higher Q_{10} value) than on Gray's medium. Both of these observations are qualitatively what is predicted from the model.

Despite the agreement of these results with predictions from the model, there are a number of questions which must be answered before the model can be upgraded from its highly speculative status. For example (1) the Q_{10} of protein synthesis itself has not been measured in our systems either in vitro or in vivo and any conclusions based on its assumed value must remain tentative. (2) In the Neurospora cycloheximide experiments only growth rates were measured, not rates of protein synthesis. Any extrapolation from one to the other is particularly dangerous in the case of the clock mutant since its growth shows some unusual responses to temperature (Sussman et al., 1966). (3) Although the data are quanlitatively consistent with the predictions, quantitatively there is some deviation between predicted and observed. This could result either from minor errors in our assumptions about rates of protein synthesis or from minor modifications which need to be made in the model itself. It could also be, of course, that the model is simply wrong.

We are impressed by the correlations between Q_{10} of a rhythmic system and the effect of cycloheximide on its period length. However, the primary usefulness of the model of the moment is in its heuristic value and it must be considered highly speculative unless confirmed by other types of experiments.

REFERENCES

Berliner, M. and Neurath, P. (1965). J. Cell Comp. Physiol. 65, 183.

Brinkmann, K. (1966). Planta 70, 344.

Brinkmann, K. (1972). In Friday Harbor Biochronometry Symposium (M. Menaker, ed.). In press.

Brown, F. A. and Webb, J. H. (1948). Physiol. Zool. 21, 371.

Bruce, V. G. and Pittendrigh, C. S. (1956). Proc. Nat. Acad. Sci. 42, 676.

Ehret, C. F. and Trucco, E. (1967). J. Theor. Biol. 15, 240.

Feldman, J. F. (1967a). Proc. Nat. Acad. Sci. 57, 1080.

Feldman, J. F. (1967b). Ph. D. Thesis, Princeton University, Princeton, N. J.

Hastings, J. W. and Sweeney, B. M. (1957). Proc. Nat. Acad. Sci. 43, 804.

Jerebzoff, S. (1965). In Circadian Clocks (J. Aschoff, ed.) North-Holland Publ. Co., Amsterdam, P 183.

Pavlidis, T., Zimmerman, W. F., and Osborne, J. (1968). J. Theor. Biol. 18, 210.

Sargent, M. L., Briggs, W. R., and Woodward, D. O. (1966). Plant Physiol. 41, 1343.

Sussman, A. S., Lowry, R., and Durkee, T. (1964). Amer. J. Bot. 51, 243.

Sussman, A. S., Durkee, T. L., and Lowry, R. (1966). Mycopath. Mycol. Appl. 25, 381.